PRAYWELL

A HOLISTIC GUIDE TO HEALTH & RENEWAL

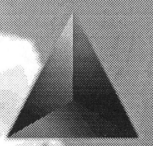

BY WALTER L. WESTON

PrayWell

A Holistic Guide to Health and Renewal

by Walter L. Weston

Published by: **Transitions Press**
P.O. Box 618
Wadsworth, OH 44281

1-800-886-5735

Edited by Julianne Stein
Illustrated by Angela Berlingeri
Cover photography by Kurt Shaffer
Author's photograph by Patricia J. Shaffer
Cover design and art work by Angela Berlingeri

Book store classification: Alternative Medicine or Self-Help
Library Cataloguing: 615.5 or 158.1

Weston, Walter L.
P r a y W e l l -- A Holistic Guide to Health and Renewal, First Edition
Copyright 1994 by Walter L. Weston
First Printing, May, 1994
Library of Congress number 94-090021
ISBN 1-884537-06-5
$19.95 US, Softcover

Table of Contents

ILLUSTRATIONS

ABOUT THE COVER

When I first saw the cover of this book, I responded with reverence. It was far more compelling than I had ever hoped it could be. As the author, I feel a need to tell you the story of this cover.

One morning last Fall, I met with my editor, Julianne Stein, to go over changes in the text. We met between her home in Cleveland and my own in the charming village of Peninsula. I was feeling pleased because her fine command of sentence structure and words was immensely improving my manuscript.

We took a work break and I wandered alone into a neighboring gift shop, Creations Gallery. It is filled with beautiful art work from many cultures. But upon entering, my gaze was immediately fixed upon a group of framed nature photographs from the southwestern United States. They were all giving off a remarkable spiritual energy. One picture stood out. It was of a deep blue sky with splotches of white clouds. Through the clouds, the photographer had caught vivid rays of sunshine descending to Earth. It was the most awesome nature scene I had ever observed. I immediately knew I must have it for the cover of PrayWell. I asked the owner, *"Where can I find the photographer?"*

She laughed and responded, *"He is standing beside you, glowing in satisfaction at your obvious approval."*

I turned around and met Kurt Shaffer of Lakewood, Ohio. I inquired, *"How do you do it?"*

Kurt warmed up to his intuitive creativity, saying, *"Somehow I am able to capture the energy of nature in my photography. My buyers tell me that they feel sensations of calmness and peace. Some report an inner healing occurs when they look at my art. I am so glad you want to use one of them on the cover of your book."*

I gushed, *"Kurt, if my book sells well, I am going to buy every one of these pictures to add to the energy of my home."* It was to be a week later that I discovered that Kurt was my editor Julianne Stein's fiance.

My best friend, Karl Bunkelman, had found Julianne for me. Now, Karl, a people broker, found me an illustrator and cover artist in Angela Berlingeri of Solon, Ohio, a computer graphics artist and an instructor at two universities. I made only one request of Angela -- Kurt's picture must be the basis for the cover. Weeks later, Angela phoned me to say she had a cover design ready for my approval. She added, *"It came to me in a dream."* This is the cover that you now see gracing PrayWell.

I asked Angela about the meaning of the golden triangle. She responded, *"It has no meaning. It was a part of my dream. It is just an artistic means for bringing the eyes to focus upon the total cover."*

I inquired, *"Are you sure you are not into pyramidology?"*

She gave me a blank look and insisted, *"It is just an artistic design..."*

I have a suggested meaning for the golden triangle. In religion classes, triangles are used to demonstrate three religious truths. God is at the top corner, humans are on the left corner, and on the right is our means for finding access to God. In my own faith tradition, Christ is usually placed there. Here, I would suggest that prayer should be on the right corner as our means for bringing the power of God into the life of the world.

ACKNOWLEDGMENTS

I thank everyone in the fields of life energies research and spiritual healing. Without their knowledge and wisdom, the this book could not have been written.

I thank my teachers, most of whom have been my healing clients, who have passed on to me their experiences and insights.

I thank my editor, Julianne Stein, whose clarity of thought enhanced my own. I thank my illustrator, Angela Berlingeri, whose talent speaks for itself. I thank my photographer, Kurt Shaffer, for the energy inherent in his work.

I thank my friends and colleagues for their practical help on my manuscripts and for their encouragement to continue. These included Karl Bunkleman, Norma Gold-berger, Reverend Dwight Hayes, Dr. Hubert Hensel, Penny Knight, Esther Long, Cora Jean Powell, Robert L. Powers, Jean Sampson, Brother Jerry Shulte and Dagmar Talew.

The quotations at the beginning of each chapter that are marked with an asterisk (*) can be found in Christian Spirituality, edited by Frank N. Magill and Ian P. McGreal. Thank you both for your excellent reference book -- historic evidence for the perennial need of humanity to further understand God.

I appreciate my wife's patience while I wrote. Dana, thanks for your support and understanding. I was often mentally preoccupied with PrayWell and spent long hours before the computer.

I thank the intuitive-creative process that I refer to as the Presence, a divine inspiration that guided me constantly and filled me with peace, energy and joy. God's wisdom far surpasses my own.

Walter L. Weston

PrayWell

"Physical, emotional, and spiritual healing is available to us through the work of the Holy Spirit." ...Agnes Sanford*

"Therefore I tell you, whatever you ask in prayer, believe that you will receive it and you will." ...Mark 11:24

"Nothing is too wonderful to be true." ...Michael Faraday

You have picked up PrayWell to see whether it is worth reading. Scanning this *Preface* will help you decide. PrayWell provides many new and practical means upon which you can build personal health and happiness. PrayWell is a unique approach that combines twenty-first century energy medicine with the ancient practice of prayer.

PrayWell provides a trustworthy new road map for renewing life. If you or a loved one are facing a life-threatening illness, PrayWell offers a good possibility for renewed health through self-healing and touch-healing prayer. If you live with a chronic or handicapping condition, PrayWell offers resources for restoring you to physical health. If you are struggling with emotional issues or painful memories, PrayWell can bring you peace and happiness. PrayWell can renew your happiness and satisfaction with loved ones. PrayWell can improve the quality of life in your school, workplace and community. PrayWell is holistic medicine at its best.

PrayWell grounds itself in the exciting new scientific data produced by life energies research. You will learn about the qualities of life energy. You will learn how to utilize life energy. You will learn how your human energy field is the basis for your own health and happiness. You will learn how energy field interaction affects you, your family and other groups. You will learn about the forming of therapeutic group energy that bathe participants in health, happiness and satisfaction.

PrayWell empowers you through the practice of Therapeutic Prayer. The purpose of Therapeutic Prayer is to express love and caring, producing wholeness in body, mind, spirit and relationships. Therapeutic Prayer renews your personal energy field and the energy fields of others. Therapeutic Prayer empowers therapeutic group energy fields that bring wholeness and unity to couples, families and other groups. Therapeutic Prayers are a balance of the mental, emotional and spiritual energies. Therapeutic Prayer can be used by people of all religious beliefs.

PrayWell provides step-by-step practical instructions to guide you. PrayWell begins with foundations based upon science, reason and experience. PrayWell's step-by-step instructions coach you in the practical applications of life energies, energy field renewal and therapeutic group energy fields. PrayWell offers Therapeutic Prayer models so that you do not have to search for the right words.

Can prayer really improve the quality of your personal life? Pray-

Well provides facts that explain why the practice of personal and family prayer dramatically improves the happiness and quality of life. PrayWell then provides you with guidance and prayer models for your home. These include family prayer rituals that affirm every family member and rites of passage that provide meaning for the important stages of human development. Promoting God in the home, the organization Religion in American Life coined the phrase, *"The family that prays together, stays together."*

PrayWell demonstrates why this is scientifically true. PrayWell seeks to enrich the quality of family life. Because these are therapeutic prayers, they can help dysfunctional individuals and families to become whole. Through prayer, God's presence creates enduring sacred space that can bathe your home in God's transforming love and renew every person present within it. God's presence provides the optimum conditions for love and responsibility.

PrayWell provides a new road map to both God and prayer based upon information you can trust. Any religious beliefs expressed in PrayWell are confirmed by science, reason and experience. Yet, nothing in PrayWell contradicts sacred scriptures. PrayWell is able to confirm ancient religious beliefs and strengthen your own personal beliefs and practice.

Will PrayWell hold your attention? I have a curious mind and am easily bored, but researching the contents of PrayWell has kept me in a state of rapt attention and utter fascination for more than a quarter of century. I believe you will find PrayWell to be the most compelling book you have read in a long time. You will learn hundreds of helpful facts about prayer, healing, health, renewal, spirituality and happiness.

WESTERN VERSUS EASTERN SPIRITUAL STYLES

PrayWell combines two ancient and diverse spiritual traditions -- the practice of Western Judeo-Christian prayers for healing with the emphasis upon Eastern techniques like meditation and energy field balancing to restore the human energy field. The differences are not so mutually exclusive as they appear to Westerners. Prayers for healing are utilized in most religions and cultures both East and West. These prayers take on certain universal traits.

To those who have read books on healing, there appear to be sharp differences between the holistic approaches of the West and the East. The West's healing traditions, even to this day, are centered in the Christian Church, and thus, in the Christian community. They are based upon religious beliefs, testimony and practice rather than upon scientific understanding.

Consequently, most books on spiritual healing in the Western tradition are exclusively Christian in outlook and are read mainly by Christian church -goers. Readers who want to learn more about spiritual healing would neither feel comfortable with the various religious beliefs expressed in these books nor learn much about practical applications.

Other books on healing are based upon an Eastern understanding. These books are rooted primarily in the ancient Hindu and Chinese healing models, both of which utilize an entirely different approach from the Judeo-Christian-Islamic traditions. The Hindu model is based upon an intuitive scientific understanding of the universe rather than the divine revelational approach of the West. Hinduism teaches that each human being has several energy bodies composed of differing energy frequencies and that these energy bodies are empowered by energy centers called "chakras." The ancient Chinese intuitively and experientially explored the network of energy meridians or pathways that circulate energy throughout the body.

Both Eastern models, scientifically verified by contemporary researchers, view illness and wellness as related to the efficiency of these energy fields. Out of this understanding has arisen most of the healing knowledge and practice pursued in the West outside of the context of Christianity. These models are utilized by most medical researchers and healing practitioners.

Thus, those seeking to practice or to research spiritual healing have tended to utilize these Eastern models. From ancient Hindu roots came the present sophisticated practices of cleansing, balancing and energizing chakras (primary energy centers) and the human energy fields. From ancient Chinese roots come acupuncture, acupressure, reflexology and sophisticated computer-assisted energy probes, readouts and health analysis. No healing technique based upon these Eastern models utilizes prayer.

Prayer in the West is viewed by most as specifically and uniquely a part of the institutional Christian community that has ignored or been hostile to any healing techniques practiced outside the Church. Reiki, Therapeutic Touch and Barbara Ann Brennan healing, three widely practiced techniques, do not use prayer, since these touch-healing techniques are largely used in medical and other settings where prayer is suspect as a tool of Christianity. They also seek to avoid the words *"spiritual"* and *"healing"* because of their negative connotations in the public's mind.

In my practice of touch-healing prayer, I have sought to separate prayer from its religious connotations by using the term *"Therapeutic Prayer."* The purpose of Therapeutic Prayer is to express caring through bringing God's energy into the life of hurting people. Unlike religious prayer, which tends to be passive, Therapeutic Prayer uses the far more intentional and directive style practiced in most healing techniques.

During the past dozen years, I have learned and practiced most of the healing techniques that involve working with the human energy fields. They all work. Most life energies research data presented in this book utilizes a similar scientific understanding of human energy fields and an energy that heals that is transmitted through human hands. I have also practiced simple touch-healing prayer in the Christian tradition for more than twenty-five years. I make use of the scientific data because it renders my work that much more effective. Research data indicates that touch-healing prayer is just as effective as the more sophisticated energy field manipulation healing techniques.

PRAYER RESULTS EQUAL TO ENERGY FIELD WORK

Harvard Medical School wellness researcher Herbert Benson, MD, reports that when his wellness support groups are given a choice of methods for coping with stress or to accomplish self-healing, eighty percent choose prayer and the rest choose meditation, contemplation or visualization. He finds each approach produces a similarly needed energy for healing.

The power of prayer was confirmed in Pondicherry, India in the 1989 Chouhan-Weston Clinical Studies in which I used touch-healing prayer. By touching cancer patients only on the forehead and neck during prayer, I transmitted healing energy to both the fingertip, as the bioelectrography videotape verified, and to the pelvic area, where medical tests confirmed that the symptoms of cervical cancer had disappeared. By a similar touch, a viral cold and chronic spinal pain were healed. These effects did not require any complicated technique focused upon assessing, repairing and recharging the energy fields. The energy fields of the entire body were transformed by simple touch on the forehead and neck.

Previous evidence using Kirlian still photography, which images the energy aura around the body, had already verified that touch-healing completely transforms the energy fields. This is one scientific basis for my confidence in healing prayer. It is also a reason why I can with integrity commend its use by others. From a religious viewpoint, Christianity for twenty centuries has believed that it could transmit the power of God through a simple touch during baptism, confirmation, ordination, weddings and healing. It has maintained that this sacred touch transforms believers in body, mind and spirit by filling them with the presence of God. Billions of believers have subjectively experienced this sacred transformation.

We now know through scientific data that a believer's energy field is transformed, renewed and made whole through the use of touch in sacred rituals. According to researcher Bernard Grad, this sacred energy, the life energy, bears information that acts intelligently to produce wholeness. In the case of Christians, the beliefs of Christianity are transmitted into the energy field through simple touch. This is the power and significance of sacred touch. It is also the basis for the significance of spoken touch-healing prayer.

Billions of humans petition God through prayer. Prayer is used by most religions and cultures. Hindus, Muslims, primitive and tribal religions, along with Christians and Jews, pray for healing. When prayer is offered for healing, those prayers take on certain universal characteristics that bridge the gaps of religious diversity. That is why PrayWell is able to offer every-one Therapeutic Prayers for wholeness and healing.

In addition, Therapeutic Prayer is vital for renewing individuals, couples, families and communities as it restores individual energy fields and pro-duces sacred group energy fields that stimulate processes leading to an enhanced sense of health and happiness in both individuals and groups.

John Wesley, an 18th century English Anglican priest and a founder of the Methodist movement, believed that, *"God does nothing but through prayer."* There is a big difference between simply believing that God exists and doing something about it by being a partner with God in bringing the power of God into the life of the world.

Prayer is a means by which we express our faith in the power of a God who created and continues to recreate and make all things new. PrayWell expresses this faith through scientific evidence, experience and practical new prayer applications. PrayWell provides practical hope for hurting people who desperately desire health and happiness. Like *Star Trek's* fictional crew of the Starship Enterprise, you are invited to *"boldly go where no one has gone before"* to explore a new universe of knowledge that offers renewed hope for every human on our troubled global village Earth.

DETERMINING THE TRUTH OF WHAT YOU READ

Some have criticized my approach. A woman friend, who read an early draft on the scientific data, angrily denounced me, saying, *"It is a lie! It is all a lie! This cannot be true! I can never believe this!"*

A beloved family member, who is a genius at repairing anything, sadly shook his head and said, *"Walt, if you were describing how an engine worked, I could accept it. But, I cannot handle a scientific description of how God works through prayer. This cannot be the basis for my beliefs."*

A supportive colleague in the healing ministry stated, *"Walt, I would like to accept the scientific data. But, as I read it, I keep wondering if it is all true. Why don't you describe the experiments in fuller detail?"*

This book may not be for everyone. The primary purpose of PrayWell is to help the hurting become healthy and happy through prayer. The second purpose is restoring all humanity and the Earth to wholeness. Other purposes include objectively demonstrating to the skeptical that God physically heals through prayer, as well as enabling those who already practice healing to be more effective, and increasing the reader's faith in the power and practicality of actively living with God. I have already had enough positive feedback on the three guidebooks produced from PrayWell's text to feel confident that PrayWell will deliver what it promises. Hearing dozens of first hand-stories about how helpful parts of PrayWell have been to various people, I have become more and more appreciative of a Presence (God) who appears to be inspiring me.

How do you determine the truth of what I write? You can discern the truth in several ways. First, the full details of the experimental scientific data take up most of the space in one of my filing cabinet drawers. It would take several volumes to list it all. Because PrayWell is written for general readership, I have been extremely selective in my choices and very brief about details. Unlike most mass media books, PrayWell footnotes each scientific statement. You can depend upon other specialists in the field to keep me honest. In addition, you can look up the reference details in a library. All the experiments can be inexpensively and easily replicated. The scientific data produces a consistent picture of what is occurring in the healing encounter.

Second, you can look for consistency throughout PrayWell. Everything fits together into a consistent whole that should come through as basic common sense to the reader.

Third, anyone involved in healing will find the contents making sense in the context of their own personal experience. Some will exclaim, *"Aha! Now I understand what is happening! That explains it well!"* Others may say, *"Yes, that is true!"* A Charismatic Christian with the gift of healing noted, *"Dr. Weston. Thank you. I approached your writings with a lot of suspicion. But, everything you wrote rang true to my experience. I now clearly understand the healing encounter. This has helped me to be more of a blessing to others and has strengthened my faith."*

Fourth, the most convincing evidence of the truth is your own application of Therapeutic Prayer and the positive results. Did PrayWell assist in your own self-healing? Did PrayWell help you bring healing to the hurting? Has PrayWell been a helpful resource for restoring you, your marriage, your family, a support group, your community? Has PrayWell deepened your faith in God? Does PrayWell enable you to bring wholeness and renewal into the world?

Fifth, is PrayWell consistent with scriptures? I began with an open mind, determined to accept the objective results of scientific research data as a trustworthy basis for my beliefs about the practice of prayer. I discovered the final picture to be consistent with what we know of Jesus' healing ministry. In contrast, the evidence in PrayWell contradicts most current popular beliefs about prayer and healing. Note the difference between these two bases of understanding as you read.

HOW TO USE PRAYWELL

Few readers will choose to read all of PrayWell. This is a how-to-do-it encyclopedia of prayers for health and renewal. Because PrayWell is an entirely new approach to prayer, the fourteen chapters of *"Part One, Preparations"* are necessary for providing the scientific and theoretical basis of what follows. These are meant to build understanding, respect and confidence for the new prayer procedures. The rest of the book, the practical applications, are written in simpler user friendly terms.

If you simply want to use the prayer sections, I ask that you read at least chapters 1, 2, 6, 8 and 9. If that is too much, read the summary at the end of each chapter. Those who read all of PrayWell will be richly rewarded in their understanding and practice of Therapeutic Prayer.

The rest of PrayWell provides practical applications. You are likely to choose only those applications you need. If you are seeking self-healing, use all of *Part Two.* You are encouraged to read chapter twenty-two for the skills needed for the rest of the book. The last chapter provides optional actions you can take to promote prayer and healing. An index at the back helps you to find specific topics and prayers.

ABOUT THE AUTHOR

This book could not have been written by a specialist. It could not have been written by a person who was only a scientist, only a religious historian, only a counselor, only a group facilitator, only a marriage and family specialist, only a prayer specialist or only a healer. In other words, PrayWell needed to be written by a generalist using a multidisciplinary approach. That describes today's clergyperson, educated in theological school to be a specialist in a dozen fields and, therefore, forced to become a generalist.

I hold a liberal arts bachelor's degree in psychology. My graduate theological degree includes specialties in pastoral counseling and small group work. In 1991, I received a Doctor of Ministry degree in spiritual development and healing research. My practical experience includes thirty years as a United Methodist parish minister, twenty-seven years of healing prayer research and practice, and a quarter-century in the marriage and family enrichment movement. I have been involved in the personal growth and human potential movement for thirty years, and am a life-long human rights activist who believes in the sacredness and immense potential of every human being.

I am an idealist and dreamer with an interest in science and practical applications. I am an outgoing "people person." I grew up in the Christian Church and am grounded in Jesus Christ. I have friends in other faith traditions whose beliefs I honor. I am a husband, a father and a grandfather.

While researching healing, I studied and observed healing as practiced by churches of the Roman Catholic, Orthodox, mainline Protestant, evangelical, fundamentalist, Pentecostal, charismatic, spiritualist and holiness Christian traditions, as well as such healing techniques as Therapeutic Touch, Reiki, Lawrence LeShan healing, Touch for Health, kinesiology, Oriental energy balancing, spirit healing and Hindu healing. My faculty advisor for my doctoral studies was Dr. Bernard Grad, a research biologist at McGill University and the world's foremost healing researcher with over two hundred plant and animal studies.

During this degree work, I had the privilege of studying with researchers and healers from England, Russia, the Philippines, Czechoslovakia, Poland, Thailand, Australia, India, China, Japan, Brazil, Canada and the United States. These included deep trance intuitive Dr. Marilyn Rossner, religious historian Dr. John Rossner, religious sociologist Dr. Peter Roche de Copens, transpersonal psychologist Dr. Denise Roussel, paranormal researcher Dr. Douglas Dean and parapsychologist Dr. Stanley Krippner of the Saybrook Institute. In this context, I studied the scientific data, beliefs, theories, practice and history of healing in the United States, other cultures and the world's religions. These studies have permitted me to look more objectively at the practice of healing prayer.

In 1989, I participated as a healer with Ramesh Singh Chouhan, MD, in the Chouhan-Weston Clinical Studies at JIPMER hospital, Pondicherry, India, which scientifically verified a dozen theories involving the practice of prayer for healing. The videotaping of changing energy fields during the touch-healing encounter provided answers for many troubling questions, creating a helpful new picture.

Throughout my research journey, I have been consumed by the need to know all I can about prayer and spiritual healing. I have shown little caution on the journey. My whole life has been focused upon the subject matter regardless of personal and professional sacrifice. On the surface, my journey would seem to be obsessive in nature. It has been as if I had no choice. I have personally felt that if I stopped searching, I would literally die.

From a religious viewpoint, the journey has been quite different. It has been a joyous faith journey. For throughout, I have felt sustained and guided by God. This portion of my faith journey began at a seminar at Albion College in Michigan in 1978 when the leader, the Rev. Henry Rucker of Chicago, from intuitive insight, commented, *"Walt, someday you are going to write a book about healing which is going to be a best seller and will convince the world of the healing reality."*

I laughed and commented, *"Not me! I know almost nothing about healing. Let God find someone else who is far more qualified."*

A few years later I awoke at two o'clock one morning with all kinds of new understandings of healing running through my mind. The information rudely persisted in keeping me awake so I was forced to arise and write it down. This process continued until the twenty-first straight night when I complained upon returning to bed, *"Lord, I am exhausted. What is this all about?"* I was shocked when the question was answered.

While I was sleeping, a loud, commanding voice shouted in my head, *"Walter, this is your Heavenly Father. I have given you information on a book about healing which I want you to write. It will convince the world of the healing reality, renew the Church and restore the planet Earth."* By the time the voice stopped, I was wide awake. I leaped up and sat on the edge of the bed, and the voice repeated the same message.

Was that experience due to a subconscious suggestion produced by Rucker's statement, or my own higher mind or God's actual voice speaking to me in terms I could humanly understand?

The Voice spoke to me again during sleep three years ago. The brief message was this, *"Remember the word, 'praywell.'"* A year later, I had forgotten that dream message when half-way through the first draft of this as yet untitled book, I found a note I had written to myself in my desk with one word on it, *"praywell."* I immediately recognized it as the most appropriate title for this book.

That same Presence continues to guide me. The Presence is with me as I type these words. Without the Presence, I would never have had the motivation, discipline, inspiration and insight needed to complete PrayWell.

My mind is at one moment skeptical and cautious, questioning the value of what I am producing. The next moment I am caught up in the Presence and the creative flow, filled with God's peace and ecstasy. Am I a crazed fool, a spiritual Don Quixote, carried along on a delusional path to failure? Or is God actually inspiring these writings on a marvelous faith journey that will bless humanity?

Knowing that self-doubt is a part of every faith journey, I, in faith, commend this book to your care. It can be your guide to bringing wholeness to yourself and others, as well as to restoring all humanity. When your prayers bathe humanity in God's ongoing presence, the way is prepared for God to make all things new and good.

Walter L. Weston

Wadsworth, Ohio
May, 1994

Introduction *by Dr. Bernard R. Grad*

It may seem surprising that Walter Weston, who has spent his working life as a pastor, should ask a scientist to write an introduction to his book on healing. Given that many people identify this method of healing with religion, it would seem appropriate for another person of the cloth to be writing in my place. However, as you read this book, you will come to see that even religiously observant people often react with hostility when they hear of spiritual healing.

But why ask a scientist, of all people? Are not scientists notorious for their skepticism and would not their reaction to spiritual healing be even more negative than that of religious people? In my case, I met a healer over thirty years ago and spent years studying the effects of healing on animals, plants, and water in the laboratory, always applying the same scientific techniques and carefully controlled experimental designs that I used in other biological studies involving hormones, vitamins, drugs, etc.

These studies convinced me that healing by touch, at its core, was an objective phenomenon, capable of being studied in the laboratory, and that its effects were not primarily due to suggestion or the placebo effect. Moreover, I believe that it can also be investigated in clinical settings, and, wisely and appropriately applied, it could be helpful in improving the lot of many patients suffering from a variety of conditions. And so it can be said that touch healing is one arena where religion and science can meet, at least at the grassroots level. This is also apparent from reading this book.

But touch healing has been with us for millennia, and if it can be as its practitioners claim, why are not doctors using it at the present time? The answer is that the degree of disbelief, and even scorn, for the claims of touch healing is so profound in the official societies of medicine, that the investigations necessary to convince doctors of the efficacy of this form of treatment have still not been conducted.

It would be wrong to assume that such negative attitudes are more pronounced in our times than in times past because we now have a more sophisticated medicine. Indeed, the opposition was equally intense more than two centuries ago when medicine's treatment tools were restricted to bleeding, a variety of purgatives, and a horrific surgery without anesthesia. This suggests that the reasons against healers may lie elsewhere. Despite the notable advances of modern medicine, and despite problems in many countries, healers in significant numbers still persist in making their presence known.

We take touching for granted because it is so prevalent, from tapping or nudging one another to draw attention, or to make a point, or to shake hands, that it may seem outlandish to claim that touching has a therapeutic potential. However, from observations in orphanages and zoos, and from experiments in the laboratory, it has become clear that the young suffer profoundly from the lack of sufficient touching by a caring parent. And many older people also realize how important the embrace of a beloved may be for their health.

This suggests that touching has a potential for healing, but the healer's touch is not essentially that of a nudge or a handshake. Nor is touch healing the same as a good bedside manner in consoling patients and helping them develop confidence in the doctor. It is true that sometimes this is enough to promote healing, but more often it is not. A healer's touch may also console the patient, but its primary objective is to diminish the illness. That is, the patient's disease provokes a process in the healer that is transferred to the patient by touch and in turn provokes healing processes in his body. The physical reactions to touch between healer and patient are discussed in this book and have also been described by myself and others elsewhere.

How long the healing session takes will vary with the healer and with the disease of the patient. Such details are discussed in the book, but generalizing from one healer to the next may be difficult. For example, in this book prayer plays a primary role in healing. However, in the healers with whom I worked in the laboratory, consciously spoken prayer was not apparent. Each healer has his/her own healing style and may even have his/her own special types of illness with which they are most successful. What a healer may learn from working with people may not apply with animals.

With about 500,000 physicians in the USA, it is inconceivable that a sizable proportion of these should not also be capable of carrying out the healing procedure to a useful degree. Some are surely doing so already, but quietly. Other professionals, notably nurses, are also using Therapeutic Touch within the limitations which the present health system allows. For example, Dolores Krieger, Janet Quinn, and others have already described their experiences in print.

Osteopaths, chiropractors, physiotherapists, the people practicing massage therapy of one form or another, the clergy of various religions, and even non-professionals who in the course of their lives have discovered that they can promote healing by touch, can also be included in the role of potential healers. Of course, all the necessary precautions to protect patients from the dishonesty of the unscrupulous should be taken.

Experiments conducted in the laboratory and innumerable anecdotal reports over the decades, and even centuries, indicate that such healing procedures have the potential of complementing existing medical treatments. For example, they can prepare high-risk patients for surgery, radiation, or drug treatment, shorten the time for recovery, reduce the number and intensity of side-effects and, in some cases, possibly make such procedures unnecessary. This book provides more information on this point.

I don't wish to give the impression that touch healing is a cure-all, but its potential can be assessed by giving it a full and unbiased assessment in clinical settings. Many of us who have worked in this field for many years are hoping that this opportunity will come in our time.

Bernard R. Grad, PhD

Montreal, Quebec, Canada
May, 1994

PRAYWELL

PREPARATIONS
FOR THE JOURNEY

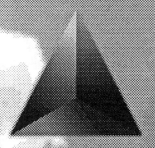

PART ONE

DEDICATION

Dedicated to life energies researchers -- scientists who face ridicule and professional ruin for exploring a new frontier -- yet dream, as a result of their quest, an impossible dream that humanity might someday be immensely blessed by improved physical, mental and emotional health and a spiritual renewal producing unprecedented peace and justice.

The Impossible Dream

To dream the impossible dream,
To fight the unbeatable foe,
To bear with unbearable sorrow,
To run where the brave dare not go.

To right the unrightable wrong,
To love, pure and chaste from afar,
To try, when your arms are too weary,
To reach the unreachable star.

This is my quest,
To follow that star,
No matter how hopeless,
No matter how far.

To fight for the right
Without question or pause;
To be willing to march into Hell
For a heavenly goal.

And I know if I'll only be true,
To this glorious quest;
That my heart will lie peaceful and calm,
When I'm laid to my rest.

And the world will be better for this,
That one man scorned and colored with scars;
Still strolls with his last ounce of courage,
To reach the unreachable stars.

Man of La Mancha

Chapter One

The Most Important Chapter

"Nothing is so firmly believed as what we least know." ...Michel Eyquem de Montaigne

"Derision will never help in the development of true knowledge." ...Abbe Alberto Fortas

"Love your enemies, do good to those who hate you, bless those who curse you, pray for those who abuse you. To him who strikes you on the cheek, offer the other also...." ... Luke 6:27b-29a

---

As you absorb PrayWell, you will need to understand the issues presented in this most important chapter. These issues make this the most difficult chapter of the book. These issues provide perspective on the author's approach and analysis throughout PrayWell. They involve the overwhelming human rejection of the massive body of evidence that prayers for the sick can produce significant healing results. As Bernard Grad states:

"...the degree of disbelief, and even scorn, for the claims of touch-healing is so profound in the official societies of medicine, that the investigations necessary to convince doctors of the efficacy of this form of treatment have still not been conducted. It would be wrong to assume that such negative attitudes are more pronounced in our times than in times past because we now have a more sophisticated medicine. Indeed, the opposition was equally intense more than two centuries ago... This suggests that the reasons against healers may lie elsewhere."

This opposition to those who practice healing has been present throughout history. The historic records show that healers have been feared and have drawn the anger of humanity to the extent that millions of those who practice healing have been persecuted and killed throughout the centuries.

HOW TO USE PRAYWELL

Few readers will choose to read all of PrayWell. This is a how-to-do-it encyclopedia of prayers for health and renewal. Because PrayWell is an entirely new approach to prayer, the fourteen chapters of *"Part One, Preparations"* are necessary for providing the scientific and theoretical basis of what follows. If you simply want to use the prayer sections, I ask that you read at least chapters 1, 2, 6, 8 and 9. If that is too much, read the summary at the end of each chapter of *Part One.* Those who read all of PrayWell will be richly rewarded in their understanding and practice of Therapeutic Prayer.

You are likely to choose only those practical applications you need. If you are seeking self-healing, use all of *Part Two.* You are encouraged to read chapter twenty-two to acquire the skills needed for the rest of the book. An index at the back helps you find specific topics and prayers.

It is as though ten thousand years ago humanity was programmed with an Eleventh Commandment: *Never, ever, accept the reality of the healing encougter. It must always be considered to be a lie, no matter how massive the weight of the evidence.*

Most people alive today do not believe that God physically heals the sick through prayer. Even those who practice healing, myself included, are sometimes skeptical about reports of healings they have not personally witnessed. Long ago, I concluded that spiritual healing is the most unbelieved, misunderstood and ridiculed subject of our time. It certainly produces consistently irrational, negative responses from otherwise fair and intelligent people.

Tolerance of other races, nationalities, religions and lifestyles is publicly and privately talked about and debated. No such conversations are being held about healing prayer. There is either acceptance or dismissal. Most people display mysterious psychological responses.

MY OWN INTRODUCTION TO THESE ISSUES

Had I waited for religious beliefs to convince me of the truth of spiritual healing, I would never have believed that God physically heals the ill through prayer. My estimate is that about ninety percent of church-going Christians, who have spent a lifetime hearing the stories of healing described in the Bible, do not believe that God physically heals through prayer in today's world. I was no different. I am rooted in the Christian faith, having experienced a moving conversion experience at the age of ten and believing God called me to the ministry as a teenager. As a well-educated professional clergyperson, I had laughed at any possibility that God heals. Scriptures and religious belief persuade few people that God heals. Spiritual healing remains the most unbelieved subject of our day.

My belief came only after witnessing the objective reality of physical healings through prayer. This is true of most persons involved in spiritual healing. I refer to my first encounter with healing prayer as God's poetic sense of humor, a little joke played upon me at my expense.

It happened this way. As a young pastor serving my first church, I was praying with a dying man. Peter had had surgery for a ruptured appendix and a peritonitis infection had set in. His doctor cautioned me that Peter had but a half hour to live. In the midst of the prayer, I had a peak experience of God and felt an energy descend upon my head and shoulders and flow down my arm into Peter's hand. I was shocked by the results. Not only did all of Peter's symptoms of peritonitis disappear during our five-minute prayer, but his three-day-old surgical wound was completely healed. Peter, the doctor and I were all shocked, but we did not discuss it. I told no one of the healing, not wishing to appear foolish.

Here is the first major issue facing healing prayer. It is the inability of skeptics to accept and be convinced by any kind of evidence that healings do occur through prayer. If I had told my wife, she would have thought I had become mentally ill. If I had told my congregation about that first healing, and had included scriptural and historical proof, I would have met total rejection. As I cautiously approached my clergy colleagues with my healing story, they told me that they thought I could no longer be considered competent.

Put yourself in my place. That first healing was followed by a consistent trail of further healings that have continued to this day. At first, I didn't believe in healing, yet the healings persisted. That is why I call this God's little joke upon intellectual, liberal me. God still appears to be laughing. What would you have done? My later personal testimony persuaded no one to believe that my healing experiences were true. Spiritual healing remains the most unbelieved subject of our day.

Realizing that I was being forced to live with this phenomenon, whether I wanted to or not, I felt a need to know more about what was happening in the healing encounter. Any time I prayed with the sick, dramatic healings might occur. I spent the next dozen years exploring the history of healing and the present beliefs and practices connected with it. Tradition contained many beliefs about why God did or did not heal, many of them contradictory and none of them were helpful for my journey. Tradition simply said: *"God heals!"*

How? Tradition is not interested, implying that how God heals is a mystery that humans are not to ask about nor explore. I was urged just to proclaim the Good News that God heals and be satisfied with that explanation. I remained consumed by my desire to know the details of what practically takes place in the healing encounter. I do not fault the Church on this. The Christian Church has simply continued to exhibit the ancient attitude expressed in the Bible.

I had never questioned the fact that Jesus and members of the early church practiced healing. But the Bible gives no clues as to how God does it. Its purpose is not to tell *how* God works. The biblical purpose is to proclaim the story of God's power and love in people's lives. That purpose remains the central focus of the Christian Church today. The Church states that when we believe these truths, we shall experience God's transforming power. Unfortunately, this wisdom does not apply to healing. Spiritual healing remains the most unbelieved subject within the Christian Church.

On what basis might we convince skeptics of the truth about spiritual healing? Do they believe the biblical truth that God heals? No! Do they believe the witness of others? No! Do they observe a healing themselves and then decide it is real? No! (We will be discussing this issue later in this chapter.) Do they take an opinion poll and let the majority opinion convince them? That is hardly the basis for objective truth. We are left with only one possible option, science.

It took me a long time to understand the implications of my quest. I wanted to know what happens during healing. That is an objective question. It can only be revealed through the scientific method. Does modern science possess the necessary tools for exploring a religious question? Yes. Are people willing to accept scientific answers about what is occurring in the healing encounter? That question must still be decided.

That decision will be based upon your willingness to explore the many unexplained human barriers to understanding. The barriers involve more than just a bias or a prejudice. Even healers are caught up in the mind games surrounding healing. Let us begin by exploring my wife's response upon discovering my involvement in healing.

MY WIFE'S INITIAL RESPONSE REFLECTS THAT OF HUMANITY

I had mixed emotions about sharing the knowledge that I was a healer. I wanted to protect my professional image and personal friendships. But another part of me was excited and wanted to shout the news joyfully for all the world to hear. I had discovered something that I had not believed existed. Prayer heals! Accompanying the satisfaction of each healing encounter was also a sense of holy bliss. My heart bubbled with joy during and after each healing but with an uncharacteristic caution, I remained a "closet healer." I did not tell my wife about it for four years. Her knowledge came by accident.

The day my wife, Dana, found out was one of most painful moments in our marriage. Arriving home for dinner that evening, Dana laughed as she told me about some nut who kept phoning and shouting, *"He healed me! He healed me!"*

At that moment, the phone rang and that *"nut"* joyfully shouted into my ear, *"You healed me!"* I had closed a marital counseling session with Madge that morning with a prayer for wholeness, knowing nothing of her medical condition. I listened on the phone as she told her story. On the way home, Madge had filled a prescription for a salve that her physician had said would take months to heal her eczema. At home, standing before her mirror with the salve in hand, she was amazed to observe that her skin surface was perfect. There were no lesions nor blemishes. She had linked this to our prayer.

As I hung up the phone, my wife was looking at me, her face registering a shifting mixture of fear, confusion, anger and concern. My worst fears were being realized. She could not handle it. I had never seen her so upset. We had always shared everything. So along with the awareness that I was somehow involved in healing, came a painful sense of betrayal because I had kept my practice of healing a secret from her.

I compounded the situation by confessing everything all at once. I began telling her about one healing after another. Then I fell silent. Dana looked as if she could not decide whether to hit me, cry, call a psychiatrist or run. We could not talk about it! A wall had risen between us. If she had charged me with being unfaithful, we would have at least talked. The silence was extremely painful.

As she told me much later, she wanted to be respectable, comfortable and safe with the way things had always been. My self-imposed four-year silence, as well as the difficulty my wife and I experienced in talking about it, illustrates the immense barriers that human beings have erected against dealing with healing. The fear, anger, confusion and concern that initially swept across my wife's face, mirror our cultural response to spiritual healing. A few years later, like others who have learned to practice healing, Dana became competent and accepted the reality of healing's existence.

SHAME AND DENIAL ARE THE USUAL RESPONSES TO HEALING

In 1989, Hubert Hensel and I became friends. Hearing me at a public lecture, this retired medical doctor invited me to practice healing on his arthritic knee in order to avoid knee replacement surgery scheduled for the following month. I placed my hands around his left knee and prayed. Dr. Hensel timed it. Twelve minutes. He reported that an hour later all symptoms of his painful knee condition were gone.

Dr. Hensel had never heard of healing but he now became eager to learn and practice it. His story could be told by any healer. His first client was a lifelong friend in her seventies, a well-educated woman. We will call her Maude. Dr. Hensel knew that Maude had two arthritic knees. Maude agreed with his experiment to practice healing only on the left knee in order to have a later comparison of the results. Afterward, Maude agreed to report the results. After hearing nothing for two weeks, Dr. Hensel phoned Maude, asking, *"How is your left knee?"*

Maude responded, *"It feels fine."*

Hensel asked, *"How about coming over and we'll heal the other knee?"*

Despite the evidence of her own healed knee, Maude responded, *"What do you think I am, ignorant? We all know healing is impossible! I am not interested."*

Hensel humored her. He said, *"Let us not call it healing. You just come over and we'll see what can be done."*

Maude agreed but insisted, *"Now, you are not going to do healing on me, are you? I will never be able to believe in healing, no matter what happens."*

Dr. Hensel, over a period of several months, practiced healing with Maude for four different medical conditions. To this day, Maude insists that Hensel has done nothing and she would have gotten well anyway, even though each condition was chronic and each healing produced a dramatic alleviation of symptoms. I have observed this same response in hundreds of my own healees. Denial, shame and embarrassment are common responses to successful healings. A few healees respond with anger and may reject any future relationship with the healer. Some of this may be due to fear.

These reactions occur in other contexts. Following healings in prayer groups, family members of healed participants may force the healed to quit the group because, *"We do not believe in that junk."* Again, the healed person provides objective evidence for the family's eyes. Many of my healed clients will attempt to refer loved ones with life-threatening or chronic illnesses to me. Only about ten percent come. Many people with whom I have had a good relationship would rather die of a terminal illness than let me pray with them. Shame and embarrassment are typical human responses to healing.

Because healing is not considered to be respectable, many people who discover they have the ability hide it, becoming *closet healers.* Being a healer can ruin vocations and marriages. I know a number of health care professionals and clergy who are closet healers. Having developed several means for identifying healers during casual contact, I have privately approached a number of suspected closet healers. Their predominant response is, *"Of course I know I am a healer. But you do not think I would let anyone know about it? It would ruin me professionally."*

EYES GLAZE OVER: THE SUPPRESSANT FACTOR

Filled with joy and excitement following a healing, I often abandoned my professional caution. Because most of the healings took place while I was praying with hospital patients, my irrepressible need to share was the greatest on these occasions. Dozens of times I met individual professional colleagues in the hospital pastoral care office and would spontaneously spill out the story of a healing that had just taken place. As I attempted to share the encounter, their eyes would glaze over, their bodies would betray their desire to depart and their silence was deafening. They would walk out without a word. On our next meeting, they would be characteristically friendly. Upon being questioned, none admitted that they remembered having heard my healing story at the hospital.

Often there is amnesia. My first healee, Peter, though he immediately told his wife the details of the healing, had no memory of it one hour later. A hospital patient named Jim experienced a dramatic healing during our touch-healing prayer. Later, Jim had no recollection of the hour I had spent with him. His wife was present and possessed normal memory of the event.

The glazing over of the eyes and the amnesia occur with regularity among skeptics. Psychoanalyst Carl Jung labeled this the *"suppressant factor."* It is caused by the mind's intense denial of the reality of an unexplainable event. If you are a person who has never believed that a miracle of healing can occur and one occurs in you, then your mind must do some mental gymnastics to protect your belief system. You may be forced into an altered state of consciousness like hypnosis or trance.

Recently, I was unprepared for the response of a friend. Sam had attended my seminars, practiced healing and been appreciative of my writings. I was sitting at a table in a restaurant with two of my healees, when Sam unexpectedly joined us. One of the healees, Jean, was telling Sam of her own dramatic healing when Sam's eyes glazed over and he appeared to be in a hypnotic state. The three of us immediately noted Sam's condition. When Jean completed her story, Sam arose without a word and walked away. Jean laughed and commented, *"Walt, that is the kind of incident that you described in your book."*

The following day, I phoned Sam. He volunteered that he had sat with us and met my healee friends, but he had no recollection of Jean's story nor of how he had left us. Healers can respond in the same way as skeptics. It is not uncommon for healers to be skeptical upon hearing someone else's healing story, myself included.

HURTING ENOUGH TO NEED A MIRACLE

Ernie Pyle, a World War II news correspondent, observed, *"There are no atheists in a foxhole."* In a similar way, a health crisis opens people to the idea of seeking alternatives to death, even divine miracles. This is called *"a state of miracle readiness."* In this state, pastors find most people are open to healing prayer. When the prayers result in healing, it brings a sense of deep relief and thanksgiving. For most, this is only a temporary state. Afterward, there may be a sense of embarrassment or shame about being so vulnerable to belief in God and the healing miracle. This may result in anger and distancing from the one who had prayed with them.

There is also a distinction made between prayer and healing prayer. During a medical crisis, prayers are offered to God for healing. Afterward, most people deny that they had used healing prayer, saying, *"We were just praying for God to rescue our loved one. It was not healing prayer."* This is denial and embarrassment concerning the healing reality.

MAGICAL THINKING

I have observed a lot of magical and superstitious thinking about God and healing prayer. In magical thinking, God is like a rabbit's foot good luck charm. *Rub a rabbit's foot just right and your luck will magically change for the good.* Or, *just have faith and everything will turn out all right.* I do not think how God works is at all like the way the Genie granted those three wishes to Aladdin.

I recall the response of a young woman who had just experienced a dramatic healing. I asked her, *"How do you suppose God did that?"*

As we stood in a drug store, she looked at me in disgust and said, *"Rev. Weston, you are not supposed to ask questions like that! God just does it any way he chooses to do it! That is a mystery best left unprobed."*

I had touched a religious taboo. Human beings are curious about how everything works but God. When I see a magician pull a rabbit out of a hat, I am curious. I want to know what is going on behind the scenes. (I still do not know.) When we are not curious about how God heals, I think we are caught in magical thinking or superstition.

God heals not through magical thinking but because humans take action. Society has worn blinders in failing to observe that a human being always stands between God and the healing results. Everyone in the spiritual healing movement knows this. Are you not the least bit curious about the human role? When we pray and healing does not result, the scientific evidence indicates that God is not at fault. His healing power is ever present and available. It is human ignorance that is at fault. Might not some scoffing and unbelief be due to the absurdity of magical thinking about prayer?

MAKING EXCUSES FOR GOD

Magical thinking causes us to make excuses for God. When prayers are not answered and death comes, we have all heard someone make a remark like, *"God in his infinite wisdom must have had a reason for not answering the prayer; for not being with the sufferer."* This makes both God and spiritual wisdom sound absurd. Do we really need to make excuses for God? This is the same kind of excuse that loved ones embarrassingly make for an alcoholic family member not being responsibly present at an important event. I believe God is consistent in wanting to grant all persons his love, goodness, wholeness, healing, and justice. Scientific evidence supports my beliefs, as we shall see.

I once heard a noted biblical scholar say, *"God is God and He acts however He chooses to act."* To which the gathered clergy smugly nodded their heads in agreement. To maintain that God acts however God chooses to act certainly keeps God at the top of the universe's power structure, making him almighty. But it also makes God sound like one of the unpredictable gods of the ancient Greek Mount Olympus or like a spoiled child. Could I worship a god, who, in his immaturity, behaves with no concern for how his actions affect others? Could I worship a god who is described as being seemingly inconsistent, favoring some with healing while unfairly denying healing to others?

What must humans do to be the most effective channels for healing? What is happening when prayers for healing are answered or go unanswered? To give theological answers to these scientific questions blocks rational inquiry. *"The greatest obstacle to discovery is not ignorance -- it is the illusion of knowledge"* (Daniel J. Boorstin).

IF YOU HAVE NEVER EXPERIENCED IT, YOU MAY BECOME HOSTILE

While I was serving as president of an urban clergy association, my colleagues asked me to speak about spiritual healing. I was naively confident I could win some support for healing. I had their respect as one who had led them in counseling seminars and to whom they referred their parishioners for counseling. I arranged for a panel composed of Roman Catholic, Nazarene and Church of the Brethren clergymen who practiced spiritual healing. In our brief presentations, we each told about God's healing. I also gave specific case histories of physical healings.

In the ensuing question-and-answer session, my thirty-five colleagues were not only skeptical, they were extremely hostile. After a half hour of gently fielding their questions, I asked, *"You asked me to present this program on spiritual healing, so why are you so upset with me?"*

Two concerns summed up their responses. First, they had imagined that the term spiritual healing referred only to assisting the sick spiritually and emotionally. After all, I was a pastor like them and we shared a common core of professional education, skills, experiences and beliefs. Yet any talk about the sick actually being physically healed through prayer did not make sense to them. This was the same cultural response with which most persons greet healing.

Second, each having prayed with as many sick persons as I had, all claimed that they had never observed anyone physically healed through their prayers. What I reported did not fit their experience. That is valid logic. I can understand the skepticism of those who have never observed nor experienced a dramatic healing. But, why is it that I am considered a competent witness when I talk about any other subject, but not when I talk about healing?

Why had these thirty-five clergy never observed healing in their own prayers with the sick? I can only speculate. Like other professionals, they are educated in consensual reality. In this case, consensus holds that healing is impossible. If healings had occurred in their ministries, they may have been blind, unable to recognize or accept them. As you will learn, those who can accept the healing reality and those who heal -- possess specific personality traits that these clergy may not have possessed. Yet, this I have trouble believing. I have also observed that closet healers, like closet gays, are not likely to admit their experiences in a public gathering.

Statistically, five to ten percent of those clergy should have possessed the personality traits that would make them potential healers.

HEALING REQUIRES A NEW WAY OF VIEWING REALITY

One summer, I was attending a continuing education seminar for clergy held at a college. Following an evening session, two colleagues and I decided to enjoy a night on the town playing video games. On this particular evening, one of the clergymen was suffering pain from an injured leg and the other had a severe headache. They were annoyed at being unable to locate any pain medication in the dormitory. I asked if I could offer a prayer to heal their pain. The first friend flatly turned me down, saying, *"No way!"* as he made a stiff arm motion toward me.

The second responded, *"No, thanks! I do not believe you can heal my headache by praying and if you did, I do not think I could handle it."*

My friend with the headache was being truthful. Our culture has this enormous block about spiritual healing. God may have sought to part the veil about the truth of the spiritual reality in the Bible, but the veil is still there in human minds. The belief is that God just does not work that way! To be able to handle the idea of healing would require radically altering one's perceptions of reality, including all that one has been taught or has believed throughout a lifetime.

A colleague approached a physician friend about giving touch-healing prayer an experimental chance. *"Give Dr. Weston a patient you cannot help and see what happens."*

The medical doctor angrily replied, *"You do not expect me to believe any of that garbage!"*

My colleague replied, *"I am not asking you to believe. I am asking you to take part in an objective medical experiment."*

The medical doctor responded, *"If Weston can do this healing, I would have to retire from medical practice. It would destroy all that I have believed throughout my years of practice."*

These responses to spiritual healing might best be explained by M. Scott Peck's book, <u>The Road Less Traveled</u>. In a section on dedication to reality he writes: *"The process of making revisions [in our view of reality], particularly major revisions, is painful, sometimes excruciatingly painful. What happens when one has striven long and hard to develop a working view of the world, a seemingly useful, workable map, and then is confronted with new information suggesting that this view is wrong and the map needs to be largely redrawn?*

"The painful effort required seems frightening, almost overwhelming. What we do more often than not is to ignore the new information. Often this act of ignoring is much more than passive. We may denounce the new information as false, dangerous, heretical, the work of the devil. We may actually crusade against it, and even manipulate the world so as to make it conform to our view of reality. Rather than try to change the map, an individual may try to destroy the new reality."

CONFORMITY TO RELIGIOUS BELIEFS REQUIRED

Since ancient times, healers have been scrutinized closely by the religious community and usually have drawn their distrust, scorn or rage. Every healer has been and still is asked the paranoid question: *"What is the source of your healing power?"* Meaning: Does the healing come from God or Satan? From Goodness or Evil? The healer is further probed about his theological beliefs. These must conform to the most conservative and rigid religious doctrines of one's particular religious community or culture for the healer to be acceptable. This remains true in the Western Christian Church of our day.

Bernard Grad recalls that when he began healing research in the 1950s, Christians believed that only Jesus Christ could be the source of healing. Any other healing source had to be evil. What Christians may be expressing is their fear of the perceived powers of the healer. *"If the healer is of my faith tradition, then I can trust him and let go of my fear."* It is not too difficult to speculate that Jesus was crucified because he was a healer and the stated source of his power was not acceptable to the religious authorities.

Many today may still insist, based upon religious belief, that only the God of their particular religious group heals. Is this the objective truth? Most American Christians know that Native American shamans are healers. Religious historians will tell you that basic to every religion in the world is the belief that God heals. Objective data reveals that healing is practiced in every religion and culture on Earth. Regardless of these beliefs, life energies researchers have proven that every healer emits the identical 7.8 to 8.0 hertz frequency of healing energy.

More startling is the observation of researcher Bernard Grad that the healers he used in over two hundred clinical studies did not use prayer. They simply intended to heal and it happened. We will be exploring this more completely throughout this book. My observation: God is love and any person who loves can become a channel for healing.

SOCIAL STATUS REQUIRED OF HEALERS

Healers have historically frightened and angered people. Part of this may be the linkage of healing to God's power and the resulting religious fervor. Is there an innate human prejudice towards the practice of healing that has somehow been carried through into the twentieth century? Throughout the Church's history, healers have emerged. Most of the great church leaders -- reformers, theologians or saints -- were healers. Their healing miracles typically have not been reported in history books, but can be found in their personal journals. Why have both the church and society been embarrassed, skeptical or fearful of healers, often persecuting them and attempting to destroy them during their lifetimes, while later generations could look back and respect their accomplishments?

What is it that those labeled as "witches" in Europe and the Americas did which has caused them to be so thoroughly denounced and vilified? Historians say it was their heretical beliefs in witchcraft rather than Christianity. Yet, in America in 1775, church historians report that only one in fifteen citizens was Christian. Witch hunts must have been supported by non-Christians if whole communities participated. Healing historians report that the main reason a person was labeled a witch was for practicing healing. Why?

Healers have always been perceived as needing high social or spiritual status in order to do their healing work. Society continues to believe that God only works through people of high social and spiritual status. A farm woman who offered healing did not have that status. She would be dealt with as a witch and burned for the heresy of loving someone back to health. While men, grounded in reason and physical reality as their world view, were creating modern science and building the basis for our technological society, women were being executed without due process of the law for practicing healing.

The fact that there were no trials makes these events resemble the mob rage of racial or ethnic murders. The violent reaction and hysteria about healers were so pervasive that this may have left a genetic imprint, conditioning humanity with the collective memory associated with the shame and embarrassment reaction and the subconscious suppressant factor reaction of today. Were those witch burnings related to a male fear of empowered women that still pervades us today?

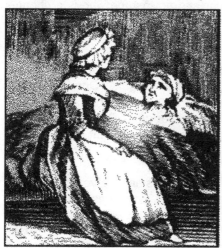 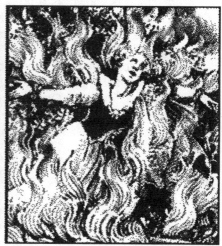

Figure 1. *Low status woman caring enough to nurse a sick person back back to health with dramatic results.*

Figure 2. *Same farm woman being burned at the stake for being a low status female touch-healer*

While low status women were being persecuted, male royalty was practicing touch-healing without fear of harm. If a culture believes that one receives political power from God to rule, then that king is somehow God's representative on earth. European royalty once held that deity-empowered image. They ruled because God supposedly had decreed their rule and thus people could accept healing through God's representative here on earth. Thus, England's King Charles II (1660-85) is reported to have healed one hundred thousand of his subjects by the Royal Touch of his hand. King George II

(1727-60) had attributed to him three hundred thousand healings by a similar Royal Touch.

THE CHURCH CHANGES THE RULES FOR HEALERS

The Christian Church plays a crucial and ambivalent role in the public attitude towards healing. In the New Testament, the Apostle Paul describes the spiritual gifts in First Corinthians 12-14. Scripturally, spiritual gifts are considered special abilities granted directly by God's Spirit. Supposedly, one does not possess these gifts until God grants them.

There are observable reasons for believing this today. I have observed Pentecostal and Charismatic Christians, filled during a worship service with the power of the Holy Spirit, instantly speaking in tongues and receiving the gift of knowledge or guidance or become healers. My own first healing occurred while I was filled with the Holy Spirit. The Church regards these gifts with special reverence, though most branches of Christianity would rather ignore them.

Paradoxically, the gift of healing is revered far above all the other gifts. Among the churches with healing ministries, there is no such term as *"healer."* One having the special ability to heal is considered a *"channel for healing."* Other spiritual gifts are regarded far differently. One who has the gift of preaching is known as a preacher and not as one who is a channel for God's preaching. One who has the gift of teaching is known as a teacher and not as a channel for God's teaching. The rules have been changed for healing.

One needs some of these gifts to become a candidate for ministry; then the seminary educates students in developing these gifts. One is taught to become a better teacher. One is taught to be a better preacher. One is never taught to practice healing, as with the other gifts. Could both the fear of healing, as well as misunderstanding, foster these different approaches?

SIX CONCEPTS EXPRESSING A FAULTY VIEW OF HEALING

First, Christian tradition views the healing ability as being given by God in a unique and unspecified way. The healer may be viewed as being God, as in the case of Jesus of Nazareth. Or, he may be viewed as having been given the ability because he is closer to God than others. Or, the suspicious may believe his power comes from Satan. (That is impossible because all healing comes from God's love.)

Second, of all the many spiritual gifts, only healing is perceived as resulting from God's direct intervention. In this view, God does all the healing while the human healer is considered to be only passively involved as an unthinking channel.

Third, this healing by God is perceived as being the instantaneous consequence of God sending a mysterious healing projectile, like an ancient god hurling a lightning bolt. This attitude is akin to magical thinking.

Fourth, healing is sacred, because God is doing it. Therefore, healing is a uniquely religious phenomenon, which is only permissible within the setting of organized religion. It may also be used as proof of the validity of a particular religion.

Fifth, the healer has other special spiritual or psychic gifts that authenticate his healing prowess.

Sixth, in the Christian tradition, only God in Jesus Christ heals. All other healings are evil or the result of the evil angel, Satan.

These six concepts may have contributed to your image of a healer. But, in the light of existing evidence, these beliefs appear to be wrong. The word *appear* is not hedging. Future scientific approaches might yield data to support some of these six concepts. But, the fact remains that healings can and do occur outside of these six categories, as we shall see.

FACTORS THAT EMERGE FROM CURRENT EVIDENCE

The existing evidence gives rise to an entirely new and far more useful image of the healer. The ability to heal is a biological and personality trait, just like physical traits, intelligence, athletic or musical abilities. It is the healer's personality and brain-wave qualities that enable the special healing ability to manifest.

God is involved in healing's empowerment, but healing is also empowered by the human capacity to express compassionate love. The creation of the healing flow is directly related to the human capacity to love. My own personal belief is that God is the source of all love and that the physical creation is an intelligent and purposeful expression of love. Therefore, any time human beings love, they become divinely empowered, regardless of religious belief. God is love and he who loves is of God, and, therefore, capable of expressing God's transforming healing energy.

There is a healing energy emitted by human beings that can be stored indefinitely in water or cloth. This does not match the traditional image of how healing occurs. Yet, according to the research data, healing reflects qualities which religions have attributed to God, including an intelligent and purposeful action that recreates and restores people to health and happiness. The healing energy explains the qualities attributed to historic holy relics. Holy relics -- the bones, clothes, and personal objects of saintly persons and places -- have been reported to bring healing to the faithful who touch them. Holy relics and healer-charged articles would seem to produce the same phenomena.

Another link is described in clinical studies of plants nurtured by Holy Water that have grown sixty-seven percent faster than the control plants. The historic depicting of saints with white or yellow halos about the head has a parallel in the increased energy fields during healing encounters which energy photographs have documented.

One need not invoke God's name to heal. As you shall see later, Lawrence LeShan's healing technique does not even involve a reference to God. In both Reiki and Therapeutic Touch, one only quiets the inner self. Like healings in the New Testament, many persons can practice healing by simply saying, *"Be healed,"* or by intentionally touching. I have done this. The principle underlying such healings may well be based in the love that flows from healer to healee. Expressions of love gather, accumulate, attune and transmit a healing energy.

A future chapter explains how a shift in consciousness can produce healing. Not all of these shifts in consciousness involve references to God. My guess is that shifts in consciousness cause healing by altering the qualities of both the brain and the mind, producing optimum functioning. Mentalist and Hindu healings appear to operate this way. They may alter the brain and the mind through what might be called God's Healing Mental Energy. This is an unexplored frontier for research.

HEALING AND THE SPECTACULAR

Healing is shrouded in the spectacular. Let us beat drums and shoot off fireworks and watch the sky for shooting stars and flying saucers! These fulfill the exotic stereotype. Many faith healers play this role to the hilt. In order to be recognized or accepted as a healer by the general public, one is expected to display other special gifts.

I have had clients who will not reveal their condition, saying, *"If you are a* **real** *healer, you will instantly sense what is wrong with me."* Another approach is, *"Tell me how long I have to live. As a healer, you must know these things."* Finally, *"Just touch me once and I know I will be instantly healed."* These comments reflect the cultural assumption that a healer has other special gifts that authenticate his healing prowess. These flashy attributes elevate the status and credibility of the healer in the public's mind.

The late Brazilian healer, Arigo, could not only use a rusty knife in performing spiritual surgery, he could intuitively diagnose illness and prescribe medication needs. Filipino healers are renowned and sought after because they appear to be able to reach into the body with their hands and remove diseased tissue. Their special abilities have caused scientists and the news media to elevate their reputations while ignoring the unspectacular healer who may be their next-door neighbor. Studies made by researchers have shown that effective healers are consistently distributed all across the Earth, regardless of whether or not they possess spectacular gifts.

Nonetheless, evidence that something spectacular will happen during the healing encounter remains a human expectation. Most people, even researchers and healers, are skeptical that healing will occur. I once made an appointment with the noted Brazilian healer Mauricio Panisset for my own healing. As the days approached for our session, I became skeptical of his abilities. Was I wasting my time and money? Were my hopes for nothing? And these doubts were going through the mind of a healer with almost three decades of experience! Then I met him and learned first-hand that Mauricio Panisset was everything I had heard he was. (He died in August, 1993.)

Most of us look for signs and wonders when we visit a healer. We have little trust in the competency of a healer. Therefore, most healers work with skeptical and suspicious clients. The scientific evidence and clinical studies in PrayWell are meant to build trust and respect for the healer's work.

OUR IMAGE OF JESUS HAS INFLUENCED HEALING HISTORY

The historic Jesus of Nazareth experienced every healer's irresolvable dilemma in facing the probing question: *What is the source of your healing power?* For an answer to be acceptable to the minds of the public, a healer's religious, moral and political beliefs have been required to conform with the questioner's. Could the authorities have sought Jesus' death because of anger and fear toward his healing powers and their implications? He taught a new religion and ethic based upon love. As a healer, he had no choice. Healing flows out of love. With his altruistic love, he related to all persons regardless of their nationality, religious affiliation or political loyalties. This stance alone could have been used to justify the authorities' death sentence.

Jesus did not invoke God's name in healing. He simply said words like, *"Rise!" "Walk!"* or *"Be healed!"* Or he silently touched people. The authorities saw Jesus, a human being, healing on his own authority, not through God's power. He was thus perceived as acting as God. That is considered to be religious blasphemy, a legal justification for his death.

This is also a mistaken justification used by Christianity for proclaiming Jesus to be the God-Man-Savior. Jesus healed on his own authority, not God's. Actually, it was a combination of some two dozen types of miracles, including healing, that convinced his believers that he was the Son of God. Healers today, as in all generations, have had the ability to heal without invoking God's name.

This runs counter to Judeo-Christian-Islamic religious beliefs. Since our whole culture derives from that earlier mindset, some healers today, because they can heal without invoking God's name, have come to another mistaken conclusion, *"I am God!"* when other reasons effectively explain their healing gift.

Regarding their claims of Godhood, it can be agreed that all human beings contain the divine spark. We are all sacred, spiritual beings. It can be agreed that healers can perform the priestly function of bringing the power of God into people's lives. But they remain only a reflection of God, not God.

I believe that all that I am and all that I shall ever be is a gift from God. God has always channeled his love, his inspiration and his miracles through human beings. Healers are no exception! Healing is one of several priestly functions. A priest is one who brings the power of God into the life of the world. That is what a preacher is doing. That is what a teacher is doing. That is what a caregiver is doing. That is what a pray-er is doing. That is what a healer is doing.

A LAST WORD

The issues we have covered in *This Most Important Chapter* can either help or hinder your study and use of PrayWell. You may have been repelled by many of the statements. You may have insights into some issues. As the scientific evidence and other information provide a trustworthy new road map, my statements in this first chapter will be substantiated.

It is not easy to practice healing. All the factors presented in this chapter confront a healer. Because it dealt with the struggles of a healer, the movie, *Resurrection,* deeply moved me. *Resurrection* is the compelling story of a healer played by actress Ellen Burstyn. It is not so much a story about how spiritual healing works, but rather about what happens to the one who seeks to use her gift of healing.

The story begins with the female healer lying critically injured in the hospital following an auto accident in which her husband had been killed. In critical condition, she has a near-death experience in which she sees a tunnel through which loved ones are beckoning to her. She recovers, but with damaged nerves in her legs, leaving them paralyzed. Her life is drastically changed.

This is a classic case of how a healer emerges: having a powerful traumatic or mystical experience and later discovering the healing gift. Trauma heightens awareness, so the latent healer within is awakened. Over a period of time, Burstyn's character heals her own legs and returns to a full physical life. But now she knows she is a healer, convinced by both her own self-healing and the inner knowledge that the near-death experience awakens in her. She practices healing in groups with the cooperation of her doctor, eventually being tested by scientists at a medical research center.

But the public expectations about the person of the healer are more than she can handle. She is no moral saint nor religious mystic, living unmarried with her male lover. She does not even pray to do healing. She does not rationally understand what her healing work is all about. She only knows that simply and naturally as she deeply loves people, her touch heals. The accompanying anger, suspicion, rejection and violence directed at her are more than she can handle.

So she finds her own personal solution. She settles in the middle of the desert and operates a service station. There, she quietly heals occasional customers, who, unsuspecting of her gift, do not threaten her. That is one way to handle the ability to heal. Another way may be to write a convincing book to persuade others to become open to healing, and perhaps, to teach some of those readers to offer healing themselves.

ANOTHER COMMANDMENT

At the beginning of this chapter, I offered an Eleventh Commandment, suggesting that the human attitude towards healing prayer appeared to be like a ten-thousand-year-old conditioning of all human minds: *Never ever accept the reality of the healing encounter. It must always be considered a lie, no matter how massive the weight of the evidence.*

Can we begin replacing that with another commandment? It need be nothing too outlandish. How about the words of the creator of detective Sherlock Holmes, the scientist Arthur Conan Doyle, who noted with his keen mind, *"When you have eliminated the impossible, whatever remains, however improbable, must be the truth."* Or, borrow wisdom from a pioneering scientist like Michael Faraday, who in the midst of new discoveries, said, *"Nothing is too wonderful to be true."*

CHAPTER ONE SUMMARY

1. Healing is possibly the most misunderstood, unbelieved and ridiculed subject of our day. Even healers are skeptical of reported healings and of other healer's abilities.

2. Fear, anger, confusion and concern are typical responses to a witnessed or reported healing.

3. In response to a healing story, a listener's eyes may glaze over, as if he is in a trance-like state. This is the *"suppressant factor"* caused by the mind's intense denial of the reality of an unexplainable event.

4. Recipients of a healing often respond afterwards with a sense of shame, embarrassment and denial.

5. Amnesia about the healing encounter sometimes occurs.

6. A health crisis opens people to seek divine miracles, producing a temporary state of miracle-readiness. After the healing, there is embarrassment or shame about being so vulnerable to belief.

7. During a medical crisis, prayers are offered for God to heal. Afterwards, most people deny that they had used *"healing prayer,"* claiming it was just a prayer to God, seeking help.

8. Many prefer God's actions to remain a mystery. Much of this desire is based upon magical thinking. The statement, *"Just have faith and everything will turn out all right,"* is a false assurance and a form of denial.

9. People often make excuses for God when prayers are not answered. To give religious answers blocks rational inquiry. When prayers go unanswered, it is due to human will and ignorance.

10. To be able to accept the concept of healing requires radically altering one's perceptions of reality, including the beliefs of a lifetime.

11. People possess a fear of the perceived powers of the healer. Healers have had to conform to the most conservative religious and moral beliefs of their culture or face death. Conformity calms people: *"If the healer holds my beliefs and values, then I can trust him and let go of my fear."*

12. Society continues to believe that God only works through people of high religious, social or political status. That is why simple farm women were burned as witches for practicing healing. Today "closet healers" abound, hiding out of fear of personal and vocational rejection and ruin.

13. The abilities of a world-class healer involve personality traits and biologically triggered brain-wave qualities.

14. Healing is shrouded in the desire for the spectacular, but healing prayer is a quiet and peaceful event. Even healing researchers can become caught up in the spectacular as shown by those who are attracted to studying the bizarre rather than the quietly practicing healers who live near their homes.

Chapter Two

PrayWell Tenets

"Faith is the characteristic that unites humanity." ...Raimundo Panikkar*

"Underlying the diversity of religious forms is a unified core that could be called spiritual religion." ...Elton Trueblood*

"God is love, and he who abides in love abides in God, and God abides in him." ...John 4:16b

---

A *"tenet"* expresses a principle or rule. *PrayWell* Tenets introduce you to PrayWell's unique focus and inclusiveness. These tenets reflect the realities of our scientific understanding, including an emerging spiritual wisdom as well as the new world order that recognizes all humans as sacred, precious and interconnected, brothers and sisters in a diverse global community. These tenets, taken as a whole, are new, self-evident truths.

A NEW PERSPECTIVE

Some 1993 public opinion polls provide a new perspective. Ninety-nine percent of Americans have prayed at least once, according to the National Opinion Research Center in Chicago, with 57% praying daily. According to the Barna Research Group, 69% of adults consider religion to be very important. The Gallup polls report that between 40% to 43% of Americans attend church on a weekly basis. Gallup statistics show that 60% of American households report that someone says a prayer before meals eaten at home. These polls do not appear, however, to reflect reality, being more a matter of national myth and reported religious respectability.

However much Americans may value religion and prayer in theory, other observations and data contradict these poll results. Have you ever seen the urban traffic jams created by one hundred million Americans attending church on Sunday morning? That is how many polls report church attendance, yet statistics on mainline churches show that only 25% to 33% of *members* attend church on any given Sunday. If half the population are church members, an extension of those statistics means that only 12% to 17% of Americans are in church on any given Sunday. Church sociologists report that only 10% to 12% of Americans are active participants in a religious community. Those figures more accurately reflect the traffic you and I see on Sunday mornings.

A recently reported poll shows that about twenty percent of Americans can name the four Gospels. As a pastor, I can tell you that any participating member of a Christian church knows these most elementary facts about the Bible.

Why have I brought these figures to your attention? For you to gain perspective on the nature of prayer and the religious life. When 69% of adults claim to consider religion to be very important, what are they saying? What is the relation between the importance of religion and the practice of prayer? What kinds of prayers *do* people offer? A prayer at mealtime thanking God for the food is not a deep level of prayer. In one church I pastored, most of the eighty members of a prayer chain asked for help because they did not know how to pray for healing. This appears to be true of most pray-ers.

Francis MacNutt, who annually leads one hundred thousand people through Charismatic prayer workshops, reports that only 1% of his participants had ever prayed aloud for a spouse's needs. That figure makes it appear that we have privatized prayer, doing it secretly and silently, as if with a deep sense of shame or inadequacy.

Jesus said, *"Where two or more are gathered in my name, there am I in the midst of them."* This implies, and prayer experience confirms, that God is more powerfully present when two or more persons are gathered in prayer. Yet, the evidence indicates that most prayer journeys are private endeavors traveled alone outside the walls of organized religion.

We have established taboos about sharing our prayer journeys with others. While these taboos are not written into law nor formally acknowledged, nonetheless they have shaped our attitudes and actions. We do not talk about God in our communities, schools or workplaces. We seldom talk about God or our experiences of God within our families. We seldom pray with our loved ones, except perhaps for the nominal table grace.

Contributing to the dilemma is our awkwardness about things spiritual. We lack the necessary skills for cultivating our relationship with God. We feel inadequately prepared for praying aloud with loved ones. This is one of the walls of shame contributing to taboos about God-talk. We don't know how to pray for healing in the midst of crisis. And yet prayer is the primary means by which humanity makes contact with God. Prayer is also the main tool for journeying with God. There is a power in prayer that opens the door to God's presence, power and healing. Through prayer, our hearts can find their peace in God and the power for personal health and renewal. Breaking down the walls of shame concerning our longing for God is the first step on the spiritual journey.

THE SPIRITUAL JOURNEY

Many people have known the joy of a peak experience of God. Afterwards, they may search for years for ways to recapture that peak experience, with little consistent success.

I had always hungered for more of the inner presence and guidance of God. The practice of healing prayer has made awareness of God an ongoing experience in my life. Like myself, much of humanity is longing for both personal wholeness and spirituality. PrayWell uses prayer to provide a path that leads to both. So this book is committed to fulfilling your yearnings. In the midst of this prayer journey, you will come to a deeper appreciation of the psalmist who declared, *"Our hearts are restless until they find their peace in God."*

PrayWell believes that prayers for healing offer the best means for opening the doors to spirituality, because prayers for healing produce not only the healing of body, mind and spirit but also an awareness of God's presence and peace. They bathe and fill us with the presence of God.

PrayWell provides a new road map for prayer, using scientific and experiential data. For more than a generation, books on touch healing, wellness and spirituality have emphasized meditation, visualization, centering and affirmations as the primary tools for achieving these goals. Yet, the evidence indicates that none of these is more effective than prayer. Prayer provides an energy for living which produces health, wholeness, purpose, harmony, happiness and satisfaction. Why this happens will be scientifically explained.

PrayWell seeks to unite people in companionship with like-minded others for the prayer journey. Perhaps this will eventually lead some to appreciate more fully the practical purposes of religious communities. PrayWell also enables people of diverse religious traditions to pray together wherever they are, permitting anyone to join with anyone else in prayer.

RESTORING ALL LIFE ON EARTH

The research data on the significant effects of prayer upon all living organisms strengthens religious claims that prayer is a powerful means for bringing God's power into the life of the world. The scientific data indicates that healing prayer releases an energy that promotes the optimum living conditions for all life. Through healing prayer, God is able to recreate and make all things new. Healing prayer can also strengthen family wholeness and restore caring and responsibility to all communities of people. Thus, healing prayer has the potential to bring health and wholeness, happiness and satisfaction to you, your family, your community and all communities.

I know this sounds idealistic and utopian. Prayer has been around since the first human being turned to God. All kinds of claims have been made for prayer since that time. Now, the new scientific picture indicates that prayer is capable of doing far more than even most religions have claimed.

This new perspective comes at a time of great need in human history. The world is helplessly witnessing the decay of traditional values, lifestyles and institutions and all that implies for the health and happiness of marriages, families, neighborhoods and communities. Ours is becoming the age of secular humanity. All religions see the need to bring God into the lives of everyone. As the new scientific picture takes shape, there is ample evidence that prayer is a major means by which humanity can transform people and all other life on earth to optimum living conditions.

TWO PERCEPTIONS NEED CHANGED

For this to happen, two perceptions must be changed. First, prayer must be rescued from its traditionally exclusive religious context. Modern secular culture has consigned group prayer activity to religious groups, churches and temples. We must find an acceptable social means to encourage support groups, community groups and nations to use prayer as a therapeutic tool for human health and wholeness. Because people are suspicious of prayer with people of other religious traditions, we need to find a means of removing the religious context from prayer.

Second, this means developing a religiously neutral or universal form of prayer in order to address specific crucial community needs. The lesson of the research data is that God recreates and makes all things new through prayer. To limit that good to religious groups is to deny most people access to the practical help available in daily group absent and touch prayer in home and community. Influencing people to do this is a major purpose of PrayWell. Providing people with the practical tools for doing this is the major focus of PrayWell.

For these purposes, PrayWell introduces the concept of *Therapeutic Prayer.* The purpose of Therapeutic Prayer is to express caring as a means for bringing God's power into the life of the world to heal and transform all humanity. Here are the PrayWell Tenets:

1. PrayWell seeks to promote the practice of healing prayer and wholeness in the home, workplace, medical setting, community and world. It does this by offering detailed guidance on the science, theory and practice of healing prayer. Healing prayer is part of the larger field of knowledge known as spiritual healing. God transforms and makes all people new and whole through prayer.

2. PrayWell seeks to enhance prayer competency. PrayWell will increase your understanding and practice of prayer in its many dimensions. It is based upon objective prayer, healing research data and experience. It borrows know-how from healers, prayer groups, healing services, the world's religions and spiritual wisdom throughout the planet. It rationally explains the nature of prayer. Step-by-step, it coaches you in vocal praying skills.

3. PrayWell seeks to enhance personal wholeness. In the process of coaching, it teaches persons how to practice self-healing prayer and to pray for the healing of others. The prayers of all persons who deeply care yield significant healing results. There is an energy in prayer that enhances all life, making all things new. PrayWell helps persons attain personal wholeness in body, mind, spirit and relationships.

4. PrayWell seeks to enhance spirituality. Spirituality involves an inner awareness of the ongoing presence of God. Spirituality begins through firsthand experiences of God. It is a journey that results in an inner serenity and joy, a sense of vital purpose and actions designed to express caring, fairness, cooperation and peace with justice. Spirituality is a normal side-effect of healing prayer, although it can be acquired through other intentional approaches. Daily prayer permits God's presence to abide within people and transform them. Daily vocal prayer with others greatly enhances results.

5. PrayWell seeks to restore humanity by bringing God's presence into all aspects of modern secular culture: to home, family and marriage, to school and workplace, to industry, business and corporation, and to community, national and international settings. It does this through a scientifically neutral, or therapeutic, rather than a religious approach to group prayer.

6. PrayWell seeks to restore the ecology of Mother Earth through the prayer energy produced by enormously large groups of people. God is the Creator. Through the prayer connection, God is able to restore and purify all of the Creation.

7. PrayWell asserts the fact that prayer is the primary means by which people make daily first-hand contact with God. All religions make contact with God through various rituals and songs, but prayer is the universal means by which human beings petition God to intervene in their lives. In this context, PrayWell is assuming that all persons have a direct and meaningful access to God and his power through prayer.

8. PrayWell asserts the fact that all humanity is united by its common experience of pain. In the midst of personal pain, when a human being turns to God, s/he offers a prayer of petition, asking for God's help. This appears to be a common instinctive reaction.

9. PrayWell asserts the fact that when any person prays in the midst of crisis, those prayers take on certain universal characteristics that transcend religious beliefs. When a loved one is ill, the person praying would obviously use plain words that simply ask God to grant healing. Example: *"God, my mother is sick. Please heal her."* Any prayer expressing compassionate love is able to bring the power of God into the life of the world for the purpose of bringing healing and wholeness to hurting people.

10. PrayWell asserts the fact that all humanity shares certain common beliefs about God. Religious historian John Rossner reports that all humanity shares the belief that God is the creator, sustainer, revealer, transformer, empowerer and healer. All religions believe that human beings are spiritual and are enhanced by contact with God. They also believe in the afterlife, in that following physical death, each person makes a transition into another dimension of existence.

11. PrayWell asserts the fact that all humanity shares certain common experiences with God. First-hand contact with God results in a universal religious experience of awe, wonder and oneness with the Creator and Sustainer.

12. PrayWell seeks to remain religiously neutral. The religious diversity of humanity is immense. Yet, the above assumptions make neutral religious prayers for healing and wholeness possible. In practical terms, there is no such thing among Christians as a Catholic, Orthodox, Baptist or Methodist prayer for healing. Nor are there unique Christian, Muslim, Hindu, Jewish, Shinto, primitive religion or tribal religion prayers for healing. Only God-language differences are present.

13. PrayWell acknowledges the divisions that result from religious language. In American Christianity alone, there are over a thousand separate and distinct Protestant denominations, each with its own characteristic prayer language and vocabulary. If PrayWell offered prayers in a Christian context, we'd need dozens of editions of this book just to address the diversity of specific Christian groupings and their preferred words for God. Yet, in plain everyday words, their prayers would all make similar petitions to God in prayers for healing. The same is true of the other world religions.

14. PrayWell uses a secular word in referring to the Supreme Being in order to resolve the God-language issue. In the English language, dictionaries refer to the Supreme Being as God. This is the secular, generic or neutral term for God that can be used in all religious contexts. Each language would tend to have a similar generic term for God. To remain religiously neutral, PrayWell addresses the supreme Being as God. Because all humanity shares the belief that God is the creator, sustainer, revealer, trans-fomer, these terms can also be as religiously neutral or universal names.

15. PrayWell is intended to be used within the context of your existing religious beliefs. It is meant to strengthen your own com- mitments and life style. It has been intentionally designed this way. Substituting your own preferred name for God in the prayers is encouraged when you are praying alone or with persons of your own religious tradition.

16. PrayWell's neutrality enables persons of differing religious beliefs to pray together. The language and style of PrayWell prayers are suitable for praying with persons of all religious beliefs. This lowers the social barriers that have limited persons from offering prayer in a religiously pluralistic setting. It intends to nurture the inclusion of others into your spiritual journey: spouses, family, friends, neighbors, classmates, fellow workers, community gatherings, international friends and those who are hurting wherever you find them. PrayWell's universal prayers are a suitable guide for persons of all religious beliefs in the art of prayer, wholeness and spirituality.

17. PrayWell seeks to be gender-neutral in addressing God. This arose naturally from calling God, "*God.*"

18. PrayWell is based upon scientific research. Scientific research data moves us beyond faith in religious beliefs to the objective truth about the value of prayer. The objective truth is that prayer is a powerful tool for the healing of the body, mind and spirit. Scientific data confirms the ancient religious beliefs that God heals. The objective truth is that when any person lovingly cares for another, intends to offer healing through prayer and then prays, those prayers have a genuine potential to result in dramatic healing. Worldwide research with healers has provided data indicating that all humanity transmits the same electromagnetic frequency (plus or minus 7.83 hertz) in the healing flow when making effective contact with God for healing.

19. PrayWell is grounded in practical results. God objectively heals through prayer. Hundreds of research experiments with plants and animals have scientifically proven that God uses human beings as channels for healing. Practical experiences with humans confirm this scientific data. Through twenty-eight years of practicing one-on-one healing prayer, the author has witnessed a ninety percent success rate in healing physical illness and injuries.

Of more than six hundred participants in my small prayer groups, 75% have reported being physically healed, 83% emotionally healed, 87% experienced interpersonal healings and 95% reported feeling the ongoing presence and peace of God. All of this happened in just five two-hour sessions.

These results are even more amazing when you consider that healing prayer has traditionally been met with immense public resistance. Most of those experiencing healing were skeptics. They did not believe anything significant would happen, but they reluctantly and cautiously gave the prayer healing process a try -- with noteworthy results.

20. PrayWell offers a spiritual technology. Don't let that term turn you off. Spiritual technology is not impersonal. It describes a step-by-step process. If you do "this, and this, and this" in prayer, you will likely produce "these" intended results. A recipe for baking bread represents a technology. So does advise on how to get along better in your marriage or on using parenting skills. So do directions for caring for a houseplant. PrayWell is centered in no set of religious beliefs, so we cannot call it religious practice. The term *"spiritual disciplines"* does not aptly describe PrayWell, either. PrayWell does provide practical recipes, advice and directions on how to pray effectively. In this context, PrayWell is a spiritual technology.

21. Praywell is a unique practical guide to personal prayer, spirituality and wholeness. It is based upon scientific and scholarly research data, reason, theory, observation and practical experience, rather than religious beliefs. These various components complement each other and fit into a consistent unity of the whole. Each provides proof of the truth of the others. When you see the practical results, it all mentally fits together, making common sense. PrayWell seeks practical, predictable results from the use of prayer as a tool for emotional, physical, spiritual, interpersonal and group wholeness.

22. Praywell strengthens existing religions by bridging the gap that separates religion from science, reason, every-day living and modern cultural stereotypes. It accomplishes this goal through *"spiritual technology"* -- detailed explanations and directions for prayer, wholeness and spirituality. Spiritual technology provides an additional conceptual basis for prayer and the spiritual journey built upon the cause-and-effect principles of the objective scientific model. It enables ancient theological truths to come alive with common-sense meaning for today's humanity.

23. PrayWell lowers the barriers that separate persons of diverse backgrounds and cultures. When individuals of diverse ethnic, national, cultural, racial and religious backgrounds pray for each other, the barriers of misunderstanding and distrust are lowered and new beginnings based upon unity, understanding, respect, fairness and caring become possible. In the context of PrayWell, every is sacred and precious. Thus, PrayWell offers guidance for ending human differences and building a new world of peace with justice.

24. PrayWell introduces the concept of Therapeutic Prayer. Therapeutic Prayer seeks to restore and make whole, and to bring the presence of God into the life of the world. In this sense, Therapeutic Prayers are not religious prayers. They do not seek to promote any particular religious belief. They are universal in approaching God as the Creator, Sustainer and Healer. They are practical because they seek to bring New Life into the world.

Therapeutic Prayer can be shared with any person or group needing God's wholeness and spirituality with the fear of insulting the sensibilities of another religion or seeking to win new converts. Thus, Therapeutic Prayer can be used in diverse family, group, community, vocational, national and international settings.

For several years, I have practiced Therapeutic Prayer with the general public during the practice of touch-healing and counseling. I was forced to do this because my sensitivity to the diversity of my clients' religious beliefs. I have found that it does not change the context, significance or power of my prayers. For me, Christ is just as powerful an inner presence. With Christians, I pray using my lifelong Christian style.

25. PrayWell believes that prayer is the most powerful tool available for defeating the forces of darkness and evil. PrayWell shares humanity's historic belief that an ongoing battle is being fought between the forces of darkness and evil and the forces of God's light and love. Our highest spiritual ideals and deepest yearnings remain focused on the hope of a future day when the forces of light and love are triumphant and peace with justice rules in the lives of all humanity. For this purpose, prayer programs divine purpose into chaos, producing order, cooperation, love, goodness and justice. Prayer is the primary means by which humanity can usher in this sacred Golden Age.

26. PrayWell believes that prayer is an essential component for sustaining each individual life journey. Prayer is a primary means by which humanity invites God to be at work in personal and community living. Prayer brings the presence and power of God into life. *God does nothing but through prayer.*

Chapter Three

Scientific Proof That Prayer Heals

"The basic texture of research consists of dreams into which the threads of reasoning, measurement, and calculation are woven." ...Albert Szent-Gyorgi

"An examination of the reports of religious experience discloses three general beliefs: (1) The visible world is part of a more spiritual universe from which it draws its significance, (2) That union or harmonious relations with that higher universe is our true end, and (3) That prayer or communion with the spirit thereof is a process in which spirit energy produces effects within the phenomenal world." ...William James*

"Beware of the truth. If you find a truth it can demand that you make painful changes." ...Frank Herbert

---

Part One: Preparations for the Journey is just what it says. These chapters provide information for the later how-to-do-it chapters. We will be drawing extensively from this data. These chapters also give you confidence in the unfamiliar guidance you will be receiving for prayer. After gaining practical experience in Therapeutic Prayers for health and renewal, you will find your self using these chapters as helpful sources of reference.

Chapters 3, 4, 5, 6, 7 and 8 possess their own importance. Most of this information is unfamiliar to everyone but experts in the field of spiritual healing and in the science of life energies. One of the reasons that so many false notions have gathered around the concept of spiritual healing is the public's unfamiliarity with this field of knowledge. Yet, even those with knowledge may cling to the old beliefs. Scientists, too, are slow in accepting data that contradicts their existing understanding of the universe.

AN ANCIENT BATTLE IS STILL BEING FOUGHT

Disbelief in healing was first recorded twenty-four centuries ago in the ancient Greece of the fourth century before Christ. It was then that the philosophers Plato and Aristotle disagreed on the nature of the universe and the basis of reality. To this day, a battle is still being fought over these ancient issues.

Plato believed that the material or physical universe is but a shadow or projection of the truly real world originating in the realm of the spiritual universe. The way human beings could know this reality was through the use of the inner faculties of higher or rational intuition.

Plato's student, Aristotle, contradicted his master's teachings by asserting that nothing comes into the mind that does not enter by way of the five physical senses (sight, sound, hearing, smell and touch). Thus, Aristotle laid the foundations for what is known as the materialist-rationalist point of view. This is today's dominant understanding of reality.

The difference in their understandings of the universe may have been due, in part, to the differing ways they received and processed information. We are referring to personality types. Plato's philosophical approach suggests that he had a natural ability for intuitive knowing and thinking. His personality type must have included the intuitive and feeling traits. Aristotle, on the other hand, could not accept Plato's intuitive way because he was unable to experience it. He must have been a sensing-thinking personality type, as defined by the Meyers-Briggs Type Indicator.

Throughout the centuries we can discern that this pair of personality types was the likely cause for the ongoing controversy about the nature of human knowledge. The sensing and thinking types have dominated Western history for many centuries. They tend to be college professors, scientists, physicians, attorneys and administrators. Statistically, as the Meyers-Briggs data shows, they account for 88% of the population, compared to only 12% for the intuitive-feeling types.

This 12%, the intuitive-feeling types, are the ones who are consistently aware of their intuitive-creative-feeling sensings. Throughout history, they have been trying to tell the rest of the world what they have sensed and experienced. They are heavily represented among inventors, innovators and creative geniuses of every generation. Historically, they have ended up being a small minority who have experienced many forms of persecution at the hands of the non-comprehending majority.

Today, they express their intuitive-creative-feeling abilities in such vocations as designers, artists, poets, writers, musicians, actors, theoretical physicists, astronomers and mathematicians, research scientists, inventors, innovators, teachers, clergy, mystics and healers. It is no accident that only about 12% of the population believes in healing, reflecting the 12% who are the intuitive-feeling types.

Can the 88% majority, the sensing-thinking types, ever come to understand and believe in healing prayer? Of course they can. They have accepted Einstein's thought, haven't they? Many of the creative thinkers and innovators throughout history have been intuitive-creative-feeling types. Their contributions to society are enormous. Their thought appears to become accepted when it is expressed in terms that the public will trust -- those of reason and science. Therefore, reason and science are the basic approaches of PrayWell.

IS RECONCILIATION POSSIBLE?

The great historic heresies of the Christian Church in theological doctrine involved the same tension that existed between Plato and Aristotle and their opposite views of reality. With Western thought supporting Aristotle and denying Plato's world-view, the battle culminated some seven centuries ago in the thought of St. Thomas Aquinas, the great Roman Catholic theologian, who made reason the basis for Christian beliefs.

The same conflict also underlies the foundations for the birth of modern science. Through the work of the pioneering scientists, Descartes and

Newton, Aristotle's thinking has become the basis for modern science. Medical science came to the same conclusion -- that human beings were mechanical in nature and that all disease and health could be accounted for through physical mechanisms. Consequently, our society holds the official view that only the physical dimension exists. This is reflected in attitudes of all textbooks, the mass media, and normal personal thinking. The spiritual and psychic dimensions, being empirically unverifiable, were simply dismissed. Those scientists who hold to the ancient concept of the spiritual nature of the universe are regularly denounced as unscientific.

Plato wrote that all physical matter has its basis in spiritual forms from which all physical forms derived. This approach to reality is the basis of all the world's religions. Religions state that human beings are first and foremost spiritual in nature, created and sustained by the spiritual power of God. Because of this, human beings have a spiritual body that is eternal and survives death. Platonic thought harmonizes with the theories of Albert Einstein about the nature of the universe, theories that we seemingly ignore outside of the classroom.

The tension between these two world-views did not have to exist. Western civilization has chosen to judge these two views of reality with either/or categories. If one is right, then the other must be wrong. But, Plato and Aristotle were both half-right. They are two equally valid and necessary ways of looking at the world. One approach is to see the world with the five physical senses and to measure and work in it with physical tools, as Aristotle did. The other way is to sense other dimensions of both our physical reality and the spiritual universe through the higher intuition, as Plato proposed.

Morton Kelsey, an Episcopal priest who has written many scholarly books on spiritual development, has lectured to thousands of clergy about *spiritual reality.* His thesis is that *physical reality* is just the projected small tip of a wedge of human awareness. Most of that wedge extends into the infinite spiritual universe of God, heaven, the Company of Heaven, spirits, dreams, revelation, extra-sensory perception, creativity, intuitive knowing, etc. The five physical senses give us a valuable, but limited, consciousness or awareness of reality.

Religious historian John Rossner states that we live in a multidimensional universe. He then goes on to state: *"The belief that the physical senses and sciences provide the only valid view of reality creates an immense aversion to the concept of prayers that heal or that what goes on in the mind can affect physical reality. The events of the Jewish and Christian faiths, as expressed in the Bible, could not have happened if there is only this physical reality."*

All religious life requires access to another dimension, the spiritual dimension where God dwells. There are no spiritual gifts in just a physical dimensional universe. Without the intuitive-creative-feeling process, there is no access to God and no intuitive-creative process. Einstein did not develop his theories by *thinking.* He *dreamed* his theories and the roots of his equations and then rationally developed them.

THE SCIENCE OF LIFE ENERGIES

Following thousands of years of reported healings due to prayer, few people yet believe those reports. The practical use of prayer to aid in healing is rare. It is even rarer for medical centers to utilize the benefits of healing prayer. In the same style that *Consumer Reports* tests the claims of consumer products, there remains the need to prove product-performance with prayer. Can product-performance convince the world that touch-healing prayer is a useful tool for producing wellness in the home, medical center and community? This book had been written with that goal in mind.

Chapters three, four, five and six document the performance of prayers for healing. They also deepen our understanding of how prayer works, drawing a new road-map capable of guiding humanity into more effective prayer, health, wholeness, spirituality and happiness. Scientific data can enable prayer to improve more fully the quality of life, just as do other technologies that we now take so for granted -- immunizations, antibiotics, coronary artery bypass surgery, microsurgery and laser surgery. Data cited here arises out of the work of life energies researchers.

Upon reading the research data in my first book, a clergy colleague dismissed it by saying, *"Oh, you are into metaphysics."* My only response was to chuckle silently. His was the old, easy dismissal of Platonic philosophical thought based upon a vital force that permeates the universe. Metaphysics is the *philosophy* of how the universe works. Life energies research is conducted by *hard scientists* -- biologists, physicists and health care professionals -- who have produced scientific data indicating that the universe is permeated by a life energy that is necessary for the development and existence of all life. Note this distinction.

In my own Wesleyan Christian tradition, there are four ways by which God reveals himself: the Bible, tradition, experience and reason. Most people reject the Bible, tradition and experience as convincing proofs of the truth of the healing reality. This leaves only reason, which includes science, as the last, best chance to convince the world of its truth.

During the past half-century, scientists have been exploring the healing encounter and coming up with many answers concerning how God acts. The research data draws us a clear new road map for our understanding of healing prayer, the nature of health and happiness, religious renewal, the basis for the practical transformation of individuals, marriages, families, groups, neighborhood and humanity, and the restoration of the ecology of our whole planet.

Scientists objectively must exclude belief in God from their research. They use terms like *energy* in studying the universe, life, health, prayer and healing. To study these subtle energies, biologists, physicists and health care professionals have developed a new science, the science of life energies. Life energies scientists have conducted more than 500 clinical studies on what is occurring during the healing encounter.

Their research has not gone without considerable professional sacrifice, including loss of status, promotions, and jobs and even imprisonment. Often, life energies researchers meet the same disbelief that their subject, spiritual healing, has traditionally encountered. Because theirs has been a misunderstood new science, getting research published in prestigious scientific journals has been impossible. As a consequence, researchers recently have established their own professional journal, *Subtle Energies.*

Their research has led to scientific discoveries as significant as those of Copernicus, Kepler, Newton and Einstein. Just as the historic discoveries in astronomy, physics, chemistry and mathematics set off revolutions in thought and created the civilization of today, so can life energies discoveries become the basis for the next stage in human development. These are down-to-earth discoveries that can be as practically helpful to humanity as the inventions of Benjamin Franklin and Thomas Edison.

Why has life energies research been so consistently rejected? For one thing, the discoveries contradict many deeply held personal, religious and scientific beliefs, and consequently demand a new way of understanding the universe. The issues are complex.

First, these scientists are studying spiritual healing, the most unbelieved, misunderstood and ridiculed subject of our day.

Second, they are scientifically examining a religious subject, something that is taboo in Western culture.

Third, they are examining the effects of the Platonic world-view that was discredited by the Aristotelian world-view of the most people seven hundred years ago.

Fourth, this is a new science, which, though using the scientific method, has little connection to existing scientific traditions.

Fifth, it is applying new technologies that have always been considered the exclusive property of religious institutions.

Sixth, because these discoveries cannot be packaged and retailed in slick commercial packages for megabucks of profit, there has been no investment interest displayed by corporate America and research grants for university research labs have not been forthcoming.

Seventh, because the discoveries threatened the vested interests of established institutions and professions, doors were slammed shut against the use of these discoveries.

Eighth, few people are taking the alleged immense benefits of these discoveries seriously. The discoveries call for a revolutionary new understanding of the universe and how it works, for a new road map for humanity, taking us from the troubled present into a far more promising future.

New scientific concepts have often been viewed with suspicion. During the 1950s, the new mathematical theories of Einstein were considered understandable only by geniuses. This perception was wrong. The new mathematics, physics and astronomy are not that difficult. They just require a new way of looking at the universe and so does the research data of the science of life energies. Because their perspective is so similar to Einstein's own, many have called the resulting technology *"Einsteinian Medicine,"* in contrast to traditional medicine that is labeled *"Newtonian Medicine."* These new concepts are so different from traditional attitudes that the human mind rebels to its core when confronted by the data.

YOU, <u>PRAYWELL</u> AND THE SUPPRESSANT FACTOR

You may have unusual mental and emotional reactions while reading these chapters. Here is my attempt to help you understand these reactions. In chapter one, you read about the *suppressant factor.* Psychoanalyst Carl Jung said that when people come into contact with information that contradicts their view of reality, they may exhibit the suppressant factor, a subconscious mental attempt to neither see nor remember healing data. The suppressant factor produces several reactions to healing.

While listening to a healing account, the eyes of many listeners glaze over and they enter an unknown state of consciousness. There may be an amnesia in these listeners and in those involved in a healing encounter. There is an inability or unwillingness of people to talk about healing. There is such embarrassment and shame about believing in healing that many literally would rather die than try healing prayer as an option for saving their lives. The subject of healing produces other responses, as well, such as fear, anger and confusion.

My guess is that many readers of the thinking-sensing type will exhibit the *suppressant factor* while reading the scientific data in these four chapters as well as new concepts in other chapters of <u>PrayWell</u>. One reader of this scientific data reported how the suppressant factor affected him. It took **twenty-seven attempts** for John to complete the first page of the data. John reported these avoidance tactics: the inability to concentrate, reading the full page and not remembering what he had read, falling asleep, unexplainably closing the book and putting it down, leaving the book open and pacing with a blank mind, muttering to himself and throwing the book in the corner while vowing to read no further.

Because I had warned of these possible barriers, he was intrigued by his own reactions and determined to overcome them. When he finished the book, John phoned me and reported his reactions. If you display any of these reactions, I hope you will have enough curiosity to explore yourself. If you succeed in completing <u>PrayWell</u>, I believe it will bless your life for years to come.

DIFFICULTY OF STUDYING RELIGIOUS EFFECTS SCIENTIFICALLY

When the earliest medical researchers wished to cut open human corpses, performing autopsies to examine the body's interior structure, their need to know was greeted by the public with anger, fear, suspicion, and sometimes violence. The human body was too sacred and too precious to be desecrated by a scalpel. Yet, performing autopsies allowed medical science to make enormous leaps in their understanding of human anatomy and disease processes. This knowledge eventually led to major breakthroughs in medical procedures designed to save lives, as well as to enhance the quality of life.

Many people exhibit a similar resistance to the scientific study of religious phenomena. In this context, our beliefs about God are too sacred and too precious to be probed under the scalpel of science. For most persons, *religion is religion and science is science. Let us keep them separate.* Yet, science is one historic means by which God has revealed himself throughout the centuries.

Because spiritual healing has been seen as a religious phenomenon taking place within the setting of organized religion, we have become accustomed to using religious words to describe what was happening. Religious words like *God, spiritual* and *prayer* are a part of religion's vocabulary. As we turn to the clinical data, we will be using the vocabulary of the science of life energies to describe what is happening in a spiritual healing encounter.

Researchers state that they are only measuring the effects of an energy transmitted by humans that causes healing effects. They are neutral towards the source of the energy. I know of no life energies scientist who has implied in any way that God is the source of this energy that heals. Existing scientific evidence indicates that life energy fills and permeates the whole universe.

Yet, from this believer's viewpoint, the energy studied is a result of God's ever-present existence as the creator, sustainer and healer. In the science of life energies, the religious terms *God's power* and *God's healing flow* are replaced by the scientifically descriptive term *healing energy.* As one views the scientific evidence, it closely matches the attributes of God as experienced and believed by most of the world's religions. Unfortunately, because spiritual healing attracted so much uninformed opposition, scientists in other fields have worn blinders in their unwillingness to accept the findings of life energies researchers.

This state of affairs prevails because our culture has separated science from religion in so many ways. With 88% of the population being the sensing-thinking personality type, believing only in physical reality, we have had to separate religious (intuitive-creative-feeling) thought and belief from our daily lives.

For years, I have chuckled about people *"hanging their brains in the cloakroom"* upon entering church. Many do not use their thinking-sensing skills in church or in formulating their religious beliefs, morality or life-style. This is so true that church sociologists report that fewer than half of practicing Christians use their religious beliefs as the basis for their morality and lifestyles. Sensing-thinking Christians are forced to compartmentalize their lives with one way of knowing reserved for church and another way prescribed for the other parts of their lives. As a clergyman, I have found this to be frustrating. I want people to use their thinking-sensing skills in their religious life. I am an intuitive-creative-feeling type myself, but I am equally adept at thinking-sensing. I have combined these skills in PrayWell.

I am aware of the discomfort of most religious believers when scientists describe God's actions in terms of an intelligently acting energy, but Pray-Well must do this. By describing the results of prayer in scientific language rather than religious language, we see that a more accurate picture emerges. PrayWell is able to state that if you do *"this, and this, and this"* in prayer, then certain specific results are probable. This spiritual technology adds reliability and predictability to prayer beliefs. PrayWell is not denying belief in prayer. It is seeking to strengthen this belief and encourage its more effective practice.

THE BASIS FOR EARLY RELIGIOUS BELIEFS

To put this into perspective, it may be helpful to understand the basis for early religious beliefs. All the world's religions arose from humanity's ancient past. Ancient humanity was just as curious as we are about why things happen. What causes floods? What causes droughts? In a prescientific era with no scientific answers to these questions, there was no scientific understanding of weather patterns. Only one possible cause was perceived -- God. So, the conclusion was, *"God causes the weather."* Thus, ancient humanity came up with religious beliefs to explain natural disasters like floods and droughts.

Why does someone become ill? What causes the common cold? What causes pneumonia? What causes leprosy? What causes blindness? Why are some infants born dead or defective? What causes an old man to clasp his chest, fall to the ground and suddenly die? No physicians are mentioned in the Old Testament. There was no awareness, then, of bacteria and viruses, cancer and heart disease. There was no medical science. Therefore, few medical causes were acknowledged for physical conditions.

The belief was, *"God causes illness."* In those early times, in answer to the *why,* religious explanations were offered. People would say, *"God did it. He died because he had broken God's laws."* Not until medical science performed autopsies and discovered what went on inside human bodies did thinking begin to change. Now, medical science can usually discover the cause of death. Because of this, people can say, *"He died of a heart attack induced by the blockage of coronary arteries."*

These early religious answers to scientific questions remain embedded in the ancient sacred writing or testaments that support our religious beliefs today. Though science has provided objective answers to these ancient questions, these early religious answers still hinder both our religious and scientific understanding of the universe, as well as our ability to pray effectively.

PRAYER: RELIGIOUS AS DISTINCT FROM THERAPEUTIC

We have been rather careless in our use of the word *"religion."* Religion has two meanings. One refers to *"a specific system of beliefs, in a religion like Christianity, Judaism or Islam."* This is the dominant meaning. The other definition of religion is *"a belief in God or gods."* When we think of prayer, we identify it as arising out of the context of a specific religion. In reality, most prayers are not religious in this context. Most prayers express belief in God, but not that of a religion.

As our exploration of religious practices in chapter one concluded, only about one-eighth of Americans participate in a religious community and only about twenty percent have ever formally learned any religion's beliefs. The prayers of most people do not arise from formal education in religion.

There are also universal religious beliefs that are not unique to any one religion. These beliefs about God are shared by all humanity. These universal beliefs include perceiving God as the Creator, Sustainer and Healer. From this come prayers of praise and thanksgiving for divine intervention and healing.

When people pray for healing, this is an expression of compassion. They are praying to bring the power of God into the life of the ill because they care. They are using prayer for therapeutic or caring purposes.

Why are we exploring this? We are exploring this in order to release prayer and healing from their religious confinement. In the United States, it is a social taboo to publicly pray or heal because these are perceived as *private* religious activities, best done in churches or privately. Prayer in a hospital is perceived as a partisan religious activity and is not seen in the context of an act of caring.

In reaction to the taboo against prayer in a public context, many healing techniques have recently been developed to express practical caring that does not use or refer to prayer. These include Reiki, energy balancing and Therapeutic Touch. Therapeutic Touch was specifically developed for use by health care professionals. Therapeutic Touch has been taught to tens of thousands of nurses for use in a medical setting, with many nursing colleges including it in their curricula. From this has arisen the National Nurse Healers Association. Therapeutic Touch teaches people to center their inner selves, not to pray, in practicing the technique.

Recognizing the sensitive issue of using prayer in public, I see the need to separate certain types of prayer from a religion context by using a new term, "*Therapeutic Prayer.*" Therapeutic Prayer is used as a therapy. It is offered out of concern to heal the ill and the troubled, and to restore harmony and balance to individuals, marriages, families, classrooms, work places, communities, nations and the planet. It can be used with persons holding any religious beliefs. It is an act of caring, like feeding the hungry, sheltering the homeless or working for world peace. Therapeutic Prayer seeks to bring the power of God into practical situations.

I introduce Therapeutic Prayer at this place in PrayWell in order to direct your attention to the possible practical uses of prayer. These will be detailed with the scientific data. Using Therapeutic Prayer gives humanity another practical tool for caring. It also opens many new and practical ministries for religions to practice. It is a new perspective that frees people to pray with the hurting without the limiting belief that prayer represents a particular religion. It provides a new healing technique, the practice of healing prayer. This is a primary focus of PrayWell.

THE DISTORTIONS OF FAITH HEALING SERVICES

Another issue has distorted the public beliefs about spiritual healing. The circus atmosphere prevalent in most American televised faith-healing services not only challenges religious credibility; it turns most persons off. The style, the beliefs, the judgmental and manipulative statements, the distortion of the truth, the money pitches and the wealthy lifestyles of the performers have blinded most persons to the fact that God actually heals through prayer.

Even though people may reject faith-healing services, the latter have still managed to erroneously shape our beliefs and knowledge about how God heals. For instance, most persons, though not believing in faith-healing, will still insist that (1) God heals instantly and that (2) it is due to the immense faith of the subject. Both of these concepts are faulty, as our explorations will prove.

Healing prayer is misunderstood in dozens of ways. These misunderstandings raise barriers to the acceptance of the following scientific evidence. When science challenges religious beliefs, many persons will unrelentingly cling to objectively erroneous religious beliefs.

My own residual skepticism has limited my own healing ability. To practice healing demands a suspension of disbelief. This must be replaced by a state of miracle-readiness. Shortly after a Roman Catholic healing service had again raised our awareness and faith, my wife and I took part in an effortless healing. We had been to dinner with friends with whom we discussed healing. Returning to our home, our friend, Chuck, gave us a friendly challenge. He said, *"Let's see if you are just talk. I have had a separated shoulder blade for forty years that causes me pain when I drive or play golf. Let's see you heal it!"*

Standing in our living room, my wife and I placed our four hands upon our friend's back. A few seconds into our prayer, our hands could feel the muscles rippling and the bone structure moving into normal alignment. As with most healings, we had the same sense of surprise and awe as our friends Chuck and Marcia. A month later we received a note from Chuck from Mountain View, California. He stated that he no longer suffered pain from long stretches of driving his car or from playing golf and that his physician had examined him and the separated shoulder blade condition no longer existed. He wanted to make sure I had his statement in my files.

This is one last reminder to be aware of the many ways you may use to avoid unpleasant truths as you read the following data. Discuss it with others who have read this book. Share it with those who have not read this book and observe their reactions. It takes courage to acknowledge that you are willing to openly explore this field. How honest will your conscious mind permit you to be?

BERNARD GRAD, THE FATHER OF HEALING RESEARCH

The pioneering researcher in conducting scientific experiments on the effects of spiritual healing is Dr. Bernard Grad. His career as a scientist began with honors in biochemistry and a magna cum laude PhD in experimental morphology, which led to biomedical research and a forty-year career at the Gerontology Unit, Allen Memorial Institute of Psychiatry, McGill University, Montreal. At McGill, he performed scores of experiments on thyroid function, leukemia, aging in animals and chronic brain syndrome in humans that are described in ninety-three professional journal articles.

Since 1957, he has devoted his spare time carrying out more than two hundred clinical research studies on the effects of spiritual healing, using the same careful scientific research designs that he used in his paid career. Grad admits he would have had a more peaceful life had he not explored spiritual healing. But for him, curiosity has always come first. Along with his curiosity came a scientific integrity and a personal honesty that he has always placed above social respectability.

Grad is a warm, friendly, unassuming person, yet a scientific giant, already a legend in the field of healing research. Grad retired from his post at McGill in 1985. When Dr. Grad began his studies in the laying on of hands by healers, there were two main attitudes prevalent about laying on of hands (LH). Grad states, *"One held by official bodies of science and medicine was that any effects due to LH (healing) were at best due to suggestion or hypnosis. The other attitude was that held by more or less religious people in the West, namely, that the healing effects of LH were miraculous when done in the name of Jesus. Other types of healing were the work of the devil."*

Over thirty years later, those same attitudes still dominate thinking, even though Grad's work has scientifically proven that healers emit an energy that heals living matter. He has proven to Christians, myself included, that healing can be done outside the Christian faith by persons of other religions. He has also demythologized healing as a miracle, because a miracle has no scientific explanation, but healing does.

In an unpublished paper, Grad tells of his scientific research methods: *"My contribution to this field was that I conducted the LH (healing) research not in humans but in animals, plants and even non-living things (normal saline, cloth, etc.). This was decisive in eliminating questions of suggestion or hypnosis which are usually invoked when human subjects are involved. Moreover, the design of the experiments was the same in every way as if I were conducting experiments on drugs, vitamins, hormones, etc. That is, sufficient numbers of replicates were involved to take into consideration biological variation and to permit statistical evaluation of the data at the end of the experiment. Also, suitable controls were part of each experiment and in many of the experiments, double and multiple blinds were introduced. The only unconventional aspect of the study was the LH (healing) treatment. When LH was indeed shown to have effects on* biological processes, the transmission of an energy was postulated as being the agent responsible for the effects."

THE PLACEBO EFFECT IN MEDICINE, PSYCHOTHERAPY, HEALING

The placebo effect has intrigued medical researchers. A placebo is a neutral pill with no medical value that is given to a control group in clinical studies of new medications. It was thought that those taking the neutral pill would not show any medical improvement. But it was discovered that a large percentage of patients get well with a placebo pill. They had been told that a new medication was being tested and they would be given either the new medication or a placebo pill. It is now known that when some patients believe they are taking the medication, they will get well using a neutral pill. This became known as the *"placebo effect."*

Scientific research into spiritual healing has sought to eliminate the placebo effect by primarily using plants and animals for clinical studies. Grad defines the placebo effect as *"any response attributable to a pill or potion except that due to its pharmaco-dynamic or specific properties. Some would widen this definition to include not only pills, but other procedures, such as psychotherapy."*

One comprehensive pharmaceutical study[1] reported that 40.6% of 14,177 patients with illnesses ranging from headache to multiple sclerosis obtained relief from placebo pills. This is the power of suggestion, trust, and belief to heal.

Psychotherapy can also produce healing. The best psychotherapists in one study[2] are those who bring to bear high levels of accurate empathy, unconditional positive regard and therapist genuineness. These qualities are also traits of spiritual healers.

Grad summarized the similarities between spiritual healing, psychotherapy and the placebo effect: *"Where favorable effects are claimed, there can always be found an element of faith or trust on the part of the patient in the healer or therapist, or in the pill or potion offered as a remedy. Also, there is rapport between patient and therapist, and this can only occur if the feelings of both, but especially the latter [the therapist], are such as not to stand in the way of the development of such rapport. ....unfavorable effects can be obtained if the emotions of the therapist or physician are negative. This was observed in psychotherapy, in the placebo effect, and presumably could also occur in the laying-on-of-hands [for healing]. Third, the effects by all three are usually regarded as having been produced by psychological means."* [3]

The placebo effect is used by most professionals in the caring field. The physician uses it in his bedside manner and encouragement. The psychotherapist supports and affirms people. In spiritual healing, the placebo effect can play an important role. But spiritual healing is far more than the placebo effect, as the following clinical data indicates.

FIRST HEALING EXPERIMENT: HEALER TREATING WOUNDED MICE

Dr. Bernard Grad's classic 1957 Wounded Mice Experiment[4] is a good example of spiritual healing clinical research. With a scalpel and template, Grad surgically removed a one-half inch square of skin from the backs of 48 laboratory mice, of whom 16 were treated by the Hungarian born healer Oskar Estebany, while the rest of the mice were used as controls. The wound healing rate was regularly measured with a template. After fourteen days, the healer-treated wounded mice showed a statistically significant, increased surgical wound healing rate over the control group. This experiment supplied the first scientific verification that healers produce a measurable healing effect in living organisms. This experiment was replicated by Dr. Remi Cadoret and G.I.Paul at the University of Manitoba.[5]

HEALING PRODUCES AN OBJECTIVELY MEASURABLE EFFECT

Since his 1957 Wounded Mouse Experiment scientifically verified a measurable healing effect, Bernard Grad has conducted more than 200 other clinical experiments on the effects of healers. Other researchers followed in his footsteps. As we look at what is occurring in the healing encounter in future chapters, many of these experiments will be described. For now, here is the report of one comprehensive review of healing research.

In 1990, Daniel J. Benor, an American medical doctor living in England, conducted a survey of spiritual healing research that had appeared in various academic dissertations and professional journals.[6]   His statistical evaluation of 131 controlled trials on cells, enzymes, yeasts, bacteria, plants, mice and humans demonstrated a positive effect of healing in the 56 trials, with a statistical analysis at a significance level of $p<.01$ or better with another 21 at $.02<p<.05$.

Most of the healing research studies that Benor rejected had nothing to do with negative healing effects. They were rejected because of Benor's methodology, which required statistical analysis for each acceptable study.

RESEARCH WITH HUMAN SUBJECTS

A number of recent studies have used human subjects. Here is an example of such healing research, entitled, *The Effect of Non-Contact Therapeutic Touch on the Healing Rate of Full Thickness Dermal Wounds.*[7] Daniel P. Wirth, MS, JD, had full-thickness dermal wounds incised on the lateral deltoid region using a skin punch biopsy instrument on healthy subjects randomly assigned to treatment or control groups. Subjects did not know who was being treated nor the true nature of the active treatment mode. Wound surface areas were measured on Days 0, 8 and 16 using a direct tracing method and digitization system. Active and control treatments were composed of daily sessions of five minute exposure to a hidden non-contact Therapeutic Touch practitioner or to sham exposure. There were 48 participants. On the 16th day, the statistical results indicated significant healing with $p <.01$.

The Statistical Significance of "p>.01"

Research results must possess statistical significance. When $p<.01$, it means that there is less than a 1% chance that the results are chance. Those are good experimental results. Poorer statistics represent any value over .01. When $p>.05$, it means that there is less than a 5% chance that the results are chance.

AN OBJECTIVELY MEASURABLE HEALING EFFECT

Future chapters will further verify that the practice of healing produces an objectively measurable healing effect. For those interested in detailed accounts, read Benor's comprehensive survey.

CHAPTER THREE SUMMARY

1. An ancient battle is still being fought between two different ways of perceiving the world. Aristotle's materialist-rationalist point of view dominates Western thought. Plato's view, intuitive-knowing, is the basis of all the world's religions and is the foundation for understanding prayer.

2. These two views are produced by two differing personality types. The sensing-thinking types, 88% of the population, have dominated Western history. The other 12%, the intuitive-feeling types, have sought to tell the rest of the world what they sensed and experienced, and have known frequent rejection.

3. PrayWell represents the hard scientific data of biologists, physicists and health care professionals.

4. Life energies scientists have conducted more than 500 clinical studies examining the healing encounter. Their scientific discoveries are as significant as those of Copernicus, Kepler, Newton and Einstein and are as practically helpful as the inventions of Benjamin Franklin and Thomas Edison. These new discoveries can usher in a Golden Age for all humanity.

5. Healing prayer represents *"Einsteinian medicine"* in contrast to traditional or *"Newtonian medicine."*

6. You may experience the *suppressant factor* while reading the scientific data -- being unable to remember, concentrate or absorb the data and using various avoidance techniques.

7. Therapeutic prayer expresses caring as the pray-er seeks to bring the power of God into human health and renewal.

8. Faith-healing services distort our understanding of how prayer works.

9. Research biologist Bernard Grad is the father of clinical healing research with more than 200 clinical studies.

10. Life energies research has sought to eliminate the placebo effect by using plants and animals, instead of humans, in clinical studies.

11. Grad's classic 1957 Wounded Mice Experiment provided the first scientific verification that healers produce a measurable effect.

12. In 1990, Daniel J. Benor, MD, performed a statistical evaluation of 131 controlled healing studies showing a positive effect of healing in the 56 trials with a statistical analysis at a level of $p < 1.14$. In human subjects, Daniel P. Wirth had full-thickness dermal wounds incised on healthy subjects. On the 16th day, the statistical results indicated significant healing with $p < .01$.

Chapter Four

Scientific Evidence of a Healing Energy

"The energy is informational! The energy itself is an information-bearer, self-regulating, programmed. Where healing calls for the slowing down of cell growth....development is inhibited. Where healing requires speeding up of cell growth....the process is accelerated. Slow down or speed up for healing? The same agent does both. The energy itself knows." ...Bernard R. Grad

"Great spirits have always encountered violent opposition from mediocre minds." ...Albert Einstein

"And a woman who had had a flow of blood for twelve years....came up behind Jesus, and touched the fringe of his garment; and immediately her flow of blood ceased....Jesus said, 'Someone touched me; for I perceive that power has gone forth from me.'" ...Luke 8:43-44,46

Everyone involved in healing is aware of the power of God in the midst of a healing encounter. There is a sense of love, peace and joy. There is the heat. Everyone in a prayer group practicing touch-healing senses the heat in their own hands and in the healing hands that touch them. Individuals -- and the whole room -- often become uncomfortably warm with this heat. Yet, a thermometer will register little objective change of temperature in either people's hands or the room -- about one to two degrees. Why?

Another type of awareness provides us with a possible clue. Some people feel a flow of energy in their healing hands. Sometimes, during healing encounters, I have felt a pleasant combination of warmth and energy flowing throughout my whole body, from my toes to the top of my head. My experience as a healer tells me that when a healee senses a tingling throughout the body, a complete healing has occurred. Could there be a flow of energy involved in healing which subjectively produces these symptoms? Could this energy be at a frequency that could be observed or measured using scientific instruments?

In the scriptural account of the healing cited above, after the woman touched his garment, Jesus is quoted as saying, *"Someone touched me; for I perceive that power has gone forth from me."* Do modern experiences provide any clues to that ancient statement? Will the research data help explain it?

Research must have some starting place. Those who practice healing have sensed a variety of consistent phenomena occurring during the healing encounter. They have *sensed* and *intuitively known* about some things. A few claim to be able to *see* the energy transmitted from the hands and the energy fields of people. A few have objectively proven they can diagnose medical conditions by *seeing* the body's energy fields. But, most of us are skeptical about the validity of all this subjective data. Thankfully, we have the scientific method and ever more sensitive tools for discovering the objective truth.

Healers have also developed their own theories. Theory is the basis for most scientific research. So, before we present the evidence for the existence of healing energy and seek to describe how it works, we need that with which all research begins, a theoretical working model.

A THEORETICAL WORKING MODEL FOR HEALING PRAYER

Humans possess energy fields. Our scientific working model begins with the nature of the universe. The universe is composed of two substances, energy and matter. Measurable energy fields permeate all matter, including plants, animals and humans. The human body is interpenetrated by at least seven energy fields, each operating at a different electromagnetic frequency. These energy fields radiate beyond the physical body from a quarter inch to more than twenty-five feet from the skin. The human energy fields contain information, act purposefully and are essential for life. They duplicate the biological, mental, emotional and spiritual components of human beings and interact with them. Every human function has its counterpart in the energy fields. Brain functioning exists in one of the human energy fields as the mind. Emotions exist as an energy form at another frequency. Spirituality exists as an energy form on at least two frequencies.

At the lowest human energy field frequency, every cell and organ of the physical body is duplicated. Russian researchers state that this energy field is a blueprint for the physical. They use the analogy of a gelatin mold. Each physical organ is formed and sustained, just as hot liquid gelatin is shaped in a gelatin mold, by the energy blueprint of the energy field. If the mold is misshapen, the product of that mold will be misshapen (and ill) in the same way. Energy fields shape the physical body the way a gelatin mold shapes gelatin. They also interact with the physical body, affecting the energy blueprint.

Another way of looking at this is through the effects of a magnet upon iron shavings. A simple magnet has an energy field, invisible like the human physical body's energy field. We know it exists because we can measure its effects as it either pulls metal objects to it or as it clings to iron objects, because of an energy force called magnetism. The invisible energy field of the magnet takes visible shape when iron filings are placed upon paper above it. The magnet molds the iron filings into a visible pattern that makes a picture of its energy or force field. The invisible energy field of the magnet creates form just as real as the form of gelatin in a gelatin mold. Or just as real as the organic matter of the human physical body, molded by the human energy field.

Every cell and organ of the physical body, down to the basic cell structure, is duplicated by the first energy field, the energy blueprint. Human wholeness and health are present when each energy field is operating at peak performance levels. The human physical body and the human energy fields interact and affect each other's function.

From a religious perspective, these energy fields represent the divine creative and sustaining presence of God in the universe. The mental, emotional and spiritual energy fields combined represent the religious *spiritual body* and are related to what is known as the human *soul*. From a religious perspective, the spiritual *body* survives the death of the physical body and is eternal. Scientifically, the spiritual body is composed of energy fields operating at specific electromagnetic frequencies. When God's Spirit transforms a person and the new Divine Life is present within the energy fields, the frequencies of the energy fields change. This transformation causes wholeness, and the religious state of salvation. The energy fields contain information, including religious beliefs. The level of one's physical, mental, emotional and spiritual health is present in the human energy fields as various information-bearing frequencies.

This is a scientific model for the human energy fields. This understanding of the human energy field model provides half of the working model or answer about how prayer and healing work. The other half involves a praying human being. God works invariably through human channels to do his healing.

How Prayer Produces Healing. When a person makes contact with God in an attempt to bring about healing in what we refer to as an act of prayer, the way God heals is not explained by religious belief except to say that God heals. The scientific model offers an objective explanation that, as you will see, research data verifies. In the objective model, a praying human is emitting a healing energy at a specific electromagnetic frequency that works by transforming the human energy fields, causing physical, emotional or spiritual healing to take place. A religious explanation states that in prayer, God and a human being are working in partnership to transmit God's healing power or energy. Anytime humans turn in a caring way to another, they can intentionally and naturally accumulate, attune and transmit healing energy.

In absent prayer, the prayer message is sent on an electromagnetic carrier beam that contains the energy within the carrier beam itself. Clairvoyants report their observation that this beam is being emitted from the heart area, and not from the brain, as a white laser-like beam of light.

This energy is able to influence living organisms because all living organisms have energy fields that receive the healing energy and utilize it effectively. When an energy field is defective by having a wrong frequency or by being inefficient, the healing energy restores it. The restored energy field is then able to restore the physical body, mental processes and emotions. Rather than defining healing based upon its source, God, it is more helpful to define it in terms of healing's effect. Thus, my own scientific definition of spiritual healing is this: *Spiritual healing is that which brings healing to the body, mind and spirit through its effects upon the energy fields and the consciousness of a living organism.*

EVIDENCE FOR THE EXISTENCE OF A HEALING ENERGY

The existence of a healing energy had long been claimed by healers who sensed the energy flowing from their hands into the healee. Early life energies researchers proposed the existence of an energy to explain the experimental effects of healing prayer. Aeronautical engineer and healer Ambrose Worrall observed that it acts like electricity in flowing from a high potential source to a person or object of lower potential. Bernard Grad observed that human beings act like electrical capacitors for life energy. Scientific evidence for the existence of this energy is presented in the following data:

1. Infra-red shows changes in healer-charged water. A 1986 study[1] examined the infra-red absorption spectra of water placed in sealed vials and treated by fourteen different healers. Statistically significant variation in the pattern of an infra-red spectrophotometric analysis was observed between healer-treated water versus calibration-controlled water samples. The changes were attributed to alterations in the chemical bond characteristics between the oxygen and hydrogen atoms in the water molecule. An energy had to be emitted to produce the changes.

2. Healer-charged bottled water. Grad had healer Estebany hold bottled water while emitting energy with his hands. The water was then used for his *Wounded Barley Seed Experiment.*[2] The healer-treated water caused barley seeds wounded by a one percent saline solution to grow faster than control plants watered with an untreated one percent saline solution. Grad stored healer-treated water for two years adjacent to other bottled water. It did not decrease in healing strength and did not contaminate the adjacent bottled water. Robert Miller[3] discovered similar effects in healer-treated water as a research chemist in Atlanta, Georgia. Charging of the bottled water with healing energy is the only explanation that accounts for the increased plant growth.

3. Healer-charged cotton and wool. In Grad's *The Healing of Induced Goiters in Mice Experiment*[4] mice were deprived of iodine and fed the goitrogen thiouracil to induce goiters. Two healers treated the experimental group of mice through touch-healing, preventing goiters from developing, while the control group developed goiters.

In a second study, healer Estebany imparted healing energy into cotton and wool cuttings that were placed in mouse cages, producing results identical to touch-healing. In addition to proving that healer-treated cotton and wool produce a healing effect, this study also demonstrated that healing energy can prevent an anticipated disease from occurring. Bernard Grad warns that temperatures above the boiling point of water, and sunlight, are likely to diminish healing energy.

4. Healer-charged surgical gauze. Dr. Dolores Krieger[5] reports similar healing results with healer-treated surgical gauze. Applied as a wound dressing, it resulted in a faster rate of healing.

5. Healers have identical brain wave frequencies. Beginning in 1969, physicist Robert O. Beck[6] began testing the brain-wave frequencies of healers throughout the world, discovering that all healers read identical frequencies of 7.83 hertz. This occurred regardless of their society, their beliefs or their healing modality. Beck worked with charismatic Christian faith healers, a Hawaiian kahuna and practitioners of wicca, Santeria, radesthesia, radionics, seers, ESP readers and psychics.

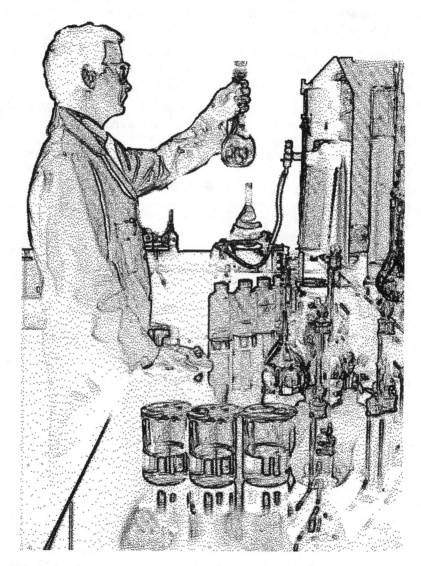

Figure 4. *Research on prayer and healing is hard science that uses the same research methodology as any other research. Science is neutral concerning religious beliefs and metaphysics. It seeks the objective truth.*

6. SQUID-measured frequency of healers' emissions. Physicist John Zimmerman[7] while at the University of Colorado School of Medicine, Denver, using a Superconducting Quantum Interference Device (SQUID), a superconducting device cooled to near absolute zero, conducted 7 investigations of healers practicing touch-healing with healees and observed discernible changes in the amplitude and frequency (7.8 hertz) of the biomagnetic fields detected by the SQUID. The healers emitted a steady 7.8 hertz frequency from the hands even when not healing. A control group of non-healers produced no changes. In an 8th investigation, the signal recorded near the healer's hands was larger during the healing than when he moved his hands towards the SQUID.

7. Infra-red shows energy emerging from palms and fingers. Zimmerman[8] also examined infra-red film photographs of healers' hands showing an energy emerging from the palms and finger pads.

8. Healers can produce more than 200 volts of energy. *Sensitives* who can *see* energy emissions have long observed that world-class healers emit about twenty times the amount of energy of other people. Now the Menninger Clinic reports significant energy discharges from healers versus non-healers.

Researchers[9] in the Copper Wall Experiments at the Menninger Clinic, Topeka, Kansas, discovered that nine world-class healers during meditation and absent healing emitted between 4 volts and 222 volts of electrical energy with a median emission of 8.3 volts. Non-healer meditators produced no surges over 4 volts. The world-class healers used Non-Contact Therapeutic Touch (NCTT). The implication here is that NCTT therapists have a different *"energy structure"* or a different *"energy handling capability"* from regular subjects.

Their new technology detected and measured electrostatic potentials and field effects in and around the bodies of meditators and NCTT therapists. The NCTT therapists produced more surges during therapy sessions than during meditation, thus, the intention to heal produced the strongest results. All NCTT therapists believed their skill could be learned by anyone.

Researchers explained that these NCTT therapists' voltage emissions were 1 billion times stronger than brain-wave voltages, 100 million times stronger than heart voltages, and 1 million times stronger than large psychophysiology skin-potential. Their effect on the human energy systems could be immense.

9. Naval physicists found frequencies that induce and heal cancer. Seven United States Navy physicists[10] discovered that when a healer placed his hands in water, the water protons began emitting an 8 hertz frequency. They then radiated mice with a 5.xxx hertz frequency, inducing cancer in them within 48 hours. When the mice were radiated with the healer frequency of 8 hertz, the mice's tumors were healed within 48 hours.

10. World-class healers at a constant frequency. Dr. Andrija Puharich[11] was the first researcher to consistently measure an 8 hertz magnetic pulse coming from the hands of healers.

When Bernard Grad recommended me as the healer for Ramesh Chouhan's clinical studies in India, Dr. Chouhan wanted to make sure I was a world-class healer. We traveled with my wife and a physical scientist to the laboratory of Dr. Andrija Puharich, a pioneering healing researcher, to find out. At that time (1988), the Soviet Union was still radiating much of the

United States with microwaves from a giant transmitter. (We, also, had a larger transmitter bombarding them with microwaves.) The microwaves broke down into three powerful, extremely low frequency waves that interfered with measuring the extremely low frequencies (ELF) emitted by healers. So, Puharich built a large shielding Faraday Cage to screen out these interfering frequencies. We all entered the steel plate cage for the test of my healing abilities.

My three traveling companions went first, each placing a hand on the sensing plate. The whole-number digital readout showed each of them emitting a rapidly fluctuating 7 to 12 hertz energy frequency. Uneasily, I placed my hand on the plate. This was a moment of truth. The digital readout was a steady 8 hertz. I was scientifically validated as a world-class healer. Puharich explained that world-class healers emit a steady 8 hertz at all times while the rest of the population emits that variable 7 to 12 hertz.

DOES HEALING ENERGY EXIST?

The scientific evidence indicates that *something* is being emitted by human hands that produces healing effects. That *something* emerges from the palms of the hands and finger pads as photographed with infra-red film. That *something* was measured by a SQUID at 7.8 hertz frequency and changed the amplitude and frequency of existing biomagnetic fields. That *something* changed the pattern of water, according to an infra-red spectrophotometric analysis. That *something* can be imparted to water, wool, cotton and surgical gauze which then are able to cause healing effects on their own. That *something* is emitted from healers' hands at all times, at about a 7.8 frequency, which is the same frequency as healers' brain-waves of 7.8 hertz. That *something* has all the scientific attributes of an observable and measurable energy that caused statistically significant healing effects in 56 different scientific studies.

ADDITIONAL QUALITIES OF HEALING ENERGY

Not all the following qualities are substantiated by scientific data. Many of the qualities were derived from the observations of trained observers. These qualities contribute to a consistent and helpful new picture of what is occurring during the healing encounter. They provide a helpful road map for the practice of healing.

11. The energy is informational and acts intelligently. From his research data, Grad draws the conclusion: *"The energy is informational! The energy itself is an information-bearer, self-regulating, programmed. Where healing calls for the slowing down of cell growth, as in the goiter experiments, thyroid development is inhibited. Where healing requires speeding up of cell growth, as in the wounded mice tests, the process is accelerated. Slow down or speed up for healing? The same agent does both. The energy itself knows."*

12. Life energy produces the optimum conditions for life. A bean experiment by SPINDRIFT[12] in Salem, Oregon, graphically demonstrates that prayer produces the optimum state for life. Three trays of beans were prepared. One contained beans that had been dried out by oven heat. The second tray had been soaked to increase water content. The third was the control with untreated normal or healthy beans. In a series of runs, persons prayed for the beans. This resulted in all three trays of beans consistently developing the same moisture content. The prayer effects added water to the dried-out beans, reduced water content in the soaked beans and had no scientific effect on the normal beans. The effect of the healing energy of prayer was to restore the treated beans to their optimal state of being. This finding agrees with Grad's conclusion that the "*energy is informational! The energy itself is an information-bearer, self-regulating, programmed.*"

13. Healing increases the amount of oxygen in the blood by up to 12%. Dr. Dolores Krieger,[13] professor of nursing at New York City University and one of the developers of Therapeutic Touch, learned that Grad had measured increased chlorophyll in plants treated with healer-charged water. Krieger noted that hemoglobin *"is an iron-containing protein and, as do all proteins, it is able to act either as an acid or a base, depending upon the medium it is in. This ability...would appear to make it an appropriate vehicle for the balancing of the positive and negative currents of life energies during the healing process as postulated by Eastern literature."* In each of three different sophisticated tests of touch-healing, the results increased oxygen in hemoglobin by up to 12%. This data on increased oxygen in the blood could account for some of the more rapid healing rate effects induced by healer-treated surgical wounds. It implies that healers could treat patients who need more oxygen in their blood or could treat blood plasma before it is transfused. This effect, in itself, would increase the healing rate of most patients.

14. Healing energy can be transmitted through electrical wiring. I heard Olga Worrall report this healing study to a group at the Holiday Inn in Boston Heights, Ohio in 1985. Her story began with a physician's wife weaving wiring into two vests whose wiring systems were connected by two hundred feet of electrical cable. Olga wore one of the vests while an ill woman, whom she had never met, wore the other in a hospital room down the hall. Physicians used instruments to monitor the flow of energy in both rooms as Mrs. Worrall emitted healing energy into the vest. This caused the ill woman to become well. This experiment indicates that healing energy can be transmitted through wiring. This opens the possibility that healing energy may someday be dispensed to the ill in the same fashion as hosed-in oxygen.

15. Through prayer, healers impressed their brain-wave pattern upon healees, resulting in physical healing. This is another verbal report by Olga Worrall for which documentation must somewhere exist. Olga and her healing client were both connected to a brain-wave machine (EEG). As Olga began healing, her brain-waves slowed to the alpha range of about eight frequencies a second. Holding her hands about four inches from the healee's head, she tried to transmit a healing energy and succeeded, im-

pressing her brain-wave pattern upon the healee, so that both brains reso-
nated on identical brain-wave frequencies and patterns. The waves pulsed
in complete harmony and oneness, qualities that many healers subjectively
report sensing during healing encounters. The healee became well during
this process.

Two conclusions can be drawn from this study. First, Olga Worrall
transmitted an energy with her hands that caused the effects. Second,
some healings occur because the healer is able to change brain-wave patterns. This implies that something as yet undetected or considered insig-
nificant in the brain-wave pattern may help to cause or to maintain physical
health or illness.

Dr. Edgar Wilson[14] produced identical results with Israeli healer David
Joffee, who impressed his brain-wave patterns upon a healee, causing the
alleviation of illness symptoms.

**16.   The physical health of persons with multiple personalities
changes with the shifting of personalities.** This data is related to the
story above. Dr. Frank Putnam of the National Institutes of Health has
found that electroencephalograms (EEGs) show that the brain-waves of
people who go from one personality to another in multiple personality disor-
der will change as dramatically as though the electrodes had been taken off
one person and been placed on another. Their brain-wave patterns vary
widely from one personality to another, a phenomenon previously thought
biologically impossible.

In the same physical body, one personality will have asthma, but when
control is shifted to another personality, the asthma does not exist. Various
studies have shown these changes with personality/brain frequency shifts:
one personality will be left-handed, another right-handed; one will wear
glasses and be myopic while another personality will have normal vision;
one will have diabetes and another not; one will be allergic to a drug and
another not.

Dr. Lee Poulos[15] of Vancouver reports other significant data. In multiple
personalities, with a shift to another personality there is a shift, as above, in
chronic medical conditions. Poulos discovered wide fluctuations in psychological test results, one personality being blind and the other having 20-20
vision, up to 60 points difference in the intelligence quotient, and different
religious beliefs. Within two seconds of shifting to another personality, the
eye irises can change color, for example from brown to blue.

Multiple personality studies present a biological dilemma. Inhabiting the
same physical bodies with one identical pattern of genetic material, the different personalities instantly produce different biological brain-wave patterns, allergies, iris color, biological impairments and illnesses. This
strongly suggests that a number of personality factors are responsible for
biological traits. It also possibly explains why a healer's changing of brain-
wave patterns can cure an illness. The role of personality obviously is important to the wholeness of persons.

**17. Only the brain-waves of a woman who was being prayed for rec-
ognized the healing energy entering her.** While a cooperating physician
was recording a woman's brain-waves, her prayer group prayed for her.

The woman remained unaware of the prayers for herself, but her recorded brain-waves dramatically changed. In the process, the symptoms of the medical condition for which she was seeing the doctor disappeared. This is another piece of the puzzle that suggests that the brain plays an important role in some spiritual healing results.

18. The healing energy is extremely stable. The qualities of the healing energy in healer-treated substances are different from any known energy source. The energy does not dissipate nor contaminate adjacent bottles of water. Healer-treated water and cotton cloth continue to emit healing energy for up to two years (Bernard Grad). This means that isolated healing energy is the most stable, storable known form of active energy. Sunlight and heat at over the water boiling temperature diminish healing energy.

Religiously, the healing energy acts as do holy relics, which are the bones, clothes and possessions of noted religious persons. Holy relics are attributed with the power to heal. The healing energy also has the attributes of holy places and spas that are known for their healing potential. Subjectively sensed, God's religious presence has qualities identical to that subjectively sensed in healing energy.

19. Healing energy dissipates when imparted to living organisms. When healing energy is imparted to living organisms, it is rapidly utilized and diminishes in quantity. When Ambrose and Olga Worrall[16] in Baltimore offered absent prayer for a blade of rye grass in Atlanta, it rapidly accelerated growth for 11 hours to a maximum of 830% of normal. This growth-enhancement then diminished for the next 36 hours, reaching a low of two times normal growth rate, where it remained for two weeks. This is similar to how some medications perform.

Grad reports that the healing energy imparted to laboratory mice was so rapidly used that a healer had to hold the mice for an hour at a time to maintain the necessary healing threshold of energy. This was attributed to the rapid metabolism of mice.

From experience, I have observed that imparted healing energy appears to be at its highest strength for about 48 hours in surgical patients and for trauma injuries. This is consistent with the evidence of the emotional side-effect of most healing encounters, an inner sense of calmness or well-being lasting about 48 hours.

When seeking to heal a chronic condition like scoliosis, I have found that a series of 3 to 5 daily healing encounters is required to maintain the threshold of energy needed to restore the spine's normal curvature. The same is true with hearing losses, arthritis, genital herpes, eczema, ruptured discs, Crohn's Disease, heart muscle regeneration and brain tissue regeneration.

In healing acute illnesses, the energy appears to dissipate as quickly as in lab mice. The healing energy must be either continually imparted or be supplied in huge quantities. This holds true for persons in hospital intensive care units, in major trauma and with specific illnesses like cancer, multiple sclerosis and Lou Gehrig's Disease. Huge quantities of properly-attuned healing energy can accelerate the healing rate of any disease or medical condition. Most huge quantities must be produced by group healing efforts or by immense amounts of love, caring and unity. The energy's effect behaves in similar fashion to that of an antibiotic and most other medications, where repeated doses are necessary to alleviate all symptoms.

20. All human-transmitted energy is not healing-quality. All persons can intentionally learn to emit an energy through their hands but this energy is not necessarily healing-quality energy. Some persons can do more harm than good. Just because one competently practices a particular healing technique does not mean that one can be helpful. To be competent, one must transmit healing-attuned energy.

Bernard Grad[17] asked two depressed patients in a psychiatric ward each to charge up a bottle of water for healing. A psychotic man's treated water retarded plant growth, while a depressed woman, happy to be useful, treated water which accelerated plant growth.

Gerald Solvin[18] injected mice malaria into mice and asked three volunteers to handle them for healing. One of the handlers, a scoffing nonbeliever in healing, was the real focus of the experiment. This unbelieving volunteer produced statistically significant negative healing effects in the mice ($p < .021$).

An extension of this scientific fact must be included in any valid research design. It has long been known in the practice of healing that one unbeliever or cynic can obstruct the healing efforts of a small group. Such an obstructive person would appear to *"untune"* healing energy. Any healing study in a medical setting might best be done secretly, with only those having to know being included in the design.

I have had my own first-hand experiences of destructive energy. Following a healing service, a well-meaning woman asked if she could offer me healing. I agreed. Within seconds of her placing her hand upon my head, I had an extreme headache and a feeling of oppression. I was this woman's therapist and knew that she was filled with anger and hatred. In another case, a depressed woman took my hand and offered me a prayer. During the prayer, I could sense her depression entering me and my own energy being drained.

Another time, a Russian physicist, experimenting with what he thought was healing energy, bathed a group with frequencies between 500-1200 hertz emitted by a thin violet fluorescent light. During the five-minute experiment, the three healers present were most susceptible. I felt my stomach become queasy from the first frequency, a headache from the second and an acute intestinal pain from the third. It took more than an hour for the three healers to restore energy-field health to the two dozen participants.

WARNING! **Do _not_ bathe yourself or anyone else in an electronically generated frequency of energy whose healing capability has not been clinically documented.** I have permitted myself to be bathed in the energy frequencies of several such psychotronic or radionic devices. In all cases, the energy felt coarse, unlike healing energy, and destroyed my own inner sense of peace and well-being. Any untested energy frequency is more likely to cause illness rather than health. Energy frequencies produce powerful effects on the human body. Psychotronic or radionic devices that enhance the operator's energy for the purpose of healing, are safer -- if the operator is a proven healer.

The existing evidence suggests that the quality and frequency of any emitted human energy are dependent upon specific biological, emotional, mental and spiritual factors. The prayers and touch of some persons can make an illness worse rather than better. It has been observed by healing practitioners that generous love for a person appears to naturally produce a frequency which results in healing energy being accumulated, attuned and transmitted.

All persons emit energy. Those who advocate hugging believe that four hugs a day (which share energy) maintain health. Newborn infants can die if not touched by human hands (passing them energy). It is reported that cocaine-addicted infants gain more weight when massaged several minutes a day. Part of this is likely to be due to the passing of a healing energy. Elderly men in many third world cultures sleep with teen-aged girls, not for sex, but in order to be have their energy levels restored. Psychologists talk about a touch-hunger suffered by people who are not touched.

Human touch can pass a healing energy that results in a sense of inner well-being and replenished energy. Throughout human history, parents have held their ill children for many hours at a time. Because of their love, parents have naturally imparted a healing energy, possibly saving millions of children's lives. The flip-side is that parents who are angry, resentful, anxious or depressed may pass an energy that has negative effects upon their children. The effects of parents passing negative energy to infants may include colic, fussiness, diarrhea and irregular sleep patterns.

21. Some man-made electromagnetic frequencies of energy are harmful to living organisms. As earlier reported, a 5.xxx hertz frequency induced cancer in mice within 48 hours. (I will not report the exact hertz frequency for cancer because it could be used as a weapon to cause disease.) A later 8 hertz frequency healed the induced cancer in mice. Other extremely low frequencies cause mood alterations such as depression, anxiety, aggressiveness and calmness. This validates the theory that the transmission of an energy at a healing frequency by a healer or pray-er can bring health to another person or an animal or plant. It can also moderate emotional levels and the resulting behaviors. It is reported that the former Soviet Union once bathed millions of workers in a 10 hertz energy field in order to maintain their calmness and energy.

The harm that can be done by low frequency electromagnetic waves is in the process of being established. Orthopedic surgeon Robert O. Becker (The Body Electric, 1985), a pioneering researcher and leading expert in the field of biological electricity and regeneration, reports that several Russian and Polish groups have established that prolonged exposure to a 50-hertz, 130-gauss magnetic field produced stress system changes and depression.

Becker's Veterans Administration research team discovered that extremely low frequency waves produced by high-power lines are linked to tumors in mice, slowed heartbeat in fish and chemical changes in the brain, blood and liver of rats. Another study demonstrated that depression and suicide occur more often in those exposed to high-tension power lines.

The greatest harm to organisms is thought to be in the 35-to-100-hertz frequency electromagnetic bands. A 1979 study by Nancy Wertheimer and Ed Leeper of the University of Colorado Medical Center on childhood cancer and 60-hertz power lines, statistically linked a doubling of the childhood death rate due to leukemia, lymph node cancer, and nervous system tumors to high-current wiring configurations.[19]

In his most recent book, <u>Cross Currents</u> (1990), Dr. Becker suggests a direct correlation between the mounting levels of electromagnetic frequencies in which humans have been bathed during the past generation and the similar increase in the number of cancer cases and the emergence of new diseases. A study by Dr. Samuel Epstein[20] of the University of Chicago Medical Center reveals some shocking statistics. Since 1975, there has been a 100% increase in lymphoma, myeloma and melanoma, a 31% increase in breast cancer, 97% increase in testicular cancer, a 20% increase in pancreatic cancer, a 142% increase in kidney cancer and a 63% increase in colon cancer.

Becker links exposure to man-made electromagnetic fields to the diseases of the Electromagnetic-Hypersensitive Syndrome, Chronic-Fatigue Syndrome, AIDS, Autism, Fragile X Syndrome, Sudden Infant Death Syndrome, Alzheimer's Disease, Parkinson's Disease, Cancer, and Mental Diseases.

Related to the enormous annual increases in exposure of humans to electromagnetic frequencies in our environment, Becker cites a 1984 study of the National Institutes of Mental Health that people under the age of forty-five have twice the rate of mental disorders than those over forty-five. In a 1986 editorial in the New England Journal of Medicine, Dr. Leon Eisenberg of the Harvard Medical School wrote that *"between 1950 and 1977, the suicide rates for 15-to-19-year-olds rose precipitously -- fourfold for males, and over two fold for females."* These rates continue to climb during each five year span in time. Could this effect also be causing the increasing gun violence throughout our nation?

Becker[21] states that any biological effects on humans are produced by extremely low frequencies (ELFs) in the 35-500 hertz range. Any steady human exposure to these frequencies at a strength of 3-milligauss magnetic field level produces detrimental biological effect (illness) that may only be reflected by the onset of an illness after many years of exposure.

Becker defines the effects of such exposure, saying that all abnormal, man-made electromagnetic fields, *regardless of their frequencies,* produce the same biological effects. These are:

1. Effects in growing cells, such as increases in the rate of cancer-cell division
2. Increases in the incidence of certain cancers
3. Developmental abnormalities in embryos
4. Alterations in neurochemicals, resulting in behavioral abnormalities such as suicide
5. Alterations in biological cycles
6. Stress responses in exposed animals that, if prolonged, lead to declines in the immune-system efficiency

7. Alterations in learning abilities

All these effects are cancer-*promoting*, not cancer-causing.

Becker then states that in urban environments, the ambient-field levels often exceed 3 milligauss; in the average suburban home, they range from 1 to 3 milligauss; and in rural areas they are generally less than 1 milligauss. The greatest exposures are caused:

1. By **television sets** *(stay at least 42 inches away from all sides of a 13 inch TV screen, and even further away from larger screens)*
2. By plug in **electric alarm clocks** *(keep at least 3 feet from body)*
3. By **personal computer video-display terminals** *(at 1990 radiation levels keep the keyboard at least 30 inches away from the screen)*
4. By **florescent lights** *(a 20-watt tube over office workers produces a field greater than 1 gauss over office workers)*
5. By **cellular phones and CB radios** *(no statistics)*
6. By **high power lines and power transformers** (limit to 3 gauss)
7. By **TV and FM/AM radio antenna transmissions** *(no statistics)*
8. By **microwave transmissions** *(no statistics)*

Becker[22] examines the need for all living organisms to be regulated by the Earth's normal geomagnetic field. Anytime man-made electromagnetic frequencies interfere with this geomagnetic frequency, living organisms become ill. Becker concludes, *"In my opinion, this knowledge is probably the single most important discovery of the century. It provides us with a key to the mechanisms by which all electromagnetic fields produce biological effects. These discoveries can give us yet another world, if we explore them properly."*

This data scientifically establishes the fact that electromagnetic energy has an effect on people. For our purposes, the fact that electromagnetic frequencies have an effect on human health strengthens the case for a helpful electromagnetic energy being transmitted during human healing encounters. It also suggests that healing encounters counteract the effects of man-made electromagnetic exposures.

22. The intentions of the healer are present in the transmitted energy. If the intention is to heal, the transmitted energy reflects that intention so that healing occurs. If the intention is to harm, the transmitted energy contains information that harms. The human transmitter is attuning the energy by his intentions. Yes, I am saying that mental intention and emotions attune the frequency of the energy emitted by humans. It is agreed within the field of spiritual healing that compassionate or generous love is the main emotion necessary for attuning the energy to the needed healing frequency. Thus, those who have a compassionate love for the sick naturally attune the energy to the healing frequency.

There is also evidence that a oneness with the person needing healing becomes a part of the attuning of the healing energy. Oneness can occur in a number of ways, all of which may be equally valuable. Healer and healee can be united through love. They can be united through the deep empathy of the healer for the healee's pain or identity. They can be united through the natural interpersonal unity that comes from close human interaction. They can be united by their mutual understanding of the medical condition.

A knowledge of both physiology and illness may improve the quality of the healing energy. This implies that health care professionals may be the best candidates as healers. It could be that a surgeon who is a latent healer unknowingly transmits a healing energy that guides his hands during surgery and contributes to tissue health and regeneration.

However, transmitted healing energy also acts intelligently on its own to heal. I have discovered that while I am intending to heal one condition, another condition may be healed, with or without the healing of the originally targeted condition. Here are some of my own experiences: a) While I intended to heal an injured finger, a woman's scoliosis was healed instead. The injured finger was later healed by traditional surgery. b) During counseling, I prayed for the healing of a marital relationship. The marital relationship was healed but in addition the woman's eczema was healed, even though I was unaware of the skin condition. c) Twice, I effectively healed a targeted illness but also unknowingly healed genital herpes in young women. This reinforces the observation that the healing energy seeks to create the optimum condition for life on its own.

Grad states that only about one healing in six hundred is instant and less than one percent of those seeking instant healing are healed at large faith healing services. These results are due to the fact that spiritual healing is a process, taking place over a period of time during many healing encounters. Researchers have observed this for years, designing their experiments for multiple sessions of touch-healing. Like an antibiotic, healing energy must be administered at necessary therapeutic levels over a period of time until the desired results are achieved. The scientific data indicates that the healing energy can initiate healing in conditions resistant to medical treatment and speed up the normal healing rate.

The healing energy acts somewhat like an antibiotic. For an infection, an antibiotic is administered so many times a day for so many days, because the antibiotic is used up by the infection and dissipates with the passage of time. The same is true of healing prayer. The healing energy is only being imparted while prayer is being offered. The charge of the healing energy then is used up by the recipient. For someone who is chronically or acutely ill, soaking them with prayer over a period of time is the only means by which healing can be accomplished. With most illness, healers need to recharge a person with healing energy every twenty-four hours.

The 1989 Chouhan-Weston Clinical Experiments used videotaped bioelectrography to observe the healing encounter. It took about ten minutes for me, the healer, to transform a cancerous energy field into a healthy one and cure a cancer patient. The healee's energy field remained a steady blue-white for almost ten minutes. Then, instantly, like an explosion, the energy field changed, becoming about three times larger and intensely white. This experiment confirmed the theory that the transmitted healing energy needs to accumulate in power, reaching a specific threshold of power before it can transform the unhealthy energy field. No healing would have occurred if touch-healing had stopped before ten minutes. This implies the need to soak people with prayer over a period of time in order to produce health.

A Practical Application. Hypothetical Alicia has cancer. Assuming that the healing energy is properly attuned and there are no barriers in the sending and receiving of it, Alicia needs a specific number of healing energy units to be alleviated of all symptoms. As an example, Alicia needs to accumulate 500 healing energy units to initiate the healing process. To continue the healing process, these 500 healing energy units must be maintained for 48 more hours before she becomes symptom free, producing a restored human energy field that can maintain her new health. Theoretically, this may call for maintaining an imput of 500 healing energy units per hour, for a total imput of 24,500 healing energy units during those 24-hours.

Alicia can receive all 24,500 healing energy units during one healing service. This may alleviate all symptoms of cancer and heal her, or she may not have a complete healing as all of these energy units are used in the first hour, needing to be replaced to maintain a healthy human energy field for an additional 48-hours.

Alicia can also receive the initial 500 therapeutic level of healing energy units through the touch healing prayers of a loved one. Say each minute of private prayer accumulates 25 healing energy units, it would take 20-minutes of prayer to reach that threshold level of 500 energy units. To maintain that threshold level may only take 10 more minutes of prayer every 3-hours for 48-hours. Healing charged water or cotton towels may also be used to maintain that healing threshold. This is a theoretical example that only clinical research can confirm.

24. There is no correlation between the size of a healer's energy field and healing effectiveness. Previous research has assumed that there is a direct correlation between the large size of the healer's energy field and the healer's effectiveness. But emerging data refutes this contention. In preliminary tests during the Chouhan-Weston Clinical Studies, the five hospital staff members were all younger than myself, the healer, by seventeen or more years. The healer's energy field was the smallest of the six persons present and grew even smaller during healing encounters. This implies that the attuned quality of healing frequency is more important than quantity in determining healing results. If, during a healing attempt, the quantity of the transmitted energy filled a whole room or a whole sports stadium, no healing would occur unless that energy had been attuned to the necessary healing frequency. A properly attuned healing frequency is the first requirement of any transmitted energy that heals.

25. Healing energy can be transmitted from any distance. Prayer can produce healing results from any distance. The earlier mentioned classic Rye Grass Experiment by Ambrose and Olga Worrall demonstrated that these two healers' prayers caused rye grass 600 miles away (from Boston to Atlanta) to increase its growth rate by 830 percent. From my own observations, absent prayer from groups in worship, prayer groups and prayer chains is extremely effective. A Russian healer successfully performed absent-healing in clinical trials. We do not have much experiential evidence that absent prayer from groups in worship, prayer groups and prayer chains is extremely effective.

A BOLD DEFENSE OF THE CLINICAL DATA

Olga Worrall freely permitted scientists to examine her abilities as a healer and a clairvoyant. She was used as the subject of more than 50 clinical studies. Olga was a no-nonsense woman who did not mince words. When her biographer questioned a specific healing result, she defended the truth as she had experienced it throughout a long lifetime in which she healed thousands of the ill throughout the world.

Olga Worrall firmly stated,[23] *"Perhaps YOU can't [accept healing] but many can. How can anything like spiritual healing or clairvoyance be proven conclusively in a material way? In the greatest feats of clairvoyance, there are always those who refuse to believe what they see and hear, who insist that only coincidence or fraud can explain what has been shown to them. In the most spectacular instance of spiritual healing, the same responses hold, the verdict is that he would have gotten better anyway. If he isn't improved, then that is used to discredit all spiritual healing.*

"People have eyes but don't see; they have ears but won't listen. When I made my commitment to spiritual healing, I was fully aware of the skepticism and ridicule and occasional hostility it would entail. But healing is God's gift to me -- and I will not bury the talent he has given into my keeping. And not only will I go on healing, but I will also go on working with scientists in the hope and faith that by dint of the sheer weight of the accumulated evidence, someday, somehow, the limitations of this physical world will be manifest to all and a glimpse of the other world will shine through."

CHAPTER FOUR SUMMARY

Infra-red spectrophotometric analysis show changes in healer-charged water, and healer-charged bottled water, cotton, wool and surgical gauze produce healing effects. Healing energy can be transmitted through electrical wiring. Healing energy is extremely stable, being storable in bottled water for at least two years, but dissipates when imparted to living organisms. A threshold level of healing energy is required and must be maintained.

A Superconducting Quantum Interference Device (SQUID) observed discernible changes in the amplitude and frequency (7.8 hertz) of the biomagnetic fields of world-class healers during healing and when not healing. World-class healers emit a constant plus or minus 7.83 hertz frequency at all times while others emit a rapidly fluctuating seven to twelve hertz. All world-class healers possess the identical brain-wave frequency of 7.83 hertz. Infra-red film photographs of healers' hands show an energy emerging from the palms and finger pads. Healers can produce up to two hundred twenty-two volts of energy.

Healers can impress their brain-wave pattern upon healees, resulting in a physical healing. Healing energy is informational and acts intelligently to produce the optimum state for life. Healing increases the amount of oxygen in the blood by up to twelve percent.

Chapter Five

Evidence of Human Energy Fields

"Mystery is but another name for our ignorance; if we were omniscient, all would be perfectly clear." ...Tryon Edwards

"The cell is a machine driven by energy. It can thus be approached by studying matter, or by studying energy." ...Albert Szent-Gyorgyi

"It is sown a physical body, it is raised a spiritual body. If there is a physical body, there is also a spiritual body." ...I Corinthians 15:44

This chapter is not about religious beliefs, philosophy or metaphysics. What we are exploring is scientific and experiential evidence that the human energy fields exist. How can healing energy produce such dramatic effects? What mechanism permits healings in which a shortened leg grows three inches within a few minutes? Would the existence of human energy fields best explain it?

Personalities of the intuitive-feeling type have often claimed to sense subjectively the presence of the human energy fields. A healer can teach most people to feel the human energy fields with their hands in order to assess the state of health. Dr. Norman Shealy's studies determine that some healers can accurately and consistently diagnose illness through their awareness of the human energy field. They can see or sense the human energy field. Let me step out on a limb. Let us begin proving the existence of human energy fields with a respected clairvoyant therapist and healer of the intuitive-feeling type, Barbara Ann Brennan.

THE HUMAN ENERGY FIELDS AS SEEN BY BARBARA BRENNAN

Barbara Ann Brennan's scientific credentials include a master's degree in physics and NASA staff experience. But, this New York City psychotherapist and healer is also a clairvoyant. She presents a comprehensive look at human energy fields through her own clairvoyant eyes. Though clairvoyant knowledge is not considered evidence by scientists, Brennan's working model has been proven accurate by the thousands of people who have successfully used this model in their practice of healing. If this were a theoretical working model, then the theory has been proven in practice. Logic would then conclude that as a clairvoyant working model, it has proven to be valid in practice.

Brennan[1] has *seen* nine layers of interpenetrating human energy fields (HEFs), but focuses upon a model based upon the first seven layers that make up the auric energy field. Through studying research data and the practice of counseling and spiritual healing, she has grasped the function of each of these HEFs. She reports that each of the seven auric energy fields has its own particular color, brightness, form, density, fluidity and function. The function of each energy field is unique. Starting with the first layer and going outward, these energy fields are associated with **(1)** physical functioning and sensation, **(2)** emotional life and feelings, **(3)** mental life and linear thinking, **(4)** love and the emotion of love, **(5)** the divine and the power of the Word, **(6)** celestial love, and **(7)** the higher mind of knowing and integrating the spiritual and physical make-up.

Brennan then states: *"There are specific locations within our energy system for the sensations, emotions, thoughts, memories and other non-physical experiences that we report to our doctors and therapists. Understanding how our physical symptoms are related to these [energy] locations will help us understand the nature of different illnesses and also the nature of both health and disease. Thus, the study of the aura can be a bridge between traditional medicine and our psychological concerns."*

THE HUMAN MIND AS AN ENERGY FIELD

Brennan[2] clairvoyantly offers us a new way of looking at the mind. She *sees* the mind in the energy fields, not in the biological brain area of the head. If we consider the mind as just another name for the biological brain, we cannot understand further explanations of the HEFs. Evidence indicates that the mind is not focused in the brain area of the skull.

She is saying that human beings function through both a biological brain and an energy field called the *"mind."* The brain is physical. The mind is, religiously speaking, spiritual, and scientifically speaking, an energy field. The mind does not exist in the physical area of the brain but is contained in various energy fields. Brain researchers use instruments that only measure known biological functioning. Exploring the interaction between the physical brain and the energy-field mind may open the doors to a golden age of human wholeness, longevity and evolution. And, tongue-in-cheek, it could be stated that, if you understand these concepts, then you will know that you are *"out-of-your-brain"* far more often than you are *"out-of-your-mind."*

GERBER'S HUMAN ENERGY FIELD (HEF) MODEL

A recent scientific model of the human energy field has been carefully developed by Richard Gerber, MD.[3] His thesis is that most orthodox approaches to healing are based upon the Newtonian viewpoint that the human body is a complex machine. Gerber's alternative is the Einsteinian viewpoint based upon Einstein's mathematics. This is what he refers to as *"vibrational medicine,"* which *"sees the human being as a multidimensional organism made up of physical cellular systems in dynamic interplay with complex regulatory energetic fields."*

He provides evidence that energy field number one is the template (blueprint) that carries information for the growth, development and repair of the physical body. The various human energy fields are composed of matter of higher frequency than physical matter. He compares these frequencies to the octaves on a piano keyboard. The lowest frequency octave is the physical; then come the etheric octave, the astral octave and the mental octave, each at a higher frequency. He refers to all these as matter, whether physical or subtle. *"Matter of different frequencies can co-exist in the same space, just as energies of different frequencies (i.e. radio and TV) can exist non-destructively in the same space."*

NASH: ELECTROMAGNETIC EFFECTS ON THE BODY

Neurologist Dr. Robert Nash, MD,[4] thinks that medical science will be relying more on electromagnetic approaches to health and less on the biochemistry that has dominated medical practice of the past century. Nash states, *"Many of the traditional academicians and teaching centers, as well as research scientists, have difficulty in comprehending that the prime cause of health, and probably disease, is some sort of energy pattern modulated by electromagnetic fields. These are both endogenous* [meaning within ourselves, such as our thoughts] *and exogenous* [meaning from the environment].

"I believe that electromagnetic homeostasis [the balance of blood pressure, heart rate, and respiratory rate] *of the brain is probably the most important aspect of the human body. This brings neurotransmitter combinations into balance, enhances the immune response and leads to health. It appears at the atomic level that the electromagnetic fields, rather than chemical events, shape signal flow and energy transmission in biomolecular systems."*

ADEY: A HUMAN ENERGY FIELD LINK TO CANCER

Dr. Nash reports that Dr. W. Ross Adey,[5] of Loma Linda Veterans Administration Center, proposes that cancer may be caused by the breakdown of the gap junctions that allow cell-to-cell communications. Cancer would thus prevent daughter cells from communication with the mother cells.

Nash states, *"By exposing cancer cell cultures which are surrounded by normal tissue to certain* [electromagnetic] *frequencies, cell-to-cell communication can be re-established from the normal cells to the cancer cells. This in turn stops the growth of the cancer, and actually redifferentiates the cancer cells into normal tissue. The work is preliminary and needs further elucidation. However, this is probably the most exciting work in progress in the field of energy medicine today."*

This preliminary research data indicates the role that the electromagnetic human energy field may play in cancer. It also reinforces the scientific, theoretical working model for touch-healing prayer in restoring life.

A BRIEF HISTORY OF HUMAN ENERGY FIELD RESEARCH

Throughout history, religious mystics have claimed to *see* an aura of energy surrounding living organisms including humans. During the Middle Ages, artists depicted religious saints with halos or auras of energy about their heads. Chinese acupuncture and acupressure are based on an ancient knowledge of a system of energy meridians that pervade the body. Blockage of those energy channels causes disease. Clearing the meridians and enabling energy to flow freely is the basis for the practices of acupuncture and acupressure.

Medical researchers have discovered variable energy readings along these meridian lines and have mapped out the meridian energy system. Some American health care professionals are now using sophisticated computer-enhanced readouts of the body's meridian energy system in assessing and diagnosing disease. They then balance the energy system using an energy tool about the size of a large pen. When I ask health care professionals who use this human energy field technology for scientific data to prove the existence of human energy fields, they laugh, because no such proof is necessary. These practitioners possess no such data because their technology assumes the electromagnetic nature of the human body, and the technology designed to restore the electromagnetic field works.

Ancient Hindu mystics clairvoyantly *saw* seven major energy chakras plus minor chakra systems. These chakras whirl in motion perpendicular to the body, like the cone of a tornado. When a chakra is whirling the wrong way or is blocked and weak, illness can result. Using their hands, healers can both assess chakra movement and make the appropriate repairs. The whole chakra energy system has been mapped out by health care professionals.

Ramesh Chouhan, MD, has screened twenty-five thousand women with bioelectrography prints of the human energy field, and can now diagnose cancer and arthritis months before their physical appearance through identifying the unique energy signature of these two diseases.

Here, we have described three different models of body energy systems as seen in meridians, chakras and bioelectrography. PrayWell will be focusing on bioelectrography.

EARLY EXPERIMENTS WITH PLANTS AND ANIMALS

During Kirlian photography, the subject is placed in direct contact with the film and 20,000 to 50,000 volts of electricity are run through the film negative while the picture is taken. This produces an energy picture showing an aura, like the sun's corona, around the subject.

In 1966, Victor Adamenko of the former Soviet Union cut away a small portion of a leaf and used Kirlian photography to take an electrophotograph of the remainder. The developed photograph showed a shadow image of the cutaway portion, as if the entire leaf were still present. This became known as the *"phantom leaf effect."* This can be interpreted as meaning that a leaf has an *energy field* or *aura* that persists in the empty portion that had been cut away, an energy image projected after physical death.

Many scientists have rejected any attempt to use electrophotography to prove anything because of a dozen difficult-to-control variables present in every experiment. In 1976, John Hubacher and Thelma Moss of UCLA, tightening the research design, reported on a dozen *phantoms.* The phantom leaf effect was obtained about five percent of the time.

This was recently confirmed in humans by Dr. John Pierrakos, founder of the Core Energetics Institute, NYC, whose client felt the energy field of her severed leg underneath her buttocks, where the surgeon had last placed it before removal. Barbara Ann Brennan concludes that the human energy field exists prior to the physical body, creating the physical body.[6]

Other Soviet electrophotography experimenters discovered that a plant's energy field showed visible signs of its disease weeks before the plant showed any outward physical signs of being diseased and dying. They discovered this when comparing two leaves of the same species that had produced different energy prints. The problem was solved when it was discovered that the one showing a weak white leaf energy image had come from a diseased bush that later died. Initially, the bush had shown no visible signs of disease. It was only weeks later that the disease became visible. The weak energy field became a predictor of later plant disease.

During the 1930s, biologist Harold Saxton Burr of Yale University conducted energy research with salamanders, worms, tadpoles and reptiles. These lower life forms are capable of regenerating severed limbs. The question biologists were asking was why aren't older members of these species able to regenerate limbs? Dr. Burr amputated the limbs of salamanders and measured an energy of 1.5 to 2.5 millivolts around the missing limbs. When the energy reading fell below that, the salamander could not regenerate a limb. He discovered a direct correlation between the energy level and age. Salamanders had difficulty regenerating a new limb when they were older and displayed a weaker electrical energy field. The energy-rich young could easily do this. This demonstration showed that a certain threshold level of energy was needed to create a physical form.

Recently, I read a newspaper article by a medical doctor stating that human children under the age of ten can regenerate the severed tip of a finger if medically permitted to do so. He cited over two hundred recent cases of such regeneration. This extends the implications of Burr's work with salamanders. In human beings, also, the young have stronger energy fields than do older ones, enabling the young to regenerate tissue more easily.

During the 1960's, Soviet clinical researchers claimed to have proven the existence of a human energy field and described its importance. The Soviet researchers established that each organ of the body has an energy field, which they called *"an astral blueprint."* The astral blueprint, which is an intelligent-acting energy field, forms a mold for each organ of the physical body.

THE BODY RESPONDS AS THOUGH IT HAS ENERGY FIELDS

The effect of the healing energy upon human beings show characteristics typical of energy-field activity. As decribed in chapter four, the healing energy's effect is a process working over a period of time. It needs to reach a certain level or threshold of energy to have an effect, and it needs to be replenished as it is used up. That describes how a human energy field would need to work in healing.

The healing energy can initiate healing in medical conditions that have proven resistant to medical treatment. Only if the human energy field is indeed the blueprint mold for every organ of the body can we account for and explain healings like the regeneration of arthritic bone joints. In such instances, the healing energy is operating on the genetic level, achieving something resembling genetic engineering.

As we saw in chapter four, the healing energy can prevent an anticipated disease from occurring. Healer-treated mice did not develop chemically induced goiters because their energy fields were strengthened to the extent that their genetic mold, or code, maintained the cells normally rather than permitting them to develop goiters. As will be described, Dr. Ramesh

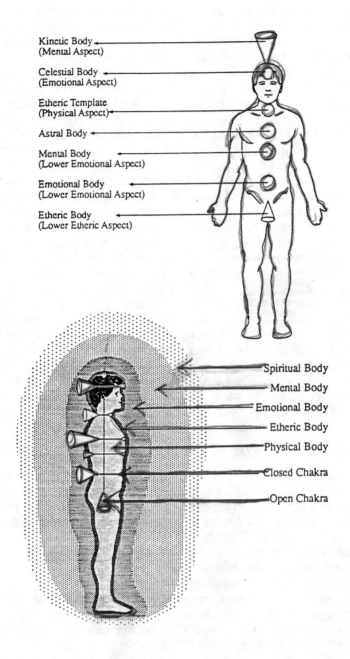

Figure 4. *The ancient Hindu chakra energy system along with their five different frequencies of energy fields that encompass our physical bodies.* **Top:** *Frontal view of the chakras.* **Bottom:** *Side view including the five energy bodies. Today we know there are at least seven and maybe as many as nine energy bodies.*

Singh Chouhan can diagnose an anticipated disease because the disease appears in the energy field before it is evident in the physical body.

Absent prayer can be transmitted to any place in the world and have a healing effect. Because its effects are identical, we can surmise that absent prayer must emit an energy frequency similar to the 7.8 to 8.0 hertz frequency which healers emit by touch. It is common sense to conclude that absent prayer, therefore, is operating through its effects on a human energy field.

These were some of the assumptions I took with me when I was invited to India to participate as a healer in the Chouhan-Weston Clinical Studies. I arrived with modest expectations. I just wanted to prove scientifically that touch-healing produced an effect that could be verified in human beings. It came as a surprise when our limited clinical studies verified most of my assumptions.

THE HUMAN ENERGY FIELD HOLDS DIAGNOSTIC INFORMATION

During the 1980s, Dr. Ramesh Singh Chouhan, a young physician at JIPMER, a modern regional government hospital in Pondicherry, India, pursued energy photography research in his bioelectrography laboratory, under a research grant from the Indian government. His resulting data is based upon fingertip bioelectrography negatives of twenty-five thousand screened women. With this advanced form of Kirlian photography, he is photographing the aura of what appears to be the first of seven human energy fields.

Chouhan measured the depth and the density of an energy aura made visible by running twenty-five thousand to forty thousand volts through fingertips, creating an ionized energy picture. In the early screening, he used X-ray negatives to record the bioelectrographic image of all five fingertips of both hands. The cost of screening was only twenty-seven United States cents per person.

Chouhan was able to make medical sense out of the immense data base available to him. He identified consistent energy patterns or signatures for several medical conditions. This produced four diagnostic breakthroughs that are non-invasive, radiation-free, inexpensive predictors of biological conditions. Most important of all, the process can predict three medical conditions earlier than any other existing diagnostic method. Here are Chouhan's four medical breakthroughs:

1. The Early Diagnosis of Cancer. His data establishes that characteristic cancer signatures appear in the body's energy field prior to the appearance of cancer in the physical body. He is able to diagnose cancer three to six months before it can be detected by any known medical procedure.

In the case of cervical cancer, surgeons, seeing bioelectrography evidence of cancer in the energy field, would remove suspicious cervical tissue. Then, while the patient was still in recovery, a second bioelectrography picture would be taken. If all pre-cancerous cells had been removed, the energy field would already have returned to normal. If cancer cells were still present, the fingertip bioelectrography negative reflected this. Then, the surgery would continue with the removal of more cervical tissue.

The implications for cancer screening, for post-surgical assurance and for evaluating the need for other treatments are revolutionary. This diagnostic procedure has one limitation. It can only diagnose the presence and the extent of cancer. It cannot provide information on where and what kind of cancer is involved. Chouhan has patented a computerized model in which a hand is placed upon a sensing plate and the energy field scanned for the cancer signature.

2. The Early Diagnosis of Arthritis. Chouhan's second diagnostic breakthrough detects arthritis six to twelve months before it can be diagnosed traditionally or its symptoms appear in the patient. Medical treatment can begin immediately, while the initiation of spiritual healing can prevent both cancer and arthritis from occurring in the physical body.

3. Pregnancy Diagnosis. A third breakthrough involves the energy field diagnosis of pregnancy moments after conception. A massive energy shift occurs that can easily be observed in the female bioelectrography negative. This pregnancy test is extremely important for women in developing nations because the test results are available within minutes and cost little.

4. Pinpointing the Optimum Moment for Conception. The fourth medical breakthrough involves Chouhan's work with infertile couples. Bioelectrography has proven to be the most accurate means for pinpointing the optimum moment for conception as a graph of daily energy field changes indicates.

Chouhan states that his research data proves that not only is there an energy field within the bounds of the physical body, but that the energy field also reflects and can predict the state of health of the physical body, whether it concerns arthritis, cancer, conception or fertility.

WHAT THIS TEACHES ABOUT THE HUMAN ENERGY FIELD

Chouhan's data indicates that the illnesses reflected in human energy fields took three to twelve months to affect body tissue in the cases of cancer and arthritis. Whatever caused the distortions in the energy fields acted slowly in causing illness. In contrast, the body has the ability to quickly change the energy fields, as noted in the immediate change in women's energy fields due to the physiological changes of pregnancy. As you will see, a viral infection can also quickly cause an unhealthy energy field.

My experience from the practice of healing is that the healing energy quickly transforms the energy fields in most illnesses, producing physical health. Once the arthritis energy signature is discovered, it takes six to twelve months before physical symptoms appear. In contrast, all symptoms of osteoarthritis can disappear within minutes or an hour of a ten-minute healing session. Since no bioelectrography studies have been conducted following the alleviation of symptoms, we do not yet know what changes take place in the energy field. Nor do we know what has biologically occurred.

Cancer's response to touch-healing is completely different from that of arthritis. Rarely do the symptoms disappear quickly. Similar cancer conditions may respond differently; one might be cured following three sessions while another stubbornly persists through two dozen sessions. The Chouhan-Weston Clinical Studies provide new pieces of evidence for a still extremely incomplete picture.

THE BARRIERS REMAIN

Following a dozen years of research and a massive volume of clinical evidence, Chouhan faces a barrier. The medical profession has not become convinced that there is a human energy field. I watched Chouhan present his findings to a group of Indian doctors. All but one doctor was hostile.

That one doctor approached Ramesh afterwards and said, *"I still have to be convinced. But, I encourage you to continue your work."* Most doctors are thinking-sensing personality types, unable to accept the existence of a non-tangible human energy field. I had expected more from them. These doctors live in the country that gave us the knowledge about energy chakras in the ancient past. Unfortunately, Indian doctors are also trained in the Western model of medicine, and reflect its dogmas.

Both Ramesh and I presented papers on energy fields and healing energy at an international yoga conference in Pondicherry. Those in attendance already believed in the spiritual body and human energy fields. Both of us received resounding standing ovations from four hundred yogi adepts gathered from twenty nations. This felt good, but it meant nothing. We were only confirming their beliefs with scientific evidence. How do we get through to the larger world?

PREPARING FOR THE CHOUHAN-WESTON STUDIES

By the time I arrived in India in January, 1989, Chouhan had designed apparatus that produced a live *visible* energy field. The apparatus consisted of a variable voltage generator and a one-foot by one-foot free-standing wooden frame with a small clear plate glass panel mounted in the center. The glass conducted electricity and was one pole of the generator. The other pole was clipped to a finger of the test subject, who placed one finger firmly against the glass panel, completing the electrical circuit. This produced the ionized energy aura of the test subject. In a light-blackened room, this ionized energy aura could be photographed with an ordinary camera or an extremely low-light one lux videocamera. With a videocamera, we could record and observe any ongoing changes in the energy aura during a healing encounter for as long as we chose.

I was accompanied by Henry Belk, III of Charlotte, North Carolina, who was our videocameraman. We thoroughly tested our equipment and procedures. Unfortunately, this was the wrong time to conduct the studies. Dr. Chouhan's research was under fire from the hospital medical staff. His unit's medical director had always supported Chouhan and given him a free hand. Upon hearing that I was coming to assist in clinical studies, the medical director had been given orders to stop Chouhan from conducting research using hospital patients. These were the pool from which we had intended to draw our test subjects.

I had recently received the same reception from an American hospital that had barred doctors from working with me on a clinical study. I had traveled half-way around the Earth to India, thinking that their medical doctors would be more open. Being supported by a research grant, Dr. Chouhan had few private patients from which to draw. Discouraged, we took time off and traveled.

Returning, our choice of research subjects remained limited. Chouhan found a woman with ten years of chronic back pain and two women whose energy fields showed the cancer signature. They both had pre-cancerous cervixes. We also had a lab assistant with an acute head cold. These became our test subjects. We had intended to use hundreds of replicates. What could we learn from such a small sample? As it turned out, we learned far more than we had initially hoped for with a hundred subjects.

THE CLINICAL STUDIES

In our preliminary trials, we learned that no matter where I touched subjects during healing, it had the same effect upon the energy field. This was a relief to me. As a minister, I practiced touch-healing by merely holding a hand and praying. This had produced consistent healing results. But, with all the research I had read and the seminars I had attended about chakra-cleansing, meridian-healing and energy-balancing, I had developed some doubts about my much simpler style of healing. I made the decision to place my hands on each subject's forehead and neck while praying aloud. No subject spoke English and I understood no Hindi. All subjects were Hindus. I calmed each subject through friendliness and touch.

I must make it clear that I would not have produced such quick results in the United States. The faith and placebo factors assisted me in India. The following elements elevated my status before the test subjects. I was a romantic and mystical figure -- an American, Christian, minister, healer working with Hindus. My physical size (6'-2", 210#) dwarfed the subjects. We were working in a prestigious medical hospital with a doctor leading a research study. Most of those factors would not be present in America where my test subjects would likely be more skeptical and suspicious.

Since this study has never appeared in a professional journal, you have many reasons for questioning my data and analysis. My only defense is to state that these studies can be replicated with equipment costing about $600 and I would be only too happy to serve as the healer in any such studies.

1. A Viral Infection Quickly Healed. The Chouhan-Weston Clinical Studies provided unexpected videotape information on the healing of a viral infection. The 21-year-old female laboratory assistant displayed acute cold symptoms, including skin pallor, a fever, runny nose, watery eyes and sneezing. The videotaped record of the healing encounter indicated that, upon touch, it took only two seconds to transform the fingertip baseline bioelectrography image of the test subject. During those two seconds, the fingertip bioelectrography image changed from its baseline blue with a white outer fringe to a pure white hue about twice as large, and remained constant. Toward the end of the 89 second healing contact, she complained of the extreme heat within her and vigorously pulled away from my hands to escape. She then explained that the heat had become too painful. About an hour after the healing encounter, all cold symptoms had disappeared.

Analysis. This experiment indicates that the symptoms of a viral infection, a cold, can be alleviated within an hour following the successful transmission of healing energy by human touch. It suggests that a healing threshold of energy was reached within 89 seconds of touch-healing contact. It validated the traditional healer observation that a sense of inner heat indicates that healing at some level is occurring.

Inner Sensings Proven Valid. Subjectively, something within me was able to sense when the cold had been cured. At about 85 seconds into touch-healing, my voice can be heard on the video-tape saying, *"She has been healed."* This was immediately followed by her escape from the heat of my hands at 89 seconds. Healers have traditionally reported such inner sensings, as had I, myself. But, I had never trusted nor acted upon this inner sensing, thinking it might be due to my imagination, impatience, optimism or the need to reassure the healee. In this case, my inner sensing was validated.

Energy Field Assessment. In the initial testing of our equipment and procedure, we had established fingertip bioelectrography image baselines. We had discovered that the normal human fingertip bioelectrography image was blue with a white fringe. Therefore, each test subject began with the normal baseline image. We had also established that a touch-healing encounter changes this normal image to a larger white image in apparently healthy test subjects. The only difference between the woman with the cold and the healthy test subjects was the sensing of heat, which became increasingly painful.

2. Treating a Woman with Chronic Back Pain. The face of the woman with a 10-year history of back pain displayed a desperate longing for help. She had traveled over a hundred miles in seeking that help. Upon my touching her for the first time, her normal energy field of blue with a white tinge changed within three seconds to a pure white field about twice as large. I maintained hand contact for ten minutes during each of three sessions. On the second and third days, she arrived with her fingertip bioelectrography image still glowing with the transmitted healing energy of the previous day. She reported no change of symptoms until the third day. In the midst of that healing encounter, she reported the complete alleviation of all symptoms.

From personal experience, I can state that this type of healing process consistently occurs with trauma injuries, back conditions and pre-surgical healing preparations. The viral condition was healed within an hour but the back injury took three consecutive days of treatments, or about 48 hours. The healing energy appears to work somewhat like an antibiotic that must be taken over a period of time in order to maintain a therapeutic threshold of healing energy to heal an infection. The healing energy must be applied consistently over a period of time. This experimental data coincides with my experience with scoliosis. External symptoms only change following three or four daily sessions. Then, the transformation occurs during sleep, when the spine either pleasantly spasms or painfully hurts, resulting in the disappearance of all symptoms of scoliosis.

3. Pre-Cancerous Test Subjects. Through fingertip bioelectrography images, Dr. Chouhan had diagnosed pre-cancerous cervical symptoms in two young women who became test subjects. Normal medical treatment would have required the partial removal of the cervix followed by fingertip bioelectrography imaging to determine the success of the procedure. Here, we were utilizing touch-healing as the primary treatment mode.

Bernard Grad and others had already established that touch-healing could prevent an anticipated disease from occurring. Aside from the fingertip bioelectrography image indicating that cancer would occur within three to six months, we had only suspicious-looking cervical tissue as evidence of possible impending cancer.

Cancer Subject One. I placed my hands upon her forehead and neck. The lights went off and I began praying in the total darkness. As in the previous studies, I would not know what was happening to her fingertip bioelectrography image until the videotape was reviewed on American based technology of color television monitor back in the States. My fingers sensed what I interpreted to be resistance to the healing flow, as if there were a wall blocking it. After about 8 minutes of touch-healing, I commented, *"She is not receiving the healing, but I will give her a few more minutes."* At just short of 10 minutes, I announced what I was sensing: *"She has begun receiving the healing flow."* I continued touch-healing for two more minutes.

A week later, my first viewing of the videotaped record of her fingertip bioelectrography image demonstrated that I had been wrong in interpreting the meaning of my finger sensings. What the videotape record showed was the normal baseline human energy field remaining unchanged for almost ten minutes. Then, like an explosion, at about 9 minutes and 45 seconds, the fingertip bioelectrography image became instantly pure white and almost three times larger. A later still fingertip bioelectrography image displayed no sign of the characteristic energy signature. She had been cured and would not develop cancer.

Analysis. This experiment raised more questions than it answered. When my fingers sensed the resistance, the healing energy was doing something, perhaps building to the threshold level necessary to cause the explosive energy field transformation at just before ten minutes. At that transforming moment, I reported she had just begun receiving the healing flow. In reality, the transformation of the fingertip bioelectrography image had at that moment registered a complete healing. As a healer, I need to reassess the meaning of my fingers' sense of resistance.

The response of the fingertip bioelectrography image of this subject was remarkably different from the previous two subjects. With the cold and the back condition, there was an immediate transformation of the fingertip bioelectrography image to the white image. Thereafter, it took time, from eighty-nine seconds to forty-eight hours, for healing to occur. These stand in marked contrast to the pre-cancerous subject. It took almost ten minutes for the fingertip bioelectrography image to change to white and with that change, the cancer signature in her fingertip bioelectrography image disappeared.

Some healing researchers think that cancer is a disease caused by a faulty human energy field that has been distorted in some way. This study hints that once an energy field has been transformed and enhanced by healing energy, cancer cells become healthy cells.

Cancer Subject Two. I was unable to view the videotapes until after the clinical studies were completed. Immediately after working with Cancer Subject One, I began touch-healing with Cancer Subject Two. Being discouraged by the first subject's resistance and not knowing about the alleviation of her symptoms, I only worked with Cancer Subject Two for about eight minutes and stopped. Her fingertip bioelectrography image exhibited no change. This implies that no healing will result with cancer patients unless the healer practices until he senses the healing flow begin. With many Americans, this might take 30 to 90 minutes of effort. At times, a cancer patient will report a heat or tingling sensation pervading the whole body following during touch-healing. Healers can know that a level of healing is occurring when they feel the energy freely flowing into the cancer patient. In addition, in all such cases, the patient reports of whole body heat or tingling have been followed by the alleviation of all symptoms of cancer.

THE EXISTENCE OF A HUMAN ENERGY FIELD

I do not know what kind of evidence is acceptable in verifying the existence of a human energy field. I now possess a videotape of the Chouhan-Weston Clinical Studies. The videotape graphically demonstrates that when I touch a healee on the forehead and nape of the neck, the healing energy affects the whole body, going to the fingertip that is being photographed. It then removes all symptoms of a cold virus in one hour, alleviates the symptoms of ten-year-old chronic back pain in forty-eight hours and removes all symptoms of cervical cancer in less than ten minutes.

The clinical evidence indicates that no matter what area I touch, the healing energy travels throughout the body to cause healing. I think the existence of a human energy field is the best explanation for how this can happen.

I also exist with a daily awareness of something that acts like a human energy. I can sense it with my hands during touch-healing assessment and prayer. I can pick up people's emotions with my hands. When I heal painful emotions, I can sense them disappearing and being replaced by calmness. When I work directly with human energy fields, even though I cannot *see* the fields, they respond the way clairvoyants who can *see* these energy fields say they should.

I have learned that I can be effective in some conditions only by working one to four inches away from the skin in what I sense are human energy fields. Every evening when my wife and I pray together while embracing in bed, we can both feel the heat of our energy chakras merging. During lovemaking, we can merge our energy fields. So, why should I go on seeking to prove the existence of a human energy field?

Because I think it is important for the future practice of healing prayer to verify what is occurring in the healing encounter. I think this can be the basis for further research. It would only take one medical center a relatively short period of time and a few thousand dollars in equipment to completely explore the healing encounter and to define the nature and function of the human energy fields.

THE SIGNIFICANCE OF ENERGY FIELDS

Life energies research data informs us that all living organisms possess energy fields that contain information and act intelligently in response to that information. For example, the plants and animals used in research studies possess energy fields, as the data on healing energy indicates. What implications can we draw from such a picture?

It means that humans can transmit healing energy to enhance the lives of animals and plants. It means that the healing energy can also affect bacteria and viruses, because they are living things that possess energy fields. It means that all cells and their genetic codes can be affected by healing energy. This amplifies our understanding and leads to many new approaches and applications of healing.

For example, years ago when I was with a mission work team building a church and hurricane shelter on top of a remote Haitian mountain, our two nurses were trying to teach the Haitians about personal and public hygiene. One problem was that the villagers often urinated upstream from where they drew their drinking water, bathed and washed clothes. Our nurses were unsuccessful in convincing them that this practice could cause illness because of the presence of bacteria. So, the whole work team met with the village leaders one evening.

They continued to laugh at our concept of invisible organisms called bacteria. We in turn smothered our laughter at their explanation of disease. They insisted that evil spirits caused disease. We were at a standstill until we used our creativity. We told them that urinating upstream attracted evil spirits that would make them ill. This, they could believe. They then established an adequate public health policy.

The point of my story is this. After later learning that all living organisms possessed energy fields, I began making connections with primitive voodoo beliefs. Bacteria possess energy fields. If certain Haitian clairvoyants could *see* the energy fields of an organism that caused disease, a bacterium, they would call the energy field of that organism an evil spirit, evil because it caused disease.

I once observed a highly educated Roman Catholic priest, Ralph DiOrio, leading a healing service. He ordered the spirit of deafness, a conscious energy field, to leave those with hearing losses. It worked. I tried the same thing. It worked. If it works, use it.

TIMMY'S HEALING

One Sunday evening my phone rang. The tense voice of a parishioner stated, *"Hello, this is Tim. My grandson, Timmy, was hit by a car. The am-*

bulance just got here. We are headed for the Emergency Room at Community Hospital."

Timmy's body appeared lifeless when he arrived at the hospital. His clothes were covered with blood. I joined Timmy's parents and grandparents in their grim vigil outside the door of surgery. A half-hour later a doctor dressed in surgical greens emerged and informed us, *"Timmy is in critical condition. Every bone in his body seems broken. There is damage to internal organs, internal bleeding, a fractured skull, and probable brain damage. We are still examining the full extent of his injuries. We have called in a neurologist and an orthopedic specialist."*

The situation appeared hopeless. And, if young Timmy survived, there would be brain damage. There was already mental retardation among this family's children. Fear and anxiety filled the area where we waited. We returned to our silent prayers. Every half-hour we would do a group hug and I would offer a prayer for healing.

As we passed through four hours of agonized waiting and prayer, physicians entered periodically. They gave us bits of hope: *"Internal bleeding has stopped." "Has fewer fractures than original x-rays had shown." "Has no fractures." "All we can do is monitor him." "His condition has stabilized and we've put him in bed to sleep."* We slept.

Four-year-old Timmy slept for sixteen hours. When he awoke, he got out of bed, ran to the nursing station and asked for something to eat. He was healthy. No broken bones. No internal injuries. No brain damage. No bruises. No abrasions. Not a scratch remained. We were jubilant.

Just for a moment take this story at its face value. Assume that it is true. How would you explain the way God could have taken the dying, bleeding, broken body of a little boy and healed everything that was hurt? Yes, we prayed and God healed. But how did that healing occur?

This chapter has explained what happened. The energy of our prayers strengthened Timmy's energy fields. Not only was his immune system stimulated -- his energy fields, Timmy's genetic energy blueprint, were restored and made every cell in Timmy's body new and whole.

CHAPTER FIVE SUMMARY

1. Barbara Ann Brennan states: *"There are specific locations within our energy system for the sensations, emotions, thoughts, memories and other non-physical experiences that we report to our doctors and therapists."*

2. Richard Gerber, MD, refers to human energy field therapy as *vibrational medicine*, which *"sees the human being as a multidimensional organism made up of physical cellular systems in dynamic interplay with complex regulatory energetic fields."*

3. Neurologist Robert Nash: *"It appears at the atomic level that the electromagnetic fields, rather than chemical events, shape signal flow and energy transmission in biomolecular systems."*

4.   W. Ross Adey, MD: "By exposing cancer cell cultures to certain (electromagnetic) frequencies, cell-to-cell communication can be re-established from the normal cells to the cancer cells.   This in turn stops the growth of the cancer...."

5.   Ramesh Chouhan, MD, with bioelectrography prints of the human energy field, can diagnose cancer and arthritis months before their physical appearance through identifying the unique energy signature of these two diseases.   Other health care professionals could also easily do this.

6.   The body responds to touch-healing as though it possesses energy fields.   The healing energy can initiate healing in conditions previously resistant to medical treatment.

7.   Chouhan's research indicates that the illnesses reflected in human energy fields took three to twelve months to affect body tissue in the cases of cancer and arthritis.   Whatever caused the distortions in the energy fields acted extremely slowly in causing the resulting physical illness.   In contrast, biological changes have the ability to quickly change the energy fields

8.   The videotaped evidence of the Chouhan-Weston Clinical Studies demonstrated that it took only two seconds for touch-healing prayer to produce a healthy energy field in a viral infection and chronic back pain, but almost ten minutes for cervical cancer.   In each case, the subjects became symptom-free.

Chapter Six

Practical Benefits of Healing Encounters

"Faith may be defined briefly as an illogical belief in the occurrence of the improbable." ...H.L. Mencken

"Meditative insight reveals to the soul a God who multiplies aid for human spiritual assistance and above all makes us ministers in mutual assistance to one another...." ...John Donne*

"Heal me, O Lord, and I shall be healed...." ...Jeremiah 17:14a

What can healing encounters contribute to your health and happiness? Four sources provide insights into this answer. The first source is religious wisdom. A second source is the scientific research data provided in the past three chapters that draws a preliminary picture. Another source would be the clinical reports coming to us from other nations where healing is practiced in hospital settings. A final source involves the first-hand observations of practicing healers. These four sources will help us explore the practical benefits of healing encounters.

PRACTICAL BENEFITS OF RELIGIOUS WISDOM

Moses proclaimed, *"...man does not live by bread alone....but by everything that proceeds out of the mouth of the Lord"* (Deuteronomy 8:3). This religious wisdom speaks to us today, telling us that the good life consists of far more than creature comforts like family, food, housing, education, health care and entertainment. It tells us that undergirding the good life is the Word of God. The Word of God is the Source of all life. It provides us with a wisdom for healthy and happy living. It tells us that this is God's universe. God permeates the whole universe with his Life Energy (Spirit) and the Word. For humans to become entirely whole, they must rely upon the power of Life that comes from God.

Life energies researchers have confirmed this wisdom of the Word. Their evidence points to a subtle energy or life force that permeates the whole universe. During the healing encounter, this life force is accumulated, attuned and transmitted by humans. Humans are capable of using this life force to bring new life to themselves and others because the life force acts to restore all life to its optimum conditions of wholeness. The life force heals body tissue, emotional pain, mental confusion, spiritual emptiness and relational divisions.

As a priest knowledgeable of the Word, and as one who has personally experienced God's transforming presence and power, I cannot read the sci-

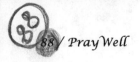

entific data without recognizing that it is describing God and God's work among humanity. God created and continues to create and make all things new through the healing encounter. God is the Source of health and happiness.

Much of the Word of God describes what it means to be fully human, mature and whole. Humans are far more than just biological tissue. The Word teaches that we are physical, emotional, mental and spiritual beings. To be whole means all four of these aspects are fully alive, interacting, complementing and balancing each other. If we ignore the health of any one of these human parts, it affects and diminishes the health, the life, of the others.

The existence of human energy fields, and their description as being many bodies vibrating at various frequencies, matches the wisdom of the Word. As the scientific data graphically portrays, when the healing energy flows into a human being, the energy fields become significantly larger and become white, like the mystic presence of God. All that is missing from this equation is the Word, God's wisdom in the life of humanity.

SCIENTIFIC EVIDENCE OF PRACTICAL BENEFITS

The scientific evidence indicates there is an objectively measurable healing effect. The evidence indicates that humans accumulate, attune, focus and transmit an energy that heals. The evidence indicates that the energy is information-bearing and acts intelligently to restore humans to their optimum condition for life. The evidence indicates that the energy works by restoring the human energy fields, including that of the mind. These restored energy fields then repair the physical, emotional, mental and spiritual components of a human being. The evidence indicates that the energy can initiate healing in conditions that are resistant to medical treatment, and perhaps perform genetic engineering.

The evidence indicates that healing energy dramatically increases the human rate of healing. As with an antibiotic, the healing energy must be constantly replenished in order to maintain a therapeutic level. The energy increases the amount of oxygen in the blood by up to twelve percent.

Healing energy has many unusual qualities. It can be imparted to water, wool and cotton cloth, and surgical gauze, and then be stored in these substances indefinitely. These then produce effects similar to those produced by a healer. This energy can be transmitted through electrical wiring. It can stop an anticipated disease from occurring. It can be transmitted through absent prayer to any location.

Healer-treated water emits a 7.8 to 8.0 hertz electromagnetic frequency, as do healers world-wide. Another extremely low frequency, 5.xxx hertz, induces cancer in mice within forty-eight hours. This induced cancer can be healed quickly with an 8 hertz frequency. Other extremely low frequencies cause emotional mood alterations both beneficial and detrimental to health and life.

The brain plays a role in the healing picture, with a healer able to impress his/her own brain-wave pattern on the healee to induce healing. Personality traits play a role in disease. Absent prayer from a group is able to affect the brain-wave pattern. All persons can transmit energy from their palms and fingers, but such transmitted energy is not necessarily healing energy.

The scientific data presents a preliminary picture of the effects of spiritual healing and the qualities of the healing energy. Physicians are in the best position to understand the full implications of this data and how the practice of healing can complement existing medical treatment. Future research must completely explore the scientific benefits of healing.

PRACTICAL BENEFITS REPORTED BY OTHER NATIONS

Healing is practiced in hospitals in England, Brazil, Russia, Poland and Hungary. Italian physician Dr. Piero Cassoli's extensive study suggests the use of spiritual healing in infections of the sinuses, ovaries and inner ear. He also recommends its use in cooperation with conventional medical care for epilepsy and malignancies.[1]

According to Soviet healer Victor Krivorotov, the list of diseases that can be cured by Pranotherapy [touch-healing] is broad and diverse. It includes both functional and chronic diseases: nervous disorders (irritation of the spinal nerve roots, skin diseases, fatigue of the nervous system, vegetative disorders, etc.), mental disorders (hypochondria, hysteria, obsessive-compulsive neurosis, etc.), internal diseases (coronary insufficiency, myocardia, respiratory disorders, gastric conditions, dyskinesia of gall ducts, etc.), and female diseases.[2]

Polish hospital clinical data on spiritual healing offers hard scientific information. It is far more evidential than subjective reporting. Barbara Ann Brennan reports this conversation with Mietek Wirkus, who worked as a healer with physicians in a clinic affiliated with the "IZICS" Medical Society in Warsaw.[3]

Mietek Wirkus reported that his clinic shows that *"bioenergotherapy or BET [touch-healing] is most effective in nervous system diseases and the diseases that were consequences of migraine, in healing bronchial asthma, bedwetting, hemicrania, nervous illness, psychosomatic diseases, gastric ulcer, some kinds of allergies, liquidation of ovarian cysts, benign tumors, sterility, arthritic pains, and other kinds of pain. BET helps to relieve pain caused by cancer and decreases the amount of pain medication and tranquilizers taken by a patient. Good effect has also been observed in treatment of deaf children. In almost every case, the doctors discovered that after BET treatment, patients became more quiet and relaxed, pain was gone or relieved, and the rehabilitation process (especially after surgery or infection) was accelerated."*

I met Evgeniya Stogny, the chief healer in one of the largest hospitals in Moscow, at a 1992 Montreal seminar. As the chief healer, she supervises a staff of two dozen healers who refer to healing as *Bio-Energy Therapy*. She says Bio-Energy Therapy improves the blood, matching American research data. Through a healing purification process, she is able to improve conditions affecting the heart, breathing and kidneys. She stated that Bio-Energy Therapy can improve all medical conditions. Evgeniya then specifically named the prostate, female problems, hepatitis, scar tissue, stomach-intestinal problems, brain conditions, disk displacement and the immune system, including AIDS. Evgeniya revealed that she is working with three new diseases that the Western nations have not yet seen. She closed her presentation by reflecting that during the dying process, the biofield folds, and then disappears at death.

This clinical evidence demonstrates the serious study and practice of spiritual healing in eastern Europe. Eastern European research data could save the United States decades of research. Russian healers have verbally shared the news that Russian healing research instruments far surpass any technology in the West. If this should prove to be true, then the rest of humanity need only inquire and receive a needed gift. The following table summarizes the specific medical conditions that respond to touch-healing as enumerated in the clinical reports from Italy, Poland and Russia:

European Clinical Reports

AIDS, immune deficiencies	allergies
arthritic pain	asthma, bronchial
bedwetting	blood improvement
brain bleeding	brain conditions
chronic illnesses	coronary insufficiency
deafness in children	disk displacement
ear infection, chronic middle	female disorders
gall bladder diseases	gastric conditions, ulcers
headaches	heart muscle damage
lung improvement	nervous system disorders
nervous system fatigue	nutritional disorders
ovarian disorders	ovarian cyst
prostate	psychosomatic diseases
respiratory disorders	sinus infection
skin diseases	sterility
spinal root nerve irritation	stomach/intestinal problems
tumor, benign	anxiety
depression	hypochondria
hysteria	stress disorders
obsessive-compulsive neurosis	

Healing functions well in cooperation with conventional medical care for epilepsy and malignancies. It relieves pain caused by cancer and decreases the amount of pain medication and tranquilizers taken by patients. After healing treatment, patients became quieter and relaxed, pain was relieved and the rehabilitation process after surgery or infection was accelerated.

AN ANALYSIS OF REPORTS FROM OTHER NATIONS

As a researcher, I look for any patterns and anomalies present in the data. In this case, we see broad differences in the reports of the types of conditions that respond to touch-healing. The four clinical reporters seldom mention the same conditions. As a healer, I have an explanation for this discrepancy. I have observed in my own practice that anything that I know can be healed, usually responds to touch-healing. I am guessing that the confidence of the healer plays a role in healing effectiveness. Having seen the above list, many healers will be able to duplicate these results. Missing from this list are a number of illnesses that have responded to my own healing efforts.

You might have noticed that touch-healing has many names. In these reports, we had Bio-energy Therapy, the current name for Russian touch-healing, in contrast to the name given by an earlier generation, "Bioenergotherapy." The Polish "Pranotherapy" sounds as if it comes from the Hindu name for life energy, "prana."

Here in the United States we also have bio-energy therapy, plus names like Reiki, Therapeutic Touch, Tai Chi, energy balancing, touch-healing, acupuncture, acupressure and Reflexology. There are dozens of other names for healing, all of which seek to restore the human energy field in order to restore physical and emotional health. Most of these avoid using the word *healing* because of its negative connotations. If you learn of a strange-sounding therapy offered by a traditional or holistic health care practitioner, ask that professional if it involves energy field work.

PERSONAL STORIES

At a May, 1992 Canadian healing seminar, Russian healer Evgeniya Stogny and I became friends. A lecturer had asked everyone to rub the back of those sitting next to us to deal with stiffness and alertness. Evgeniya and I ended up as back-rubbing partners. The next day I signed a copy of my book for her. She smiled her thanks and then practiced her considerable healing skills upon me. I felt like the real winner in that transaction.

Diagnosing my energy fields, she stated through a translator that I was in perfect physical health but at a low energy level. Using wire dowsing (divining) rods, she measured the radius of my energy fields as extending about eight feet from my body. Evgeniya assessed my chakras and found my root chakra to be weak. She passed her hands about four inches from my body, restoring this chakra. Again, using the dowsing rods, she showed my energy fields now extended to about twenty-five feet.

During this healing session, a deep sense of inner peace and well-being began filling me, reaching its peak about an hour later and lasting for about two days, a normal side-effect of most healing encounters. This was an extraordinary experience for me. I felt as if I were on the world's best tranquilizer, while feeling boundless energy and an enhanced creativity. Christians call this *"the peace of God which passes all understanding."*

Evgeniya Stogny is a devout Russian Orthodox Christian. She uses thin candle tapers blessed by a priest as a basic diagnostic tool. Lighting a taper, she passes it quickly next to a healee's body. Wherever a thick wisp of black smoke is given off, that area requires healing.

Evgeniya was born in the back country. As a child, she was considered not only a healer but also a *sorceress*. In Russia, a sorceress is highly respected because of the many psychic abilities that accompany her healing skills. Thousands of such healers work as staff members of Russian hospitals. If I should ever get to Moscow, I will look up my friend, Evgeniya.

I have observed that Russia seems to possess far more than its fair share of trained and competent healers and psychics. If these observations are true, I speculate on five reasons for this.

First, Russia did not burn five million witches during the Middle Ages, the way the rest of the Western world did, preserving this genetic stock for future generations.

Second, in the United States, many of our best psychics and healers have been nurtured in isolated rural settings. Russia possesses far more such isolated areas.

Third, Russian Christianity comes from the far more mystical Orthodox Church tradition that would tend to accept and nurture healing and psychic abilities.

Fourth, under secular Communist rule, Russia was far more open to nurturing its psychics and healers because it did not possess the constraints against research and development that faced the Western cultures with their religious and scientific taboos.

Finally, Communist Russia viewed psychic and healing abilities as possible assets to the state for defense and health purposes.

I have worked with a Moscow psychic, healer and computer analyst, Sasha Artiouchkine, whose wife is doing post-graduate work in biochemistry at Case-Western Reserve University, Cleveland, before returning to Russia in 1994. Sasha, like Evgeniya, speaks no English so his wife, Luba, is our interpreter. This poses few problems because our energy fields are in sync. Sasha is an excellent clairvoyant diagnostician. As a team, we do far better healing work than either of us can do individually, as we complement and strengthen each other's insight and abilities.

My association with Sasha motivates me to encourage team-healing, and on an international basis whenever possible. Because spiritual healing remains a most unbelieved, misunderstood and ridiculed subject, international healing teams and seminars hold the promise of increasing acceptance and respect in the field. I have found that the further I travel from home, the more respected and effective I become. In other nations, I am far more effective as the respect and status accorded me increase.

BENEFITS ACCORDING TO A PRACTICING HEALER

Over the years I have made more than ten thousand hospital and home visits to care for sick parishioners. The following data represents my personal observations about what healing accomplishes on a consistent basis during a pastor-healer's workday. Obviously my subjective observations are not acceptable medical evidence. They do, however, give you some perspective on what occurs in touch-healing.

I was initially hesitant to report this data. Citing professional observations of only one expert witness made me feel vulnerable to criticism. But having made a commitment to honesty, I placed the data in the first draft of this book. Two of my clergy colleagues who practice touch-healing, George Fisk and Francis MacNutt, critiqued that first draft. Their comments in the page margins confirmed my own data. They emphatically stated that their observations on healings were almost identical to my reported data. Both punctuated their comments with multiple exclamation marks. I gave a sigh of relief for my increased confidence.

PRACTICING IN A MEDICAL SETTING

First, let me say that I feel comfortable in a medical setting. Medical procedures have saved my life. I have turned to surgeons for surgery. I have used prescription medications. I possess hundreds of hours of clinical education in pastoral care and counseling, having specialized in counseling and small group work. Like most pastors, I averaged a dozen hours a week visiting patients in hospitals. As a pastor, I have felt that I am a part of the medical team, offering emotional, physical, spiritual and interpersonal wholeness to the ill.

Since learning in 1966 that I had the ability to offer healing, I have practiced touch-healing prayer in hospital and home. This was done by simply holding a person's hand and offering a prayer, again as most pastors do. The only difference was in the intention and directness of each prayer.

An increasing number of healers have ready access to hospital patients. Thousands of nurses practice Therapeutic Touch and are members of the Nurse Healers Association. A growing number of physicians are closet healers who hide their healing practice under other names for fear of losing their licenses, patients or reputations. The evidence indicates that thousands of clergy and nuns possess powerful latent or active healing abilities.

Medical settings are the best place to practice healing. I think the general acceptance of healing is dawning and a new day is at hand when physicians and healers will work with the ill together, as they presently do in Russia and Poland. Using healers may reduce health care costs by as much as fifty percent. This enormous savings in medical costs alone may prompt the government and health insurers to reimburse healers. The hospital where my wife works already reimburses spiritual healing in their health plan benefits. I envision working soon in a medical setting as a healer, researcher and teacher.

PRACTICAL APPLICATIONS AND CLINICAL OBSERVATIONS

1. Surgery. When I practice touch-healing prayer just prior to surgery, surgical wounds consistently heal faster with about 80% healing in half the normal time and the remaining 20% resulting in a 700% increase in healing rate. Healing also produces significantly less post-surgical pain, an inner sense of well-being and increased physical and emotional vitality. Post-surgical depression all but disappears.

In addition, prior touch-healing can lessen the severity of the surgical condition. Dozens of times, patients were diagnosed with cancer but during surgery only normal cells were found, with all symptoms disappearing.

Equally true, surgeons would find cancer filling the abdominal cavity and be forced to do nothing and a few months later, the patient would be cancer-free. Some medically untreated ruptured discs became symptom-free within twenty-four hours.

Prayer before cancer surgery yields high results, even when incurable cancer is the prognosis. Prayers offered after the patient hears surgical reports of incurable cancer have been less effective. Prayers during chemotherapy or radiation treatments have resulted in reducing negative side-effects and producing a higher rate of remission.

Touch-healing can also control vital signs like pulse and blood pressure. I can place pulse and blood pressure at any level desired simply by touching and willing it. Internal bleeding due to ulcers, vessel rupture or surgery can be consistently stopped.

One morning in January, 1992, my eighty-four-year-old father, Bernard Weston, was rushed to the emergency room of Timken-Mercy Medical Center in Canton, Ohio. When I arrived at ten o'clock, a drainage tube had already sucked a liter of green goop from my father's swollen left groin area. I practiced touch-healing prayer. That afternoon he was admitted to a surgical ward room and at two o'clock, family members gathered with me for touch-healing prayer. Before surgery, his surgeon cautioned us that with this much gangrene infection, his poor heart and advanced age, prospects for surviving surgery were not good.

Late that afternoon, the surgeon approached us, smiling. He reported finding no gangrene, only bright pink tissue that looked like a twenty-year-old's, and confirmed the successful surgical repair of a simple groin hernia. My father was released from the hospital two days later, his surgical wound all but healed.

2. Physical injuries. Trauma injuries like bruises, torn muscles, lacerations and broken bones respond remarkably to touch-healing prayer, which enhances the healing rate by two to thirty times. The earlier the touch-healing treatment is offered, the better will be the results. It seems that if we can prevent the trauma injury from being impressed upon the energy fields, then trauma healing can occur within minutes or hours, as the energy fields are enhanced and then proceed to restore physical cells. The implications of touch-healing are obvious for emergency, trauma and burn units, and for sports medicine.

3. Massive bruises. One day during my hospital rounds, I found a young man with an arm in a cast and in traction, and both legs in traction. He had been brought in that morning after an auto accident. Both legs were a blue-black from the top of the thighs to his knees. We had never met before. I told him what touch-healing prayer might do for him. He smiled and cooperated. Two days later I observed his legs were their normal color, no limbs were in traction and he was being discharged.

4. Trauma brain injuries respond well to touch-healing. This is true even with brain-dead patients. Two-thirds of the brain-dead injuries I have treated, survived, with damaged brain tissue regenerated and memory functions restored. Normal physical therapy follow-up was usually necessary. These healings were not accomplished through one simple touch. In all survival cases, I practiced touch-healing prayer within hours of the injury. I also practiced thirty minutes at a time, two or three times daily for one to two weeks. If possible, I involved loved ones in healing prayer, including first-hand touch with the patient.

5. Hearing losses can often be restored at all ages with one to three consecutive daily touch-healing treatments. The restoring may take seven or more days to occur.

6. Dental conditions respond consistently. Healing relieves toothache pain and also diminishes pain, bleeding and swelling in tooth extractions.

All the above conditions respond consistently to touch-healing. I attribute this to two factors. These are uncomplicated conditions in which the healing energy merely initiates and speeds up the normal healing process. Emotional and mental factors that might maintain a condition are also minimal. The earlier that touch-healing can be applied to a condition, the more likelihood of success.

7. Osteoarthritis. With no previous surgery, most osteoarthritis responds to one or two healing sessions, with the healee being relieved of all medical symptoms within hours or overnight. For this to occur, we are going beyond simple acceleration of the healing rate. Bone tissue is being regenerated in what common sense logic can best explain as genetic engineering. Success is achieved after initially unsuccessful results by placing the healee in a light hypnotic state before transmitting healing energy.

8. Heart muscle damage due to a heart attack is best treated in the earliest stages, but I have been able to regenerate heart muscle successfully within two months of the initial damage. Low and irregular pulse rates can be restored in one twenty-minute healing session, using two healers. I have not worked with other heart conditions.

9. Chronic lung impairment treatment has produced no consistent results. I attribute this to poor motivation on the part of the patient who has no sense of impending crisis. I also find lung-impaired people are more skeptical of the healing process than others. When I request cooperation for three or four weekly sessions over a period of weeks, they are less likely to agree than other clients.

10. Genital Herpes II can consistently be cured with a few minutes of treatment.

11. Scoliosis responds well to four consecutive daily half-hour sessions. Between sessions the healee usually experiences extreme spinal pain or pleasant spinal spasms during the night. One hurting healee consoled herself with the explanation that if the bone structure were changing shape, it would be likely to be painful.

12. Cancer, multiple sclerosis and Lou Gehrig's Disease respond unevenly. Few cancer patients are healed in one session, especially in the initial hospital setting. When wellness counseling succeeds in healing painful emotional hurts, then touch-healing produces a rapid shrinking and disappearance of cancerous tumors. If emotional hurts are not healed, then cancer is extremely resistant to touch-healing. For these reasons, cancer patients respond best to wellness counseling, a support group and touch-healing by an individual or group. If surgery is a good cancer option, I favor surgery combined with touch-healing.

I am not happy with my multiple sclerosis healing record. My observation is that multiple sclerosis is either healed quickly in three to six sessions or it will not be healed with an additional thirty individual sessions. I suspect that the placebo effect is the major factor at work in those I have healed. Because of my poor success record with this condition as an individual healer, I would recommend bathing anyone with multiple sclerosis or Lou Gehrig's Disease in large quantities of healing energy from long-term group prayer or healing services.

13. Breast lumps (benign) respond to touch-healing as well as arthritis does. My first experience with breast lumps occurred fifteen years ago when a mammogram disclosed that my wife had a lump in her left breast. Prior to the surgical biopsy, I practiced touch-healing prayer daily for a week. No lump was found during the biopsy and the incision was twice normal size because the doctor looked for it carefully. Since then, one ten-minute touch-healing session removes the symptoms within forty-eight hours for about ninety percent of clients. Though my wife responded well, those most resistant to healing are family members.

Cancerous breast lumps do not respond quickly to touch-healing. They require a daily series of twenty-minute sessions.

14. Bacterial and viral infections are most healable during their earliest stages. It seems as though when the energy field patterns have been changed to reflect the infection, there is more resistance. So healing must begin in the earliest stages before the energy fields are also infected and help to maintain the disease.

15. Emotional conditions respond well. Counseling and healing prayer can cut the grief process by two to twelve times the normal rate. In counseling persons with anger, anxiety and resentment, therapeutic insight is quickly internalized by healing prayer at the close of sessions. The same is true in marital and family counseling. It is as if we are releasing the pain from the energy fields and building therapeutically healthy energy fields that bathe the counseling client in wholeness. Radiant Heart Therapy, which is described in chapter twenty-two, produces more dramatic healing results than prayer following therapy.

Chronic depressives and those with borderline personality issues can regain a normal lifestyle with counseling and healing prayer, though this is not a cure. Continued healing energy must be regularly administered, just like a medication.

16. Counter the effects of man-made electromagnetic frequencies. In chapter four, we explored the effects of man-made electromagnetic on human beings. Robert O. Becker, MD,[4] suggests a direct correlation between the mounting levels of electromagnetic frequencies in which humans have been bathed during the past generation and the similar increase in the number of cancer cases and the emergence of new diseases. He states that these frequencies are interfering with the human resonance of the Earth

Becker defines the effects of such exposure, saying that all abnormal, man-made electromagnetic fields, *regardless of their frequencies,* produce the same biological effects. These are:

A. Effects in growing cells, such as increases in the rate of cancer-cell division
B. Increases in the incidence of certain cancers
C. Developmental abnormalities in embryos
D. Alterations in neurochemicals, resulting in behavioral abnormalities such as suicide
E. Alterations in biological cycles
F. Stress responses in exposed animals that, if prolonged, lead to declines in the immune-system efficiency
G. Alterations in learning abilities

Becker links exposure to man-made electromagnetic fields to the diseases of the Electromagnetic-Hypersensitive Syndrome, Chronic-Fatigue Syndrome, AIDS, Autism, Fragile X Syndrome, Sudden Infant Death Syndrome, Alzheimer's Disease, Parkinson's Disease, Cancer, and Mental Diseases.

Because healers appear to draw their energy from the Earth, the above conditions should consistently respond well to healing energy. Recently, I worked with Aida, who has struggled for ten years with the Electromagnetic-Hypersensitive Syndrome. By necessity, her home in a rural area possesses few electromagnetic appliances. She phoned me two days after our one-hour touch-healing prayer session to report she felt completely normal for the first time in ten years. The next day's session continued her improvement. With healer-charged towels, she has maintained her high energy levels for the past several weeks. This same response should hold true of others damaged by electromagnetic pollution.

17. Healer-Charged Materials. I give healer-treated cotton dish towels to people with physical injuries and specific chronic conditions. Those who drape a healer-charged cotton towel over arthritic joints will normally experience the alleviation of all arthritic symptoms within a few weeks.

Knowing the scientific evidence on healer-charged water, my first attempt was with Gertrude, an eighty-six-year-old woman who had spurs (calcium deposits) on her spine, for which medical science had no treatment. Her medical condition caused such pain when she walked that she became confined to a wheelchair. Because of my limited time to practice touch-healing prayer with her on a daily basis, Gertrude agreed to drink two ounces of healer treated-water four times daily. Her son-in-law, John, brought me a glass pitcher of water that I held in my hands for twenty minutes to charge. Four days later, Gertrude phoned and asked me to come over. She greeted me at the door in her finest dress. She had awakened that morning pain-free, gotten up, taken a shower, dressed and fixed the family breakfast. Gertrude lived a full life into her nineties.

In another case, for three years a thirteen-year-old named Wanda had daily suffered the symptoms of Crohn's Disease. These symptoms included nausea, dizziness, vomiting, and abdominal pain. After one healing session, Wanda was symptom-free for a week before the symptoms returned. Additional healing sessions each brought relief for about seven days. I charged water jugs with healing energy that she ingested daily at home. This routine can keep her symptom-free. Wanda has a chronic illness the symptoms of which are alleviated by healer-charged water, just as insulin relieves the symptoms of diabetes.

The use of the healing energy to enhance the growth and health of plants and animals has been overlooked. Those who might choose to practice in this area might be better termed *"life enhancers"* rather than *"healers."* Experimental data indicates that plant growth and health can be enhanced by blessing with prayer and touch. Seeds can be bathed with healing energy before planting by soaking them in healer-treated water.

Further clinical research is crucial for understanding the clinical usefulness of stored healing energy. How helpful would it be to therapeutically bathe a hospital patient in a healing energy provided through healer-charged wiring, water, cotton towels or quartz crystals, or a frequency generator?

THE POTENTIALS OF TOUCH-HEALING

We have looked at a few of the practical applications of touch-healing. The data suggests that the practice of touch-healing, in cooperation with medical and other professions, can do far more than anyone has heretofore dreamed. Here is a list of the potential uses of healing knowledge.

The Potentials of Spiritual Healing
A. Can reduce or completely curb most physical and emotional pain.
B. Increases the body's growth and healing rates.
C. Initiates the healing process in chronic illnesses.
D. Can prevent anticipated diseases from occurring.
E. Heals major chronic and life-threatening illnesses like cancer, heart disease, arthritis, hearing loss and developmental damage due to cocaine.
F. Holds the secret to how the body's immune system works, providing medical understanding of such diseases as multiple sclerosis, Lou Gehrig's disease, herpes simplex, AIDS and cancer.
G. Helps restore infants with birth defects to normal.
H. Restores damaged human body tissue and organs.
I. Heals destructive mental states, including the emotions of battered children, irresponsibility in delinquent youth, the criminal behavior syndrome, psychosis, anxiety syndrome, depression, borderline personality, stress syndromes and grief.
J. In counseling, causes therapeutic insight to be internalized, destructive emotions to be healed and dysfunctional family members to reunite constructively
K. Heals compulsive/addictive behaviors involving alcohol, cocaine, heroin, nicotine, tranquilizers, obesity, stress, gambling and consumerism.
L. Enables self-help groups to be much more effective in bringing wholeness to their participants.
M. Enhances learning and cooperation in school classrooms.
N. Offers spirituality and wholeness to couples, families, schools, the community and worksites.
O. Can form therapeutic group energy fields which transform everyone encompassed in them, aiding families, communities, and nations.
P. Can restore the ecology of Earth through planetary energy fields.

Chapter Seven

The Existence of Group Energy Fields

"Things do not turn up in the world unless someone turns them up."
...James A. Garfield

"It is only in community that a proper framework for growth in faith can take place." ...Gustavo Gutierrez*

"When the day of Pentecost had come, they were all together in one place. And suddenly a sound came from heaven like the rush of a mighty wind, and it filled all the house where they were sitting. And there appeared to them tongues as of fire, distributed and resting upon them. And they were all filled with the Holy Spirit...." ...Acts 2:1-4a

The mystery first presented itself some twenty years ago in Pittsburgh as I was reading a group of books about the healing evangelist Kathryn Kuhlmann. Two books by different authors told the same documented story. I was intrigued by it at the time and long puzzled over it.

When Kathryn Kuhlmann was leading her healing services, the stories said, people walking on the sidewalk outside the building or driving past in a car were healed. Although they had not been aware that a healing service was going on inside the building they were passing, they were healed, nevertheless. Was there a rational explanation?

Kathryn Kuhlmann did not touch persons to heal them. The healings took place in persons seated throughout the congregation. Father Ralph DiOrio also does not touch persons for healing in his healing services. How, then, do such healings occur?

As my understanding grew, I came to know that there is only one logical explanation. The only way that people can be healed when they are seated anywhere throughout a hall during a large healing service is if somehow the healing energy is able to touch them. Having sat through many a healing service, I can sense the presence of an energy throughout the meeting-place. Energy cannot exist freely outside of a field of energy. Therefore, somehow, during a healing service a large group energy field is formed. This energy field is filled with information that acts intelligently to restore humans to their optimum state for life, just as does the energy transmitted by an individual during touch-healing.

As we shall see, the healer acts as a catalyst in the forming of a *healing group energy field* that is filled with the intentions of all those present. When the healing group energy field (GEF) of the healing service becomes extremely powerful, it grows beyond the dimensions of the building, enveloping pedestrians on the sidewalk and people in passing cars. Because the

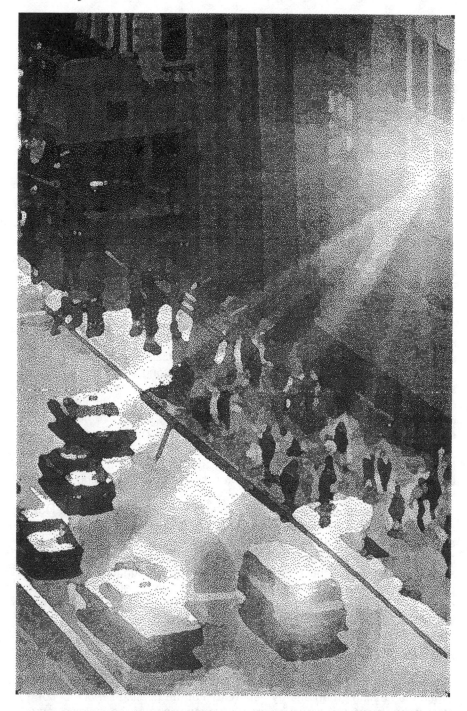

Figure 5. *During Kathryn Kuhlmann's healing services in Pittsburgh, the healing group energy field became so powerful that the healing energy expanded beyond the building walls, touching pedestrians and people in cars and producing healing effects in these unsuspecting passerby's.*

information-laden group energy field (GEF) acts intelligently, it acted to transform the energies of those within the vicinity and these people were healed. Thus, the mystery is solved.

SACRED SPACE AS A SACRED ENERGY FIELD

God is spirit. God can be described scientifically as an energy field. When people have strong experiences of God, God's presence or energy can continue to linger, permeating the objects in the area, just as healing energy can permeate water, cotton and wool.

Those in the Judeo-Christian-Islamic tradition are aware of the concept of *"holy ground"* as applied to locations in the Old Testament where God had appeared to people. Aside from the historical significance of the God-encounter, God's presence lingered after the event as an information-laden energy. People later sensed this divine presence in the lingering energy and the area literally became holy ground.

This brings us to the contemporary concept of *sacred space.* Religious congregations dedicate their worship areas to God. The worship area becomes a sacred space where reverence is shown through personal attitudes and sacred usage. But it seems to be more than the concept of sacred space that creates the reverence. Most persons *"sense"* the presence of God in these places. And, as God's biblical people, they may state their awareness by saying, *"Surely, God is in this holy place."* Again, an explanation for this is that God's presence lingers on as an energy field that permeates the area.

For similar reasons, spiritual wisdom advises people always to carry out their spiritual disciplines of worship, meditation and prayer in one place in their homes. Experienced healers do all their healing in one particular healing room, even placing healees in the same chair. People can *"sense"* the holiness in such rooms. God's presence has formed a sacred, information-laden energy field in those places, making further contacts with God easier.

When I was to be interviewed by a potential new congregation, I would first go up to the altar area of the chancel. I would stand quietly, seeking to discern the presence of God. I wanted to be sure that I could sense God in this holy place before I accepted any invitation to be the pastor.

THE POWER AND CONTENT OF GROUP ENERGY FIELDS

For years, I have heard that the healing power of prayer was the square of those gathered in prayer. Later, the scientific theory of this will be provided. If ten thousand people gathered for a Kathryn Kuhlmann healing service, the power generated and the size of the resulting healing group energy field would be enormous. It would represent 100 million individual praying units of intelligently acting healing power. That is why a passerby, with no expectations, could be healed outside a Kuhlmann healing service.

Any time two or more people gather together, they form a group energy field whose information is filled with their identity, intentions, actions or words. I discovered this truth through the following mystery.

A HEALING CIRCLE PROVIDES ANOTHER MYSTERY

We are assuming that a healing service's group energy field (GEF) carries within it God's power to heal. This energy is intelligent. It bears information that heals. Are other GEFs similar in their ability to carry information within them? The following story provides our first clue.

My first reaction in the group was one of surprise. I had been expecting God but I was enveloped by another enormous power. There was none of the familiar holy presence of gathered Christians; there was no sensing of a holy presence or of love, joy or peace. My surprise quickly turned to curiosity. What was going on?

This occurred during the late 1970's. I had been invited by a group of strangers to take part in a healing circle. The leader, Jim, led twenty of us in an unfamiliar chant to *"raise the healing vibrations."* I had expected to experience the familiar sense of God as I did in Christian church gatherings. But I did not. Instead, an enormous neutral power, an informationally neutral GEF, filled the little room and enveloped us. It was a pliable power. It appeared as if those present could use it in any way they chose. The emotional levels stayed neutral. We silently directed this power to persons needing healing.

That night, I spent several sleepless hours, seeking to make sense of the anomalous experience. I recalled the Old Testament's First Commandment, *"You shall have no other gods before me"* (Deuteronomy 5:7). Was that enormous neutral power in the healing circle God? Or had I come into contact with another god, other than my Heavenly Father? No, that was no god. What was it? I knew I must explore this further.

The next week, I was again part of the healing circle. Before going, I surrounded myself in the Creator's presence. In doing so, I wanted to protect my human energy field (HEF) from outside influences. During the healing circle I now sensed nothing unusual. There was only the Creator within me. I had unknowingly surrounded myself with the biblical *"breastplate of righteousness"* (Ephesians 6:14). I had gathered with a group of persons who said they were creating divine power to heal, but the group energy field (GEF) they had created did not include qualities of my God. I had another mystery to store until more information brought understanding.

GOD'S POWER DURING HEALING SERVICES

In the years since, I have participated in numerous gatherings whose purpose was healing. Each time a *"power"* is present within the group energy field. I had once called that *power* God, the Heavenly Father. Now I did not know what to call it.

I have the ability to sense the different qualities present in GEFs. For religious gatherings, my baseline is my own experience of God in the Christian context. During worship, I had always sensed the fruits of the Spirit. (*"The fruits of the Spirit are love, joy, peace, patience, kindness, goodness, faithfulness, gentleness and self-control."*...Galatians 5:22.) I had thought that I would always feel these qualities of God in the same way. By now, the phenomenon was occurring in more than just that healing circle. When I visited various healing services, God felt different in each. Certain traits were missing. Often, one trait predominated, like peace or love or holiness. In many services, I sensed only an enormous power or energy, as in that first healing circle. This was often tempered by a pervading sense of peace. What was the significance of this?

Another clue can be found in giant healing services. A long period of preparation, usually hours, passes before the service begins, as the congregation arrives early to find the choice seats. During this period, I discern a changing of feeling levels. First, there is a boredom, then an annoyance at the delay and a letdown just preceding the service. Finally, an air of expectation quickly builds. The large congregation is becoming unified as a group. This is followed inevitably by the build-up of living energy, an enormous power. It feels thick, like a warm fog. Sometimes it comes through as oppressive and clinging, like honey. If you have been to such services, you are already identifying with this description. I had always thought this to be the presence and power of God. But is it?

AN ANOMALY NOTICED AMONG HINDU YOGIS

In 1989, hundreds of yogis from twenty nations gathered for an international yoga conference in Pondicherry, India. These were some of the most developed yoga adepts on earth. Yoga is a Hindu meditation style designed for developing the self mentally, physically and spiritually. Those who have mastered yoga are called yogis.

During the four-day conference, I experienced almost a dozen yogi devotional moments in which the yogis sang their sacred songs and mantras. I did not understand their language but I could sense the spiritual qualities of the gathering. The sacred group energy field they created through their religious ritual was completely devoid of all feelings. This was another anomaly. I sensed no love, joy, peace or holiness. What I did sense was pure intellect. It was disconcerting at first. But then I remembered the goal of Hinduism. It is to become totally devoid of feeling. It is to become pure intellect so one can be united with the Pure Intellect that is God. I sensed the same qualities at a Hindu worship service at an ashram.

GOD POSSESSES DIFFERING RELIGIOUS QUALITIES

How can the one God possess differing religious qualities? Could it be that I had been sloppy in my thinking? Perhaps I had been mistaken in believing that I sensed the essence of God in GEFs. But what other explanation is there?

The revealed image of God is different in each religion. The qualities people sense in God's Spirit vary with the religion. Hindus experience God as pure intellect and devoid of emotion. Christians and Jews experience God as having emotional qualities like love, joy and peace. So, could there be a link between what people believe about God and the GEFs they form?

John Rossner, a religious history professor at Concordia University, Montreal and a Canadian Anglican priest, states that every religious tradition is expressed in four identical developments. **First** is a God who reveals his/her own nature. This is the revelation of the nature of the divine to human beings. The **second** development is a God who transforms believers into his/her own revealed divine nature. **Third** is a God who empowers believers with the ability to perform divine miracles. **Fourth,** God empowers his/her believers to be channels for divine healing. All religions share these developmental stages in common.

There is one anomaly in these four developmental stages. It is something that does not fit. It makes one of the stages different from the others. What is it? The last three developments are true of all religions. God transforms the believer into his/her image, empowers him/her to do miracles and enables him/her to offer healing. The anomaly is the content of the divine revelation.

There is one God of us all. But the revelation of the image of God is different in each religion. The revelation tells the believer the nature of God. The believer seeks to become transformed into the image of the qualities revealed to be in God. For the Hindu, this means to become pure spiritual intellect during spiritual moments. For the Muslim, this means faith and submission to Allah's laws. For the Christian believer, it means to be transformed into the revelational image of God as seen in Jesus, the Savior.

THE REVELATIONAL IMAGE OF GOD

At this point, we must make a distinction between two concepts, the true image of God and the revelational image of God. Most religions claim that their particular revelation of God is the only true image of God. For instance, some Christians claim that the only way to salvation and eternal life is to be transformed into the image of God as revealed in Jesus the Savior. They believe Jesus has given humanity the only true image of God. Some Christians believe that their particular branch of the Church holds all the truth, and, that all other branches of the Church possess false beliefs.

It is scientifically questionable whether any of Earth's existing religions reflect, objectively speaking, the true image of God. All revelational images of God tend to pertain to the human culture from which the revelational image emerged. Believers have no choice but to accept the revealed image of God of their religion. As believers are learning these from scriptures and traditions and are immersed in the group energy field during worship and prayer, the information-laden group energy field is acting intelligently to transform them into the revealed image of God. The beliefs of believers are present in the information-laden sacred group energy field. This information, the revealed Word, acts intelligently in transforming and molding their minds.

This transformation into the revealed image of God is the second universal stage of development in all religions. I can sense the qualities of the fruits of the Spirit being emitted by mature Christians. I can also sense a common peace of God being emitted by believers of other religious traditions.

When believers gather together, they begin emitting their individual revealed image of God and form a sacred group energy field filled with those revealed images of God-qualities. When they are subsequently bathed in the information of the formed sacred group energy field, it fills them with these divine qualities that act to transform them further. The power of God fills them. In this context, I have heard hundreds of parishioners comment, upon leaving the worship service, *"God charged me up for another week."*

The encouragement to participate in gatherings of one's particular faith tradition thus has a purpose beyond enabling the worshipper to act as a loyal believer. In building community, one is also building religious unity. The highest quality sacred group energy fields would be formed by believers who have religious education, commitment, spiritual experiences, and a life reflecting these. Religious rituals, songs and prayers strengthen the content and power of the sacred group energy field.

MAKING SENSE OF THE HEALING CIRCLE ANOMALIES

During the healing circle noted above, where we chanted to create energy for our group energy field, we produced the pure energy we had intended. It did not contain Christian qualities, because we were performing an intellectual exercise. These were not practicing, believing Christians; therefore, their individual energy fields contained no revealed image of Christianity. So their GEF was only capable of creating pure mental energy. I felt uncomfortable in the group because my energy field contained a different and discordant religious content.

AN EXPLANATION OF THE HINDU WORSHIP ANOMALY

This also explains how I discerned the information of the Hindu yogis in their devotional rituals. The revelational image of God into which they had been transformed by the practice of yoga was present in their sacred group energy field. I sensed the pure divine intellect of their revealed image of God. The sacred group energy field that they created contained qualities representing their image of God that they embodied in each of their individual human energy fields while in contact with God.

This does not mean Hindus are not loving. They are loving in their personal lives. But while in religious ritual, they embody the revealed image of God of the divine intellect. Hindus practice healing, but they do so in the context of their revealed image of God. Their healing is, most likely, mental healing, rather than the spiritual healing in the Western context. Healing effectiveness might increase if compassionate love were introduced into their healing practices.

LARGE HEALING SERVICE ANOMALIES

The revelational image of God also explains the emotional anomalies that I have sensed in large healing services. People in large faith-healing services seldom worship. They are not a religious community. They are strangers to one another. Even if they do worship, their primary role is as spectators waiting for God to act. Their expectations, their needs and hopes, their spiritual being, plus other factors, are emitted from their personal human energy fields to become a part of the content of the giant healing group energy field. The main sensed quality of that group energy field is God's power. God is present in all his great power. Just as we are partners with God in healing prayer, we also are partners with God in creating the group healing energy field.

THE HEALER AS A GROUP CATALYST

Earlier I described what I experienced in large healing services. The qualities present in the healing group energy field were different from those found in any other Christian rituals. Certain traits were missing. They were often dominated by one trait like peace or love or peace and holiness. In many services, I sensed only an enormous power or energy. This was often tempered by a pervading peace. Much of this I attribute to the diversity and singular intent of the group. If they are not a worshipping congregation, but present to observe or to obtain a healing, the group energy field reflects this.

The healer presiding over a large healing service is doing something very special. The healer not only heals. Before healing can be offered, the healer must first be able to form a group energy field. The healer's presence and charisma act as a catalyst, and the expectations of the gathered crowd contribute to this process as a healing group energy field is formed. And just as in the individual practice of healing, the healer must attune the energy of the whole healing group energy field to the healing frequency. This the healer accomplishes automatically.

As a leader of both worship services and healing services, I intentionally fill myself with God's presence and then mentally seek to spread this holiness throughout the gathering. Only measuring instruments could tell me if I am actually doing this or whether some unknown factor is involved. Within minutes, I can sense the sacred or healing group energy field being formed. My belief is that the intentions of all the individuals in the group are the major contributing factor. My role and ability involve creating a cohesive group energy field.

Healers appear to be hampered in creating a truly plus or minus 7.83 frequency healing group energy field. The energy in most services feels coarse rather than fine-tuned. Ten thousand people squared produces one hundred million person-units of prayer power, yet less than one percent receive the healing they seek. Alone, with my relatively extremely weak healing energy, I am more than eighty percent effective in healing people. The difference is that my individual energy is easier to attune than a group field.

During a recent large healing service conducted by another healer, I decided to fine-tune the group energy field frequency around me to a purer healing one. I was just sensing this occurring when the healer shouted, "Stop." He was pointing at me. Describing my appearance, he then said, "Leave my healing service alone. You have your way of doing things as a healer and I have mine. Mine works for me. Stop interfering!" I stopped. After the service, I apologized to the healer. His face was radiant with love as we embraced.

In large healing services, some healers appear to be in an altered state of consciousness similar to the hypnotic state but more accurately described as a trance state. In this trance state, the healer is believed to be inspired either directly by God's Spirit or by a guiding spirit from the Company of Heaven. Kathryn Kuhlmann had no memory of the service afterwards, a quality engendered by some trance states.

In this state, the healer has the spiritual gift of knowledge in which s/he knows either who is being healed or what type of illnesses can be healed at a given time in the service. In secular terms, the healer develops a telepathic linkage with the persons who will be healed and intuitively knows that he will be attuning to the specific energy frequency to heal a particular disease, like deafness. This ability to attune to persons can be explained by the unique information present in each individual energy field.

Everyone at a healing service has access to that immense healing group energy field. But it is the presiding healer who is most effective in bringing about individual healings. The issue of attuning answers the question of why less than one percent of those seeking healing at a giant healing service are healed. Only when the healer attunes the whole healing group energy to the frequency of 7.83 hertz, or when he attunes his own energy to the unique frequency of a particular individual or a specific disease, can healing take place.

GOD AS EXPRESSED IN GROUP ENERGY FIELDS

God uses people as channels for healing. As do individual acts of touch-healing, healing group energy fields enable us to be channels for God's wholeness. This goes far beyond what we have dared to speculate. When people gather together for a healing service, the qualities of the revealed image of God in the individual human energy fields of those gathered help to create the healing group energy field, along with the healer-leader as the catalyst. This group-created healing group energy field forms the context from which the healing flows for God's miracles of healing. Then frequency-attuning takes place to make the best use of the healing energy.

Group energy fields are constantly being formed naturally, outside of a sacred context. Whenever two or more persons are gathered for a common intention or action, a group energy field is formed. When caring occurs, a group energy field is formed which has characteristics similar to a healing group energy field. You can sense the love and peace present in a caring encounter. This is especially true of support groups where people share their hurts and compassion is expressed. I design such encounters into my own healing services.

WILLIAM TILLER'S THEORY OF GROUP COHERENCE

Is there any scientific basis for my group energy field analysis? The answer, I am pleased to say, is yes. Physicist William A. Tiller of Stanford University provides a scientific theory on the power of the energy emitted by a coherent group energy field. Coherent means to stick together or to be logically connected and intelligible. A coherent human group has a common, clearly defined intent, emotion or action. Professor Tiller states that the energetic power of a coherent group is the square of the number of people involved.

The energy of one person is one. The energy of two people gathered together is four. The energy of ten people in a coherent group energy field is ten times ten or one hundred. The energy of five thousand people in a coherent group energy field is five thousand times five thousand or twenty-five million individual human energy units. A million gathered people is 1,000,000,000,000 energy units. A billion people can produce 1,000,000, 000,000,000,000 energy units through the attuned intent of their prayers.

This accounts for the energy involved in groups. The square of the number gathered will be used throughout PrayWell as the basis for quantifying the power in group healing efforts. For those who would like to examine the scientific data, the following section presents the details of Dr. Tiller's scientific theory.

TILLER'S THEORY PRESENTED MATHEMATICALLY

During the 1960s, before I had any curiosity about the nature of group energy fields, physicist William Tiller formulated his theory of group coherence. In my private communications with Dr. Tiller, he explained the basic physics of his theory, beginning with: *The energy of a wave is proportional to the square of its amplitude.*

1. On average, a single individual's energy effectiveness, **E**, for any specific application like healing, creating, working, etc., can be theoretically modeled as being directly proportional to the square of some quantity that we can call the individual's output wave amplitude, **A**, that is,

$$E < cA^2 \text{ where } c \text{ is some constant.}$$

2. On average, a group of **N** people's energy effectiveness for collective application to the same area of focus will be:

$$E < N(cA^2)$$

2a. **Destructive Interference.** If people are acting as interacting but largely independent resonators, this is because of the usual *destructive interference* that occurs between uncoordinated individual efforts, that is, their efforts are not in phase with each other.

2b. **Constructive Interference.** However, if **N** people are coherently attuned to each other, their efforts will be both cooperative and completely in phase with each other's so that *constructive interference* occurs and we have:

$$E = c(NA)^2 = N[N(cA^2)]$$

Thus, we see that coherence versus incoherence in group efforts substantially increases the energy effectiveness of the action (by a factor often significantly higher than **N**).

THE INFORMATION-LADEN GEFs OF SECULAR GATHERINGS

At every large gathering of people, sacred or secular, there is a distinctive group flavor. A common feeling pervades everyone present. All groups of people who are focused on one purpose or action create information-bearing group energy fields. Even before a music concert begins, one can feel elated expectation pervading the crowd. Then the music begins molding the whole audience into oneness -- a sharing of common thoughts and emotions, a coherent group. We can understand that and say it is caused only by the sounds of the music. But the evidence is that the performers have projected their energy into the audience. A good performance means the performers have projected their charisma -- the information from their inner selves -- into the audience's group energy field.

When fans gather for a football game, the emotional energy feels great. When the team is losing, one can feel the letdown pervade the crowd. When the team is winning, one senses an emotional high. Even persons who know little about football get caught up in the emotions of the coherent energetic group energy field. The noisy cheers are considered a home team advantage.

Another factor to consider is the effect of the home team's coherent group energy field on both teams. Also, do the emotional qualities of the group energy field at times cause violent actions and even sporting event riots? Could the aggression and anger building up in a group energy field place some persons into a mindless and violent trance state? The people gathered for any one purpose or intention are molded into a oneness of expectancy and emotion. Emotions are contagious.

Let us repeat what has been said. Every person possesses human energy fields. The human energy fields are a bearer of information -- mental, emotional, religious, moral -- according to the activity with which the person is involved. Energy radiates from the individual human energy fields and mingles with other gathered human energy fields. When the individual human energy fields merge, they become one enormous, information-bearing, group energy field entity whose power is the square of the coherent number of persons gathered.

The group energy field entity is a *"group mind"* that can overwhelm individual will when the group energy field intelligently acts on the information within it. Parapsychology has compiled impressive experimental evidence that emotions are transmittable, but the mechanism by which this phenomenon occurs has not previously been named. That mechanism is now obvious. It is the information-bearing energy fields of living organisms that transmit information to other organisms.

This provides insight into troubling manifestations of group behavior. We have always been puzzled by mob violence. Why does a group of sane, responsible persons become a mindless group entity filled with such rage that they will injure and murder other human beings? A violent mob is a merging of individual human energy fields into a coherent group energy field, expressing the fears, angers and prejudices of each individual. The group energy field takes on a life of its own, becoming an independent emotional entity. It becomes a mass mind that overpowers individual thought, caution and responsibility. No other explanation fits!

The practical implications for crowd control expand with this understanding. When law enforcement authorities seek to control a violent mob, the authorities can become just as mindlessly violent as the mob as they, too, become enveloped in the angry, information-bearing group energy field. The feelings of a group are contagious, enveloping anyone who enters the group energy field. This implies that enforcement authorities need a means of protecting themselves from the angry *vibes* of a group energy field so they can responsibly perform their purpose of crowd dispersion. Chapter fourteen offers several means for maintaining the integrity of one's own human energy field separate from a group. Also, certain individuals may be more resistant than others to the effects of a group energy field, and we will consider this, as well.

There are several possibilities for cooling a violent crowd. First, it is necessary to employ procedures to move a crowd out of the feeling-state of consciousness into the thinking-state of consciousness. That might mean getting the mob refocused on thinking and logic through obedience to authority, awareness of the wrongfulness of their actions or logical dialogue. Other possibilities involve deploying appropriate music, humor, caring and love, or prayer.

It would be constitutionally problematic, but bathing a violent mob with a calming wavelength from a frequency generator of extremely low frequency waves would work. The most likely frequencies are at the 7.83 hertz healing frequency and at the calming frequency of ten hertz that the United States Navy physicists discovered and the Soviet Union has used to calm workers.

The concept of group energy fields created by gathered individuals raises other concerns. Why do people tend to become like the company they keep? We think we have strong minds of our own. But if individual or group energy fields are information-bearing and can transfer this information to others, then even what we think and feel is being quietly changed. Be with substance abusers or criminals and their information-bearing energy fields will slowly subvert your best intentions. You will be changed against your will or knowledge. This explains the wisdom that *"you become like the company you keep."* It also explains the changes that occurred in kidnap victim Patty Hearst, who was transformed into a supporter of the beliefs and actions of her politically revolutionary kidnappers.

The implication for families is similar. The individual human energy fields of household members interact with each other. Emotional states, values and attitudes are spread to everyone. Stress and anger, or love and peace, are spread to everyone. In searching for the emotional causes of disease, medical researchers must not only look at the emotions of the ill, but also onto the emotions projected to the ill by family and others. Living in a hostile environment will destroy healthy energy fields and replace them by energy information and frequencies that cause illness and death.

There are solutions for those living within destructive group energy fields I now know that families and other groups can change the negativity in their midst through group prayer. In doing so, they are creating sacred space. A sacred group energy field bathes them in the power, love, joy and peace of God. In other words, they are being bathed in God's presence. This transforms everyone; each is filled with these qualities. Health and wholeness follow. You can learn to do this in Part Four.

There are many other examples. Many urban experts are puzzled about why residents of an entire neighborhood carry similar thoughts, attitudes, values and actions. Aside from the known factors, could neighborhood group energy fields transform residents by working on individual human energy fields, causing either similar constructive or destructive factors? And if so, can we use Therapeutic Prayer to form a neighborhood Therapeutic group energy field to bathe and transform all residents into caring and responsible persons? Part Four provides understanding and tools for doing this.

It is said that prisons harden guards as well as criminals. Placing a thousand criminals together would create a group energy field whose qualities would reflect the values, attitudes and emotions of each criminal. To alleviate this means developing a way to alter the harmful group energy field into a more productive group energy field. This can be done by making each individual separate from the group energy field through an electronic frequency shielding.

An even better way would be to teach the prisoners Therapeutic Prayers to create a therapeutic group energy field that will bathe them in qualities they voluntarily accept. Prisoners then become able to change and grow. They become no longer violent or criminal, emerging from prison as normal. Research suggests that many criminals are enslaved by rigid brainwave patterns. Prayer can heal these. This, too, is explored in Part Four.

DESIGNING GROUP ENERGY FIELDS

I have attempted to create a group energy field composed of love and peace by simply asking those present to concentrate on love and peace. This has not worked. But one can create the qualities desired in a group energy field through the activities with which the group is involved or through the intentions expressed in prayer.

When people care for and pray for each other, the group energy field becomes filled with God, love and peace. This can be done within a family, among friends, in any community group, or for a whole neighborhood, community or nation. Being bathed in such a group energy field transforms people just as touch-healing prayer or a worship or healing service will do.

Designing therapeutic GEFs for senior citizens, the grieving, the depressed, the mentally ill, criminals or crime-ridden neighborhoods could change the quality of life for a whole nation or the world. I am so confident about the enormous benefits that would result, that guidance for doing this is provided in Part Four.

Finally, the use of GEFs to restore our environment is also feasible. Imagine a GEF with one million, one billion or one trillion energy units of prayer power. Remember that healing energy acts intelligently to transform all life to its optimum condition. Polluted water and air possess energy fields upon which such a force could work. Could toxic waste sites be cleansed of their poisons? This is theoretically possible.

GROUP ENERGY FIELDS IN HISTORY

Group energy fields play an important role in the history of most religions. The Jews experienced a number of group events during the Exodus from Egypt. Christians have a group gathered in Jerusalem waiting for coming of the Holy Spirit, out of which comes Pentecost. These will be explored in chapter eleven.

Have you ever wondered how a cruel tyrant is able to maintain his power? I have no doubt that Adolph Hitler was a group catalyst. With this ability, he was able to create and maintain a coherent national group energy field in Nazi Germany that brainwashed and changed decent people into cruel and inhumane zealots. This could have been possible only if he tapped into the darker fears and angers of a sizable group of Germans. Once they opened themselves to the GEF, their transformation became complete.

One of the most remarkable recent group events occurred during 1989-90, when the communist Soviet Union and its European satellites experienced one of the most rapid peaceful political and economic revolutions in human history. Obviously these were group phenomena. The pent-up needs of enslaved people reached a critical group consciousness, exploding into revolutions that suddenly transformed their nations and shocked and surprised all of humanity. I have no doubt that these revolutions were created by information-bearing, coherent group energy fields acting intelligently to achieve their goals. I cite one example of how this occurred.

THE FALL OF COMMUNIST EAST GERMANY

In 1989, the government of Communist East Germany, also known as the German Democratic Republic, collapsed as a result of more than just political and economic forces. Since 1980, the churches of that nation had annually celebrated a peace event known as "Ten Days for Peace," during which peace was emphasized in prayer, workshops, celebrations, and correspondence with persons of other nations. Out of this grew weekly prayer services for peace in many German churches.

In the autumn of 1989, the government, believing the churches were promoting political subversion, forbade the prayer services and the demonstrations growing out of them. In October, the churches defied the order. The Communist government decided to make the Nicolai Church in Leipzig an example. Twelve hundred Communist party members arrived early and filled every seat in the downstairs of the Nikolai Church, thinking they would keep out all worshippers.

To seat the parishioners, the unused balconies of the church were opened and filled with sincere worshipers. A service of prayer was conducted. No hatred or anger was expressed. In love, they prayed for peace and justice. This created a huge sacred group energy field. This energy field contained the knowledge of their prayer content and the political and spiritual yearnings of the worshippers. The group energy field then acted intelligently, based upon this knowledge.

The results were amazing. The love, peace, light, justice and the national yearnings of those in prayer transformed the government agents. They felt at one with the church people. They became incapable of using violence against their fellow citizens. Millions of Germans began praying, creating a huge sacred group energy field that pervaded all of East Germany. The information in this energy field changed the consciousness of a nation. The government collapsed.

This example can give us a new understanding and interpretation of many seemingly unexplainable historic religious, political and military events. It can guide intelligent planning for change through the actions of group energy fields. Ten million people praying provides the enormous force of 10,000,000,000,000 energy units of prayer power.

Our awareness of the power of group energy fields gives us a tool for transforming our troubled planet. Any positive results you achieve in your family or in a small group will also work with even greater effect in a neighborhood, community or nation. So experiment, develop your skills and prepare for the larger visions.

CHAPTER SEVEN SUMMARY

How could people walking and driving by a building where Kathryn Kuhlmann was holding a large faith healing service be healed? How could people within the service be healed without being touched?

People can be healed anyplace they are seated during a large healing service only if the healing energy is able to touch them. This can only be explained by the actions of energy fields. The group energy field must contain information about healing that acts intelligently, the same as all healing energy. When the healing group energy field grows beyond the walls of the building, the people enveloped outside can be healed.

Holy ground and sacred space are places where God's presence has left energy behind in an energy field. The healing power of a group is far stronger than an individual's. Group healing power equals the square of the number present.

The individuals in a group provide the information present in a group energy field. Healing service energy fields vary in data content. The religious information in energy fields of gathered Hindu yogis and of Christians is completely different. The contents of any group energy field formed by religious ritual is determined by the beliefs and intentions of the participants. During religious rituals, those bathed in the group energy field are being transformed and empowered by information-bearing, intelligently-acting sacred energy.

The healer must act as a catalyst in forming a healing group energy field.

Physicist William Tiller provides a scientific theory and mathematical equations to support the hypothesis that the power of a coherent group energy field is at least the square of the number of participants.

Group energy fields play an essential role in crucial historic events including the Exodus of the Hebrew people, the Christian Pentecost and the fall of the government of the German Democratic Republic.

Chapter Eight

Profile of a Healer

"Science surpasses the old wisdom of mythology." ...Ralph Waldo Emerson

"A person's psychological makeup contributes to the more specific characteristics of a person's religious experiences, and this accounts for the variety among religious experiences." ...William James*

"Thanks be to God for his inexpressible gift!" ...II Corinthians 9:16

Most persons have given little thought to the human role in the healing encounter. Traditional wisdom holds that one prays and God mysteriously heals in any way he chooses. Often this belief includes a childlike image in which, during their prayer, God strikes people with a bolt of lightning from Heaven. But previous chapters have provided an entirely new picture of healing. Scientific data indicates that healing occurs *because of the existence of a healing energy accumulated, attuned and transmitted by human beings.* This healing energy possesses the ability to transform the human energy fields into optimum health, causing healing in body, mind and spirit.

Do not be shocked by this straight talk; it should come as no surprise. The human role in the healing encounter makes sense. It is just an extension of normal human caring. Throughout the ages, people have bemoaned the fact that God has not intervened to rescue them from poverty, pain, anguish, natural disaster, illness and other injustices. Those expectations do not match our current understanding of how God works.

Today, we know that God does not personally feed the hungry, care for the sick, clothe the poor, provide money for housing and stop human injustice. If caring and justice are to exist on earth, then it is caring humans who must act for God and become his hands and feet. God uses human agents to achieve these practical purposes.

Expanding on this concept leads to the leap of understanding that God inevitably uses human agents to answer healing prayers. When, out of concern, humans turn to God in prayer, scientific data indicates that they naturally accumulate, attune and transmit healing energy at a specific healing frequency. In religious terms, they have become channels of God's healing power. As in other practical works of caring, human beings are God's hands and feet.

WORLD-CLASS HEALERS

Some people possess special abilities to act as healers. These people exist in every religion and culture on Earth. It sounds elitist to say that certain persons might be set apart for their abilities as world-class healers. When it comes to abilities that are considered to be religious gifts, we like to be democratic. Throughout history, religions have resolved this elitist issue by stating that God gives certain people spiritual gifts like the gift of healing. The religious explanation is that God has chosen certain people for their qualities of holiness, faithfulness, obedience, goodness or usefulness for divine purposes.

The gift of healing can certainly be awakened by religious experiences. It is certainly empowered by persons filled with generous love. Faith, hope and expectancy are key elements of healing encounters. But rational data indicates that the healing ability is genetic. It comes at birth, like the color of one's skin and eyes. It is similar to innate abilities like learning aptitude or athletic potential.

We would possess little scientific data about the healing encounter if it were not for the involvement of world-class or professional healers in clinical research. So we turn again to world-class healers to gain insight about praying for healing.

Before we become envious of healers, it must be clearly stated that anyone can function in the role of a healer, that is, as one who is a transmitter of healing energy. Few can become the consistent healers used by researchers. Their ability is similar to that of a world-class track athlete. A world-class track athlete shows consistent performance ability at the highest planetary competitive skill levels. This athletic ability begins with an inborn genetic potential that can be recognized early by coaches. The athletic ability is then nurtured through coaching, endless practice and competition. It is the person with innate exceptional abilities who can attain to a world-class track performance level. The same is true of healers but with one important difference. We can compensate for that difference in several ways.

A. **Through love.** Immense love for the hurting empowers the healing flow.

B. **Group power.** When the power of prayer is the square of the number praying, then it is possible with five praying persons to achieve the same healing results as that of one world-class healer. This is similar to weight-lifters. Few individuals can lift the six hundred pounds of a world-class weight-lifter but five persons working together can.

C. **Through understanding and techniques.** Being relaxed and having competent skills is usually more effective than brute strength.

D. **Through intention, faith, confidence, experience.** These produce similar inner power. The greatest barrier to healing effectiveness does not involve divine power, love, group power, understanding, intention, faith, confidence or experience. The greatest barrier to healing effectiveness is being unwilling to try.

THE PROFILE OF A WORLD-CLASS HEALER

1. Healing and Personality Type. The evidence indicates that those people most likely to utilize healing are optimistic, outgoing, "people-persons." They are also the people who have the most potential as channels for healing prayer. Unfortunately, our image of healers has been molded and distorted by television faith-healing evangelists. This cultural image of healers is extremely inaccurate and does not reflect reality. Rather, people with the greatest healing potential are more like the friendly, smiling, talkative, unassuming, caring neighbor down the street.

Healers exhibit one specific personality type. Two researchers, Monsignor Chester P. Michael and Marie Christian Norraisey,[1] identified the healer personality on the Meyers-Briggs Type Indicator. Healers are the "ENFJ" type. ENFJ stands for an extroverted, intuitive, feeling, decisive type of personality. The ENFJ trait is found in five percent of the population, accounting for two hundred fifty million persons on a planetary scale. This personality type deeply experiences God and expects dramatic answers to prayer. They are natural leaders, radiate warmth and fellowship, rely on feelings, are very personal, friendly, tactful and sympathetic and place high value on harmonious human contacts. They enjoy admiring people and so tend to concentrate on a person's most admirable qualities. They try to live up to their ideals, are loyal and are unusually able to see value in other people's opinions. They have faith that harmony can somehow be achieved and often manage to bring it about. They think best when talking to people and enjoy talk. It takes special effort for them to be brief and business-like.

President Clinton appears to possess an ENFJ personality type. If so, he is a latent healer. Notice how Bill Clinton hugs people. Some he hugs for long periods of time, just as a healer would do if he were practicing healing. His best use of this ability would be as a group catalyst. This ability is discussed later in this chapter.

---

2. Healers emit healing-attuned energy at all times. These individuals are at all times emitting a healing energy that causes people around them to feel calm and trusting. Their energy is always attuned to the healing frequency. Intentional efforts to offer healing through prayer strengthen and focus their healing flow.

Physicist John Zimmerman,[2] while at the University of Colorado School of Medicine, Denver, using a Superconducting Quantum Interference Device (SQUID), a super conducting device cooled to near absolute zero, conducted seven investigations of healers practicing touch-healing with healees and observed discernible changes in the amplitude and/or frequency (7.8 hertz) of the biomagnetic fields detected by the SQUID. The healers emitted a steady 7.8 hertz frequency from the hands *even when not healing.* A control group of non-healers produced no changes. In an eighth investigation, the signal recorded near the healer's hands was larger while healing than when he moved his hands towards the SQUID.

Andrija Puharich, MD, has been a healing researcher for forty years. He researched the Brazilian healer, Arigo, who among other things, conducted surgery with a rusty knife. In 1988, I went to Puharich's home with three traveling companions. Puharich has a device with a sensing plate that measures the frequency emissions of the hand. My three friends each placed a hand on the plate, and like all non-healers, emitted rapidly shifting variable frequencies between seven and eleven hertz. I placed my hand on the plate and the digital readout displayed a steady eight hertz, like that of world-class healers. This means that world-class healers need only intend to offer healing and without any other preparation, they transmit healing energy.

3. Healers can produce more than two hundred volts of energy. Sensitive people who can *see* energy emissions have long observed that world-class healers emit about twenty times the amount of energy of other people. Now the Menninger Clinic reports significant energy discharges from healers versus non-healers.

Researchers in the Copper Wall Experiments[3] at the Menninger Clinic, Topeka, Kansas, have discovered that during meditation and absent healing, nine world-class healers emitted between four volts and two hundred twenty-two volts of electrical energy with a median emission of 8.3 volts. Non-healer meditators produced no surges over four volts. The world-class healers used Non-Contact Therapeutic Touch (NCTT). The implication here is that NCTT therapists have a different "energy structure" or a different "energy handling capability" from that of regular subjects.

Their new technology detected and measured electrostatic potentials and field effects in and around the bodies of meditators and NCTT therapists. The NCTT therapists produced more surges during therapy sessions than during meditation; thus, the intention to heal produced the strongest results. All NCTT therapists believed their skill could be learned by anyone.

Researchers explained that these NCTT therapists' voltage emissions were a billion times stronger than brain-wave voltages, one hundred million times stronger than heart voltages, and a million times stronger than large psychophysiological skin-potential. Their effect on the human energy systems could be immense.

4. Healers possess identical brain frequencies. Beginning in 1969, physicist Robert O. Beck[4] began testing the brain-wave frequencies of heal-ers throughout the world, discovering that all healers measure identical frequencies of 7.83 hertz. This occurred regardless of their society, their beliefs or their healing modality. Beck worked with charismatic Christian faith-healers, a Hawaiian kahuna and practitioners of wicca, Santeria, radesthesia, radionics, seers, ESP readers and psychics.

5. Healers are able to merge their minds with the mind of a healee. Dr. Edgar Wilson[5] produced evidence that Israeli healer David Joffee impresses his brain-wave pattern upon a healee in order to produce healing. The healee must voluntarily allow this entraining to occur. During this process, some healers place a healee in a trance state similar to hypnosis. This provides one explanation for the amnesia of many healees about the healing encounter.

Physicist John Zimmerman[6] has developed a theory based upon his data that the sense of vibration or tingling in the healing encounter is possibly due to both the introduction of the 7.8 to 8.0 hertz biomagnetic field upon the healee and the impressing of the healer's brain-wave pattern upon the healee. The sense of warmth or heat is logically explained by the infra-red radiation emitted by the entire hand of the healer and from the longer microwave emanations coming from near the center of the healer's palms.

Therapeutic Personalities Are Likely Healers

A therapeutic personality comes through as a sympathetic care-giver whom people quickly grow to trust to the extent that they share their innermost thoughts and feelings. In the presence of a therapeutic personality, people feel calm and safe, the same emotions associated with the presence of a healer. This data implies that therapeutic personalities emit the same energy as healers and are thus inborn healers, themselves.

Channels for healing are not restricted to this personality type. Anyone who is generous, self-giving, compassionate and sympathetic can offer healing. But in the present skeptical world, the healer or therapeutic personality is the most likely to attempt self-healing or healing.

Grad's experimental data[7] suggests that positive results in psychother-apy and with the placebo effect are the result of the healing energy emitted to the patients by psychotherapists and physicians when there is a relationship of rapport and trust. In other words, caregivers naturally emit a healing energy when they establish rapport and trust with those for whom they are caring.

6. A Psychiatrist's Profile of a Healer. Psychiatrist Robert Laidlaw[8] was chairman of the Commission To Study Healing at Wainwright House, Rye, New York for eight years. He developed a personality profile of a healer based upon the many healers he had met.

   a.   A healer must be one who elicits rather than inhibits.
   b.   A healer must be a resonant cavity, an instrument, an open channel.
   c.   A healer must be relaxed.
   d.   A healer's senses must be highly acute.
   e.   A healer must be a dedicated person.
   f.   A healer must be in a state of openness, of conscious or unconscious prayer.
   g.   A healer must have expectancy and faith.
   h.   His gifts often involve clairvoyance and telepathy and he is, to some degree, a sensitive.

7. The healing ability may run in families. It has already been stated that healing is a genetic trait, so of course it runs in families. That does not mean that everyone with the ability is willing to become a healer. My grandfather was a practicing healer. My parents are latent healers who have repressed this ability. I have evidence that all my brothers and sisters are healers. One has accepted that role. The others have not. In fact, two of them do not believe in the existence of healing.

Most Filipino healers were born in one specific farm district. They attribute their healing prowess to secret spiritual information that only they possess. They may, indeed, know a few special tricks of the trade. A more plausible scientific explanation is that through intermarriage in a small community, they share a common pool of genetic traits, including the healing ability.

8. Andrija Puharich's Ten Specific Healing Abilities. During his research, Andrija Puharich[9] produced a list of ten abilities that he had observed in healers. No one healer has possessed all of these abilities. The Brazilian healer, Arigo, known as the "*surgeon with a rusty knife,*" possessed seven of these abilities.

The first four abilities can be learned by most persons. These are **(a)** the ability to heal through touch (laying on of hands), **(b)** from a distance (absent prayer) and **(c)** to heal oneself (self-healing). **(d)** The fourth ability, to diagnose an illness, can be learned or naturally emerges.

(e) The fifth ability is the use of molecular medicine -- to match intuitively what is chemically wrong in the healee's body with the right chemical needed to correct it. This may involve chemicals in such substances as herbs or prescription medicines.

The next three are a package of abilities. These are the abilities **(f)** to produce anesthesia by non-chemical means, **(g)** to perform instant surgery with a knife or the hand, **(h)** to perform surgery in unsanitary conditions without resulting bacterial infections. These abilities are primarily practiced by Brazilian spiritist healers, Filipino spiritualist healers and North and South American Native Indian shamans.

(i) Ability number nine is to be inwardly guided by God, a spirit guide, a voice or intuition, which is constantly present with a healer in his work. This ability eventually develops in some persons who regularly practice healing.

(j) The tenth healer ability is to regenerate tissue, an organ, ear, eye, limb or even life itself in a person who is clinically dead. This is a comparatively rare individual gift that can be observed in healers throughout the planet. Healers with this specialized skill sometimes are unable to produce results which other healers achieve consistently. I have observed that regenerating tissue is far more common in group healing than with individual effort, possibly because of the added energy.

9. Weston's Five Newly Identified Healer Abilities. The previous ten healer abilities were identified by researchers studying individual healers. Being rooted in a religious community, I have had the opportunity of observing healing in a group context. With a background in healing research, I recognized these five new healer abilities naturally emerging from a rational grasp of what was occurring during large Christian healing services. Identifying these abilities provides answers to the most disturbing issues arising from faith healing-services. Applying our knowledge of these abilities should enable many more persons to be healed during healing services.

(a) The Group Catalyst. As stated before, every person possesses an energy field that helps to maintain life and health. This individual energy field contains information and interacts with other energy fields. Any time people gather together, their individual energy fields combine to produce a group energy field that is filled with and expresses the information of that group's intent. The most intentional group energy fields are strengthened by persons who act as catalysts. So, the first additional healing ability involves acting as a catalyst in creating and shaping group healing energy fields.

Here is my reasoning for these conclusions. I have led what I call *"A Course in Prayer"* in order to teach people to pray aloud. My prayer groups produced dramatic healing results in comparison to those led by other clergy. Why? I came to understand that my presence itself was adding to the results. What is that all about? Let us move on to a consideration of healing services.

People enter a large healing service with the expectation that healing will occur. Not anyone can lead a large healing service. Everyone knows that *a healer* leads a healing service although that healer is doing far more than most people realize. As one waits for a healing service to begin, the energy of the group is similar to that of any waiting group. Then, as the healer enters the gathering, one senses a change in the information of the group energy. The energy thickens and one senses peace and power. Within a few minutes the energy has become enormous, clinging to each person like a mist of honey. At times, it is almost suffocating in its intensity. Sometimes added components of love or heat are present. Anyone who has attended a large healing service will recognize this description. Again, what has happened?

For a prayer group or healing service to work, at least one person, usually a healer, must act as a catalyst in the creation of a group healing energy field. All ENFJs can act in the catalyst role as well as most persons with the leadership quality of charisma. Their heart chakras are dominating and controlling the quality of the energy in the room.

Those who have charisma can hold an audience spellbound by the energy they project. Accomplished politicians, stage performers and religious leaders have this ability. Each acts as a group catalyst, projecting and creating an energy field that is filled with information expressing the leader's intent. In this fashion, some healers have the ability to be group catalysts in forming a healing group energy field.

(b) The Healer-Attuner. The second identified ability is that of healer-attuner. Large healing services are usually criticized for their lack of beneficial results. The question most often asked by observers is, *"Why are so few healed?"* The more personal questions are, *"Why was I not healed?"* and *"What could I have done to be healed?"* With all the healing energy present, less than one percent of those seeking healing are healed. Why? Various religious answers have been given. Rational explanations go beyond religious wisdom in making sense of this dilemma.

The clues to rational answers are provided by another phenomenon -- the spiritual gift of knowledge. This is expressed in large healing services by the healer who has an awareness of or knowledge of which persons are being healed amongst the gathered thousands. Pointing to the balcony, the healer may say, *"There is a woman in a yellow blouse with breast cancer who is being healed at this moment. She is feeling heat in her right breast."* She is there and she is being healed. From a rational viewpoint, somehow the healer has become attuned to that particular person's energy frequency identity. Those to whom he is particularly attuned to are the ones most likely to be healed.

The spiritual gift of knowledge has another expression. At a specific time, the healer will *know* that all persons with a specific disease can be healed at that moment. *"Will all those who have a hearing loss come forward?"* What's going on here? Again, the healer has attuned to a knowing -- a knowledge, this time not of an individual but to the unique frequency of the healing energy that heals deafness.

The failure to attune is a logical explanation that makes sense out of a number of issues. Why are some not healed in a healing encounter? Because no attunement to the healing frequency, to the person or to the disease has been properly made. Some healers explain that they produce consistent results because of their *at-one-ment* with the healee. They have *attuned,* permitting the healing energy to work effectively. We see that the ability of the healer-attuner is important in any healing.

Attuning can be enhanced in the group-healing setting through the following means: Increase group unity and identity. Develop a group empathy for the ill. Sense a oneness/closeness with both God and the healer. These attunings can be achieved by singing appropriate songs with written words provided, by group prayers with words provided, by pray-along prayers, with rituals of compassion, by empathy for the ill, by involvement of the ill in the personal sharing of their anguish and hopes, and by involving the group in the practice of intentional healing.

Because research demonstrates that spiritual healing is a long-term process that requires ongoing quantities of attuned healing energy, it is essential to provide the healing energy after the healing service ends. This can be accomplished by teaching everyone present to pray daily for a month for the healing of those present. Experience teaches that the power of their prayer would likely approach the power present in the healing service. Hampering this approach are the faulty images shared by both healers and participants that only the healer possesses the ability to heal.

Major attuning occurs through compassion for the healee's condition, so that natural loving and caring produce emotional attunement and the healing of the emotional energy field. Attunement can also be made to the sacred uniqueness of the healee, with healing occurring in the spiritual energy fields. This attuning is to the deeper knowing of personality and being. Attunement can be at the mental level of knowing the physiology of the disease or condition, producing healing in the mental and physical energy fields. Or attunement can be made to the thought processes, another approach that heals the mental energy field. All persons who wish to be channels for healing must become aware of the art of attuning.

(c) The Sensitive. Another healer ability is that of the sensitive. This is a psi factor. The healer-sensitive can diagnose and heal through direct awareness and manipulation of the various energy fields. The sensitive can *see, understand, manipulate,* and *repair* each of the human energy fields. Some refer to sensitives as *psychic healers*, implying that what they are doing is not spiritual. This is a false interpretation. In their way, they are truly spiritual healers because they are working beyond normal physical awareness in the seven human energy field frequencies. The sensitive works through the cleansing of energy fields, energy balancing and kinesiology.

(d) The Energy-Enabler. A fourth ability involves energy-enabling. The power of the healing energy may be raised or boosted by non-healers. This is a very valuable role. The trigger for enabling is compassionate love. Groups can act as energy-enablers. Strong feelings like anxiety, fear and expectation generate power that can be attuned to healing. Children and teenagers are power generators. Certain adults, who are limited in energy attuning, can assist healer-attuners by boosting the power of the healing energy. I have become aware of energy-enablers during hundreds of my own healing encounters when one or more of a healee's loved ones have been present with their compassion and concern.

Four new abilities have been identified -- the Healer-Catalyst, the Healer-Attuner, the Healer-Sensitive and the Energy-Enabler. Rare is the healer who possesses all four of these qualities. It does not take much imagination to project a healing team composed of four persons, each specializing in one of these qualities, working together with the healer-catalyst coordinating their efforts. This can be done in a healing service or within a medical, therapeutic or community setting.

(e) The Prime Healer. This brings us to the final ability. That is the ability of the healer who possesses all four of these qualities. Such a person might best be called a Prime Healer. There is no research data on Primes but they would appear to be extremely rare within the population. Combining these four qualities in one person (or a healing team) produces what might be called a Reality Changer. A Reality Changer can change the nature of physical, emotional, mental and spiritual reality. The most effective faith healers are likely to be Primes. The great religious and spiritual figures of human history needed to possess the Prime qualities. I have witnessed only two Primes in action, one in a huge faith healing service; the other in a group of about four hundred.

All prayer changes reality. The energy of prayer programs order and purpose into chaos and decay. A Reality Changer is special because s/he is a catalyst for introducing massive shifts in reality empowered by large sacred group energy fields. My own fingertip aura suggests that I am a Prime Healer and Reality Changer.

IDENTIFYING THE HEALER IN YOURSELF AND OTHERS

These traits of healers can be used to identify people who have a special ability to offer healing and lead healing services. If you recognize yourself as a healer through the personality type, it may answer many baffling questions you have about yourself. World-class healers also possess the potential for all the spiritual gifts or psychic abilities. Healers also have the ability to act as group catalysts for prayer groups and healing services, meaning they are able to form, attune and maintain a healing group energy field.

Bernard Grad cautions me about some of the above conclusions regarding world-class healers, especially those of the ENFJ personality type. He thinks that others, who may not be ENFJs, may be world-class healers. I am open to additional evidence about others with world-class healing abilities, but at the time, this is where my data has brought me.

The rest of the population can still practice healing or self-healing. It just means that those who do not possess world-class gifts have to work harder at it. My wife is a competent healer even though her personality is private and introverted. These traits limit her ability to reach out boldly to help others, yet she is excellent in assisting me. Her naturally compassionate and nurturing personality enables her to boost the amount of energy created while I maintain the necessary frequency.

My experience is that other factors can compensate for the lack of a world-class healer's natural abilities. These other factors include faith, spiritual maturity, prayer abilities, concern for oneself or a loved one, technique, experience and group efforts. Concern includes fear and anxiety over someone's illness or condition. I have known many non-healers to be more effective than myself because of these traits. When a family member is in crisis, loved ones are filled with strong emotions of love. Love remains the source of all healing. We can also utilize the power of group prayer. Remember, the power of prayer is the square of the number of people praying, enabling any group to out-perform a world-class healer.

A Caution: A healer has difficulty functioning among family and friends. People have difficulty accepting loved ones and friends in the role of healer. At the other extreme, learn that a renowned healer from a distant city is coming to heal your life-threatening disease and you have increased expectations. People expect great things of those coming from far-away places. This increased stature enables the placebo effect to aid in the healing. I do my best healing over fifty miles from home.

The Mysterious Caregiver. When I have played the role of the mysterious caregiver, healing becomes much easier. I will meet a stranger with an obvious illness in an elevator, waiting room, or a social gathering. Introducing myself only as a minister, I will offer caring and a prayer. This usually results in healings, many of them instantaneous.

This occurred one day while I was waiting to officiate at a funeral. I noticed that the secretary at the funeral home was limping badly and using a cane. We were alone in the office. She told me that the arthritic condition in her knee was forcing early retirement at the end of the month. I offered a brief prayer for healing while touching her knee. The following week I entered the funeral home. She walked normally across the room to greet me with an affectionate hug. She whispered that her knee had been healed, but cautioned me not to tell her bosses, who would obviously not understand.

Self-Image Barriers. Do not let your self-image dissuade you from seeking to become an effective healer. I am a perennial workshop attender. When I began attending healing workshops, most leaders immediately reached the conclusion that I was an unlikely candidate for being a healer. A few strongly discouraged me, saying that I displayed none of the personal traits necessary. Thankfully, by the time I began attending healing workshops, I had already served many persons in the healing capacity, and thus, knew I was a healer.

I believe many leaders of healing workshops have held the wrong profile of a healer, themselves, thus misguiding others. My experience is that any person who has been spiritually transformed, who can love others with compassion, and who has unselfish motives, has the potential for being a healing channel. Development usually requires understanding, training, and experience.

Becker links exposure to man-made electromagnetic fields to the diseases of the Electromagnetic-Hypersensitive Syndrome, Chronic-Fatigue Syndrome, AIDS, Autism, Fragile X Syndrome, Sudden Infant Death Syndrome, Alzheimer's Disease, Parkinson's Disease, Cancer, and Mental Diseases.

CHRONIC FATIGUE SYNDROME HITS LATENT HEALERS

Many women with Chronic Fatigue Syndrome (CFS) fit the personality profile of a healer. Recently, I began working women who have been medically diagnosed with CFS. CFS produces such severe and chronic fatigue that patients become non-functional in every area of life. Over a million Americans suffer from CFS and it is resistant to medical treatment.

My first nine CFS women patients have similar personalities. They are ENFJs on the Meyers-Briggs Type Indicator, the same personality type as we find in the profile of a healer. They describe themselves as good care-givers-nurturers, competent at home and at work, problem-solvers, achievers, spiritually grounded, and mild-mannered people-pleasers who surround themselves with dominant people. They accept the blame for everything and everyone in their lives. They possess few personal defenses, making them easily wounded and hurt.

I have had little contact with male CFS patients. The women have medical histories of infectious mononucleosis, endrometriosis, Epstein-Barr Syndrome and other ongoing medical conditions. As a male ENFJ and healer, I have had the experience of infectious mononucleosis and Epstein-Barr Syndrome. I suffered much fatigue until fifteen years ago when I learned to protect my energy fields, but my symptoms were not chronic.

I view Chronic Fatigue Syndrome as a pure energy-field disease. ENFJs and CFS patients are empaths who absorb the pains of the world into their heart chakras. Intuitively, I see them as latent healers whose unused healing energy is poisoned by their damaged heart chakras, producing disease rather than health. At some point in time, their energy fields have ruptured, probably at the diaphragm chakra, making it impossible for them to maintain a reservoir of life energy. It is at this point that their symptoms of CFS occur. These observations suggest that CFS is an illness specific to latent healers.

My approach to treatment involves explaining this diagnosis, exploring their interactions with others, telling them they must actively express their creativity, teaching them to protect their energy fields as explained in chapter fourteen, healing their ruptured energy fields, recharging their energy fields, and teaching them to practice touch-healing and self-healing.

Early reports reveal rapid increases in health. All of this is preliminary as PrayWell goes to press. I include these observations to provide others with the opportunity for exploring this approach.

MANY GAY MEN MAY POSSESS HEALING POTENTIALS

Robert O. Becker, MD,[10] links exposure to man-made electromagnetic fields to the diseases of the Electromagnetic-Hypersensitive Syndrome, Chronic-Fatigue Syndrome and AIDS. I noticed that most of my clients suffering from Electromagnetic-Hypersensitive Syndrome and Chronic-Fatigue Syndrome match the profile of the healer, making them more sensitive to environmental electromagnetic pollution. When I saw AIDS on Becker's lists, the obvious hit me. Many gay males are the extroverted-intuitive-creative-feeling type of personality, so they, too, match the profile of a healer. With all the discrimination that gays face, they may not welcome assuming the further liability of practicing touch-healing. But, the benefits are enormous. AIDS should respond well to the application of healing energy.

CERTAIN PEOPLE MUST NURTURE THEIR ENERGY FIELDS

Extroverted-intuitive-creative-feeling types of personalities must protect and nurture their energy fields in order to remain healthy and lead a full life. Practicing healing helps to do this. Cleansing and protecting energy fields is explained in chapter fourteen. Barbara Ann Brennan provides detailed exercises for nurturing and strengthening energy fields in her book, Hands of Light. I commend this to these vulnerable personality types. Such energy field exercises could keep them from ever contracting infectious mononucleosis, endrometriosis, Epstein-Barr Syndrome, Chronic Fatigue Syndrome and many other diseases.

TWO HEALING STYLES

Psychologist Lawrence LeShan,[11] through interviews with healers, has identified two basic styles or approaches to healing. All healers assume that they are partners with God in the healing encounter. They assume the traditional role of priest. *A priest is one who brings the power of God into the life of the world.* Healers are aware that they are acting as channels for God's power. Anyone who offers healing prayer is acting in the role of priest. This new understanding makes healing efforts more effective.

In Type One Healing, *the healer enters an altered state of consciousness* (prayer, meditation or centering). From this perspective, he views the healer and healee as one entity. No attempt is made to do anything -- more than to encounter, be one with and unite with the healee. The healee is viewed in a non-physical reality of timelessness, of the unity of all being and things, of neither good nor evil, but of what just is. All is one. *The healer is focused by love and by caring on the healee.* There is a oneness of healer, healee and God. There is a spiritual empathy. One form of Type One healing is non-directed absent-prayer.

In Type Two Healing, *the healer enters an altered state of consciousness* (prayer, meditation or centering). The healer perceives a pattern of energy between his palms, a flow of energy. His hands are placed on either side of the healee's injured area. Half the healers report feeling heat in the hands and some a cold sensation. This type of healer tries to heal. He wants and attempts to do so through the healing flow. *The healer is focused by love and by caring on the healee.* Nothing exists for this healer but his hands.

We are presuming here that both types are using touch-healing rather than absent healing. But the Type One healing behavior would also be appropriate for absent-healing, while the Type Two healing behavior must be altered for absent-healing.

Both types share two behaviors in common. They *enter an altered state of consciousness* and *are focused by love and caring* on the healee. Note that traditional prayer shares these two behavioral traits. Prayer itself is an altered state of consciousness, and one prays out of concern and love for the person in crisis. The love and caring, which grow out of concern, fear and anxiety, are powerful emotions that play an enabling and attuning role in prayer.

Clinical Data on Healing Styles. The effectiveness of Type One and Type Two healing styles was experimentally explored. Larry Dossey, MD,[12] uses data from SPINDRIFT experiments in differentiating between the results of directed versus non-directed prayer. The SPINDRIFT tests used absent-healing in seeking prayer results for biological organisms.

Non-directive prayer (Type One healing) results were twice as great as directive prayer. In seeking to cause laboratory molds to grow, directive prayer produced no results. Directive prayer seeks specific goals or results through a request for healing or involves directed imagery or visualization. This is the traditional style of prayer.

Non-directive prayer excludes physical, emotional and personality characteristics and replaces them with a *"pure and holy qualitative consciousness of whomever and whatever the patient may be."* SPINDRIFT experiments do not use touch-healing. Therefore, they provide no data on Type Two healing nor is it known whether touch-healing prayer would produce the same results.

I have other reservations about these experimental results. The professional healers, Christian Science Practitioners, were trained and experienced in non-directive prayer as their only style. Directive-prayer was, therefore, unfamiliar to them. Third, my observation is that some persons may be more effective at one prayer style than another. Fourth, in directive (or traditional prayer) the element of compassionate love as an energy-enabler was not considered. Fifth, having used variations of both styles, I don't think it is possible to use non-directive prayer without having a directive intention at some level of the mind. To play it safe, I will be directing you to combine these styles in your prayers.

Having read most of their massive report, THE SPINDRIFT PAPERS (SPINDRIFT, Inc., P.O.Box 3995, Salem, Oregon 97302-0995, $25), I must express my admiration and respect for their eighteen years of research. It broke substantial new ground in our understanding of both prayer and precognition, supplying data that is unfortunately not relevant to this book's focus.

THREE DISTINCT GROUPS OF HEALERS

LeShan[13] also identified three distinct groups of healers. **Spiritual Healers,** the largest group, describe their work as prayer and believe their success is due to the intervention of God.

Spirit Healers believe the healing is done by the spirits of deceased humans or spirit guides (the Company of Heaven) after the healer has set up a linkage between the spirits and the patient.

Psychic Healers believe they are originators and transmitters of some form of energy that has healing effects. The healer has a flow of healing energy and concentrates on the healing flow entering the healee through his hands.

The source of healing energy may be either the God *beyond* or the God *within.* The evidence indicates that healers in all three groups are transmitting a healing energy at the same frequency, and their results are identical.

EIGHT WAYS TO OFFER HEALING

1. Absent-Prayer. The most common means for offering healing is through attempts at absent-healing prayers for the ill, usually a loved one. No statistics are available on what percentage of those billions of prayers have assisted the healing process. Research data indicates the best way to do this is by establishing a oneness between God, the healee and oneself.

2. Touch-Prayer. Among those who regularly practice healing, the use of touch through the laying on of hands is most common. This action is practiced in healing services, small groups and individually.

3. Psychic or Energy Healing. A third way of regularly practicing healing is the movement of the hands amidst the body's energy fields as one seeks to repair, balance, attune and recharge the energy fields that then enable physical, mental, emotional and spiritual healing to occur.

4. Non-Contact Healing in a Group Setting. The fourth way healing may happen is without physical contact, at a healing service in which a healing group energy field encompasses everyone present. Without touch, a person is healed as the healer attunes to that specific person or to the healing frequency of his disease.

5. Self-Healing through Spiritual Disciplines. A fifth way involves self-healing through meditation, prayer, visualization and touch.

6. Self-Healing through Touch-Prayer. This is my favorite way to practice self-healing. I place my preferred hand on the place needing to be healed, pray for healing and leave my hand there for ten to fifteen minutes daily until healing occurs.

7. Self-Healing through a Shift in Consciousness. Self-healing can occur through a shift of consciousness, through biofeedback theta training, hypnotism, autogenic training, meditation, visualization, an out-of-body experience, a near-death experience, the spiritual disciplines, classical music, sports, falling in love, a religious conversion, etc. Each of these can transform brain functioning or produce a healthy energy field that is then able to restore the physical body.

8. Mind-Body Work. An eighth process involves mind-body work in which one intentionally seeks to become mentally, emotionally, and interpersonally whole or balanced to the extent that one attains to personal happiness and satisfaction. The mind-body movement advocates this approach. In the context of spiritual healing, when the mind becomes healthy, the healthy mind corrects faulty energy fields that then heal the physical body.

INNER AWARENESS DURING HEALING PRAYER

Through the years, I have been a pragmatist who believes *"if it works, use it."* In the presence of each healing miracle, I am awed. I am focused totally upon the person as I pray for a healing. These are the most exciting, alive, joyous moments of my life. After the healing encounter, I can remember with sharp focus every detail of those life-enhancing moments. I have discovered several factors are often present in my healing prayers:

1. I always sense a holy presence that I acknowledge as God.
2. I am always touching the other person, with a handclasp, or hands on the injured area, or one hand on the healee's head with the other clasping one of his hands.
3. I always have a relationship with those I heal. There is caring. If I know of their hurting, there is compassion. Sometimes it is human friendship, a closeness. Sometimes there is the stimulation of persons getting to know each other at deeper levels. Sometimes there is laughter and the prayer is begun in a joyous spirit. Sometimes there has been tension between us, but as the prayer begins, an intimate bond begins joining us together and a deep rapport develops.
4. There is always a sense of merging, unity or oneness, between myself, the healee and God. I call this the Healing Trinity.
5. There is always a sense of peace with any negative awareness filtered to a vague background.
6. Usually there is yielding or accepting, a simple flowing into a beautiful new reality of timelessness.
7. I usually sense a mutual healing. I am healed, too, as if there were a mutual healing exchange between healer and healee, or because the healing is flowing through me. Any fatigue or tension is gone. If I have a raspy throat, a stiff back or a sore muscle, all are healed. After I do healing all day, I feel refreshed.
8. Sometimes my fingers will tingle and sometimes I feel heat where my hands are touching. I feel heat in my own fingers only when my fingers touch myself. Often I can sense an energy flow from my fingers, but this has no known correlation with the healing results. More recently, when I feel nothing, the healing results are better. This leads me to believe that the sensed heat during healing is not signifying that healing is taking place but is showing the resistance of the energy field to the transmitted energy. The only effective heat is that felt *within* the healee's physical body.
9. When a healee's loved ones are present, I often sense a much stronger energy flow.
10. Those whom I have healed report a variety of impressions. Some feel heat either where I have placed my hands or in a diseased or injured area. Some feel a tingling through out the body. Some sense an energy flow. Emotional factors are reported more often than physical. These include peace, love, joy, holiness and energy.

As the prayer begins, I attempt to do nothing except pray. As the prayer continues my words flow without conscious thought. When this happens at a deeper level, I am conscious of the other factors described above. I flow easily between Type I and Type II healing modes -- alternating between the oneness and the energy flow. Only rarely is there a telepathic exchange at the conscious level, yet a deeper knowing of the healee usually emerges.

THE HEALING STYLE OF JESUS

In the gospel accounts, Jesus' healing encounters are briefly described. We do not know how much the witnesses might have missed or did not think needed to be reported. The biblical purpose is to tell the story of God's power at work. Jesus performed healing in several ways.

Touch-healing. In Matthew 8:14-15, Peter's mother-in-law, "lying *sick with a fever,*" was just **touched** and the fever left her.

Expected healing. In Matthew 8:2, a leper knelt and asked to be cleansed. Jesus agreed, touched him and the man was well. The leper obviously **respected** Jesus because he knelt. The leper's very statement showed that he **expected** or **took for granted** Jesus' healing ability.

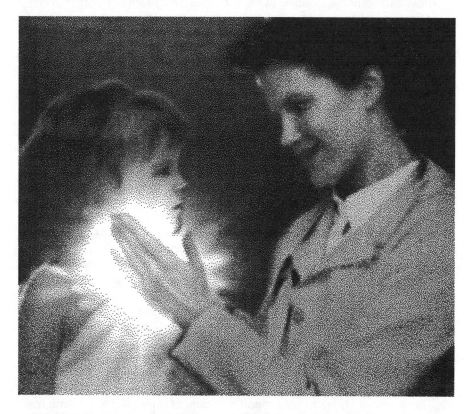

Figure 6. *Healers transmit life energy with their hands at a frequency of about eight hertz. This life energy must be applied regularly like an antibiotic and produces the optimum conditions for the health of all living organisms.*

Many transactions. In Matthew 9:2-8, a paralytic was healed. The following transactions took place. The paralytic, and those who brought him, had **faith**. Could that mean either an expectation that Jesus would heal or a belief that Jesus healed? Or is it a trust as one might trust in modern medicine? This faith seems to mean **'to put one's trust in.'** Another element is **forgiveness**. Since this is all we know of the encounter, we must assume that Jesus intuitively saw the man's obvious need for forgiveness.

The third element is a **command** to be well, in which the spoken word focused and empowered the healing energy.

Touch-healing. In Matthew 9:18-26, are two reports of healings. One tells of the hemorrhaging woman who **touched** the hem of his garment. Mark 5:25-34 says that this act immediately healed her and Jesus *"perceived in himself that power had gone forth from him."*

Today's healer would sense the same loss of power, and this affirms modern research that there is energy transmitted from a healer or from that which he has touched (a garment). In Matthew's account, Jesus **assures** the woman that *"faith has made you well."* This is the same assurance today's healer might offer to fixate the healing. The second healing was of Jairus' daughter who had actually died. Jesus took her hand or **touched** her, and she lived.

Healing as a process. Mark 8:22 tells of the gradual healing of a blind man. First, Jesus spat in the man's eyes. Is healing energy in a healer's saliva? Then he tested out the healing, just as a modern healer would do. Then he healed again, **placing his hands** on the eyes, and this time his testing showed the man had completely restored sight.

Healing as compassion. In Matthew 20:30-34, two blind men were healed by touch after Jesus had **pity** upon them. Today's word for pity might best be described as **compassion**, which is one of the qualities necessary for healing.

Absent-healing. In Luke 7:3-10, Jesus carried out absent-healing on the centurion's servant. The centurion felt **compassion** for his servant and Jesus may have channeled the healing through the Centurion (a focus for sending the healing to the servant) just as a healing group might do today.

Ungrateful lepers. Luke 17:11-19, one my favorite healing encounters, describes Jesus healing ten lepers **by command** without touching them. Only one leper returned to Jesus and gave thanks. Why? Jesus said it was a lack of religious belief. That speaks to the modern healer. Ninety percent of those healed never mention it to the healer. Partly, it is the selective amnesia that goes with a miracle. Partly, it is not believing that Jesus did the healing. (He didn't touch them; it merely happened.) Partly it is their lack of any faith commitment.

Disappointed healer. A similar event was the disappointment of Jesus depicted in John 4:46-54. Jesus had sent absent-healing to a Capernaum official. During this encounter Jesus told the father, *"Unless you see signs and wonders you will not believe."* Healees usually need to see healing as dramatic and convincing, yet healing occurs so quietly that most people do not know anything is happening. So the healer often has the healee **claim** or **acknowledge** his healing, to affix it so it won't slip away.

Healing of a misfit. The entire ninth chapter of John deals with a blind man's healing. Even before the age of modern science people did not believe that healing was possible. Here Jesus denied that the sins of the blind man's ancestors or that deeds of anyone else caused the blindness. Here is a healing of a person who was seen by the community as unfit to be healed. To the healer, no status or faith or religion was required.

HEALING STYLES IN THE EARLY CHURCH

Powerful commanding. The Book of Acts relates many healings by the followers of Jesus. The first one is told in Acts 3:2-10. This healing got Peter and John arrested. A man who had been lame from birth was healed as Peter commanded, *"...in the name of Jesus Christ of Nazareth, walk."* Peter took him by the hand and raised him up and immediately his feet and ankles were made strong. Here is a **command in Christ's name**, a **touching** and a boldly demonstrated faith action, **expecting specific healing results**.

Passing the Holy Spirit. In Acts 9:10-19, Ananias was sent as a messenger by Jesus to heal the blinded Saul and **to fill him with the Holy Spirit**. Ananias' **touch** not only healed Saul but it **passed on the Holy Spirit**. This implies that Ananias possessed the energy of the Holy Spirit within him and when Saul was touched for healing, the Holy Spirit remained, a purposeful, intelligent spiritual energy and presence.

Powerful commanding. Another story of a healing performed by Peter is found in Acts 9:33-35. Peter said, *"Aeneas, Jesus Christ heals you; rise and make your bed."* Aeneas, bedridden for eight years and paralyzed, immediately arose. No touch. Just a **command in Jesus' name**. But again, we see **the order to rise** (to act or do something) to fixate the healing results.

Believing. In Acts 14:8-11 is an account of how Paul performed a healing. But he did not even attempt it until he looked in the man's eyes and knew the man **believed** that he would be healed. Paul did not even evoke Jesus' name, or touch the man. He just **commanded** in a loud voice, *"Stand upright on your feet."* By today's standards that would be sacrilegious. Yet Christ said he would empower his people with the Holy Spirit.

Paul healed with and without reference to Jesus. As we see in Acts 14:16-18, he did **invoke Jesus' name** to cast out a spirit which had given the woman the ability to do divination.

Touch-healing. When Paul preached a long sermon, Eutychus went to sleep and fell to his death. Acts 20:10 describes how Paul **embraced him** (energy exchange) and made a shift in reality, or spoke for the expected results, when he said, *"Do not be alarmed, for his life is in him."*

Touch-healing prayer. Finally, in Acts 28:7-9, we read of how Paul went through the traditional rituals of healing for Publius' father, who had a fever and dysentery. He visited him (perhaps talking and relating), **prayed** and *"putting his hands upon him healed him."*

Summary. In Acts we see healing done by **commanding, by invoking Jesus, by touch, by demonstrating the expected results.** In all but one situation, the healing was freely **volunteered** with no talk of faith or commitment. It is the healer who must have the faith, not the healee. The suddenness and casualness with which the healings were offered did not give the healees a chance to doubt or raise resistance. It is obvious that the Holy Spirit empowered the disciples to do healings equal to what Jesus had done.

Chapter Nine

Everyone Is Qualified To Heal

---

*"A priest is one who brings the power of God into the life of the world. Anyone can be a priest. The only qualification is caring enough to offer a prayer for God's renewing power." ...*Walter L. Weston

*"Union with God can be attained by all." ...*Saint Francis de Sales*

*"Prayer is the state of the heart in which it is united to God in faith and love." ...*Madame Guyon

---

I have seen it throughout my life. You have seen it, too. Early in life, everyone feels inadequate to represent God. You would think we would get over it. We seldom do. Throughout the world, humans turn to priests to represent them before God. This is especially true in the midst of any crisis.

There is nothing wrong with this natural yearning. At times, I, myself, a priest, turn to others to bring the power of God into my life.

Yet, when one is struggling, hurting or in crisis, one may need more than a priestly figure to consult occasionally. People may need help on a regular basis. Not just daily -- often hourly. Sometimes minute by minute. The practical solution involves learning to act as a priest for yourself and others. That means learning the practice of healing prayer.

Most of us feel comfortable with practical acts of caring. A kind word of support. Providing food. Comforting someone. Working for justice. These are all means by which you and I bring the power of God into the life of the world. Yet, when it comes to spiritual things, most people feel inadequate, not good enough, not godly enough, not capable enough, not experienced enough.

This is my main motivation for writing PrayWell. Very few people possess the skills needed to pray during a crisis. Few people can find the right words. But, most of all, we feel inadequate to act in the role of a priest. That stops us cold. It keeps us from even trying.

PrayWell seeks to provide all you need to know, a step-by-step process for bringing the power of God into your own life and the lives of others through prayer. To begin, you must become comfortable in the role of a priest. *A priest is one who brings the power of God into the life of the world. Anyone can be a priest. The only qualification is caring enough to offer a prayer for God's renewing power.* Anyone who cares is qualified to practice Therapeutic Prayers for healing, self-healing and renewal.

ANYONE WHO DEEPLY CARES CAN PRAY FOR HEALING

My teachers through the years have impressed me with one important truth. The practice of healing prayer is easy. It does help to know more about this subject, which sometimes seems to be the most misunderstood subject on Earth. By this time, you have learned quite a bit, if you have read everything up to this point.

I am trying to build your confidence. Hear these words again: Anyone who cares deeply about himself or others can pray effectively for healing. Anyone can act as a priest in bringing the power of God into the life of the world. This will not be the last time you will read these words.

The following examples express everyday ways by which people act as priests.

Prayers by children. Nine-year-old Allison grew more fearful upon learning that her mother's medical condition had deteriorated at the hospital. Her father had explained that her mother's breast cancer had spread to the fluid in the lining of the lung and to the liver, and that surgery was scheduled for the next morning. Afterward, Allison cried in her bedroom, and then urgently prayed for her mother throughout the evening and into the night. The next morning, the surgeons operated, only to find no signs of infection or cancer.

This type of incident has been reported often. The child is usually eight to twelve years of age, and the prayers are for a loved one. Afterwards, a family member acknowledges the child's role in the healing. Then, it is never mentioned again to the child and the child often forgets the incident. Years later, an adult family member will tell the story.

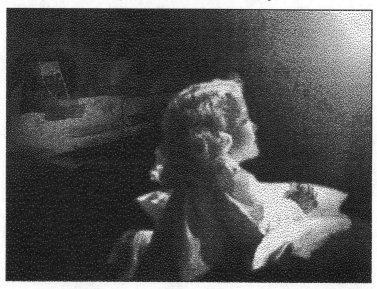

Figure 7. *Many children have saved the lives of their critically ill loved ones by praying urgently for their recovery. Above, daughter prays for ill mother who is lying in the bed in the left background.*

Family prayer for a critically ill loved one. The first time I heard of this type of healing encounter, it came from an osteopathic physician. Since then, other families have told of similar healings. Dr. Bob's elderly mother in a distant city had broken her hip. After it was set, complications developed, including pneumonia. Upon learning that her condition had grown worse and that she was nearing death, a half-dozen family members gathered at the hospital outside Intensive Care. The attending physician told the family that he had done all medicine knew how to do and it was only a matter of time before her death. Before departing, he added, *"She is in the hands of God, now."*

Dr. Bob invited his family to join him in the hospital chapel where he led them in vocal prayer for ten minutes. A half-hour later, the attending physician entered the waiting room smiling and stated, *"I do not know what you have been doing out here but it sure helped Mrs. B. She is making a dramatic recovery."*

Physical fatigue and age are no barrier. As ninety-two-year-old Oskar Estebany, the renowned healer for most of biologist Grad's healing experiments, lay physically debilitated on his death bed, he clasped a visiting friend's arm and proceeded to transmit his usual healing flow. With great satisfaction, Estebany exclaimed, *"It is still there!"* He died an hour later. Age and limited physical vitality are not detrimental factors. Even while physically and emotionally fatigued, people are capable channels.

ALTERED STATE OF CONSCIOUSNESS COMES NATURALLY

During the past three decades, hundreds of articles have been written about improving your life by attaining an "altered state of consciousness" -- an alpha or theta state of lowered brain-wave frequency -- in order to have contact with God, be healed or be creative. It is the *in thing* if you are on a spiritual journey. Many teachers have claimed that this state is similar to that induced by hypnosis.

A recent in-depth study of hypnosis and brain-wave frequencies conducted by a team of medical doctor-hypnotists disproves these alpha-theta hypnotic claims. With hundreds of subjects in the deepest of hypnotic states, none exhibited the lowered brain-wave frequencies of the alpha or theta levels. All remained within the normal range of beta, everyday brain-wave frequencies.

I still affirm the value of relaxation techniques, hypnosis, meditation and visualization. I have personally practiced and professionally used them for more than two decades and found them to be helpful. I still use them on a daily basis for my own stress reduction, wholeness, contact with God and creativity. As you will later discover, I was in such an awareness -- a peak religious experience -- during the healing of my damaged heart muscle. But, let us forget about trying to attain lowered brain-wave frequencies during healing prayer.

Throughout the day, we are constantly shifting into various states of consciousness or awareness. When reading, I become so concentrated that I do not hear my wife speaking. When painting, I dare not talk because I forget about the brush and can be messy. When laughing, I am often both loving and creative. These are automatic shifts in awareness-perception-consciousness. When I pray, I automatically shift into a state of God-awareness. With practice, you will, too. At times, Therapeutic Prayer will lift you to a peak religious experience that can quickly transform and empower you. This is especially true when praying with others.

PERSONAL QUALITIES THAT ENHANCE HEALING

We proceed here to the personal qualities that enhance healing prayer. Two primary factors were reported in LeShan's research -- *an altered state of consciousness* and *a focus upon love and caring.* These are actually similar if not identical qualities.

Any time one senses the presence of God, or calms the inner self, or intends to offer healing, or deeply cares, one attains to an altered state of consciousness from which healing can flow. My own experience indicates that we need to expand our understanding of how the healing flow is triggered.

At first, I needed to pray in order to attune and transmit the healing energy. Through the years I have become so conditioned by experience that now the healing flow can be triggered in several ways. It is triggered by intention. It is triggered by seeing a hurting person. Sometimes it is triggered when I walk into a crowd where someone is ill. My healing hand begins to tingle and I am drawn like a magnet to that ill person. My hand grows hot with healing flow when I touch ill or injured persons, even without prior knowledge of their condition. It is triggered by a friendly conversation. It is triggered by talking or writing about healing. It is triggered by love or laughter. It is triggered by a walk in the woods. The mounting evidence is that most persons who care and who intend to offer healing naturally transmit a healing-attuned energy.

1. Professional healers versus caring pray-ers. We need to make a clear distinction between the healing styles of professional healers and caring pray-ers. The profile of a healer as explored in chapter eight is most helpful for those who choose to make healing a professional vocation. Healers practice healing with many people, most of them strangers. This makes the strength of their emotions much weaker than if a loved one were ill. I suspect this is one of the reasons they need to center and be at peace during the practice of healing. This strengthens their healing ability.

In contrast, those who are praying for the healing of themselves or loved ones will have strong feelings of concern while praying. These strong feelings empower their prayers. Therefore, the prayer style of the caring pray-er need not be that of a professional healer, nor should it be. Let your love be genuine. That usually means being anxious, fearful and hurting. These are expressions of loving concern. They powerfully strengthen the healing energy of the caring pray-er. Borrow from professional healers only those techniques that you find helpful. Always remember, your anxious caring is the most powerful tool you possess.

In the midst of Therapeutic Prayer, you may find God's peace calming you. God, love, faith, and hope are capable of producing this peace. We have no way of knowing how many find God's peace in the midst of prayer.

I think of God's peace being an added bonus. It calms you. It is not necessary for prayers to be beneficial. While praying for hurting loved ones, I usually feel God's peace, even though a background level of anxiety still persists.

2. Religious practices help. Every religion uses rituals and worship to express the religious knowledge of God in meaningful ways, but they do more than this. Rituals and worship begin transforming the participant into the revealed image of God. Earlier, we discovered that every person is interpenetrated by energy fields that are information-bearing. During spiritual moments, such as religious ritual and worship, the human energy fields take on the qualities of the religious knowledge contained in the created sacred group energy field. Any spiritual journey will be enhanced by being bathed in a sacred group energy field.

Through sensing their energy fields, one can recognize persons who have been transformed and empowered by God. They radiate peace and love. These qualities are then reflected in the transmitted energy of healing prayer. So, participating in a religious community can transform and empower a person's energy fields and increase the ability to offer healing prayer.

3. Worldly barriers that block healing energy. A number of everyday barriers make contact with God and the transmitting of healing energy more difficult. Specific emotional states create blockages. Deeply religious persons in the midst of depression consistently report being troubled because they can no longer make contact with God. Many persons in the midst of grief report a similar experience. Research data indicates that other emotions like hatred, anger, fear or a sense of inadequacy create brain-wave static that becomes a barrier to attuning healing energy. With depression and grief, reaching out in love through prayer can be both therapeutic and effective. Those filled with hatred, anger, fear or a sense of inadequacy should not pray with the sick until resolving these issues, because their prayers may be transmitting an energy that makes ill people worse.

Many healers state that anyone who uses tobacco or alcoholic beverages is closed to being a channel for healing. Kent State University experiments verified that following the smoking of one cigarette, test subjects could not achieve a brain-wave shift to the alpha state of consciousness for twenty minutes. Similar barriers to a strong contact with God are likely to occur with caffeine, a chemical cousin of nicotine. One cup of caffeinated coffee has the stimulating effect of the nicotine in four modest cigarettes. Certain teas and soft drinks, as well as chocolate, contain caffeine. A final barrier is listening to a steady diet of rock music. Research indicates that the energy of rock music impedes the growth of plants while the energy of classical and easy-listening music improves growth.

4. Love, caring and spiritual compassion. Some persons find it difficult to care deeply for a loved one in the midst of a crisis. For various reasons, they are forced to withdraw their emotions rather than actively care, looking from afar as a spectator. A few persons express caring skills naturally, but most of us have to work in order to grow in our expression of supportive actions. In the painful agony of crisis, one may only feel a nameless anxiety, numbness and fear. A sense of helplessness may paralyze all functioning as the shock waves hit the brain like a sledgehammer. In this destructive state of consciousness, one's awareness is fixated on the anxiety level where clear vision, loving action and healing prayer are impaired. How do we cope?

First, identify and name the source of the anxiety and fear.

Second, focus on actively loving everyone involved. An embrace, a touch, a loving word of reassurance, a perspective on eternity; all these dull the effect of the destructive elements of the crisis.

Third, focus on God and his love by sharing a prayer with those present. This permits everyone to shift from the state of emotional pain and stasis to the more helpful state of God-consciousness. The intentional healer often feels immense pain, with deep feelings of love for the healee. There may be stress, agony, fear and tears. But when the prayer for healing is offered, the spiritual compassion empowers the coming of God's presence, peace, love and hope as the pray-er is able to transcend the moment spiritually, taking the hurting loved one with him to become one with God.

These dynamics also occur in a support group. Group members share their pain and others respond with compassion and caring. This releases an energy for healing. In this setting, without a prayer being spoken, a peace pervades everyone in the group.

THE WOUNDED HEALER

The concept of the *"wounded healer"* becomes helpful in understanding spiritual compassion. When one has been wounded, known pain, received compassion and become whole again, one has met the qualifications necessary for becoming a wounded healer. The wounded healer is naturally able to offer wholeness to others because of his own personal experience of having suffered and traveled the path back to wholeness. Thus, the recovering alcoholic is qualified to offer compassion and hope to other alcoholics. A recovering cancer patient is qualified to offer compassion to new cancer patients. Any wounded healer can offer compassion to the wounded.

Spiritual compassion requires an awareness of another's hurt. One comes by this consciousness out of the experience of having been terribly wounded and known healing. This level of consciousness knows that compassion does not wallow in the other's pain. It has reached the spiritual stance that sees the suffering person in the midst of God's love to all eternity. God is with us in life, in death, in life beyond death.

The intentional pray-er often feels immense pain, with deep feelings of love for the healee. There may be stress, agony and tears. But when the prayer for healing is offered, spiritual compassion empowers the coming of God's peace, love, joy and presence, as the pray-er is able to spiritually transcend the moment, taking the hurting loved one with him to become one with God. This opens the door to God's powerful healing energy.

EMPOWERING THE ABILITY TO HEAL

Years ago, I experienced a healing *"drought."* The energy of my prayers seemed non-existent. I observed no healing effects from my efforts. A friend, who is a Charismatic Christian, suggested I ask God to strengthen my gift of healing. I prayed for the ability to be more effective in healing prayer. This prayer resulted in a dramatic increase in the energy of my prayers that was confirmed by a return to consistent healing results.

I will not speculate on how such a simple prayer request could make me a much better channel for healing. I now repeat the request every time I practice touch-healing prayer. Because it works for me, I think it will work for everyone. Here is a prayer model, asking God to empower your healing ability:

A Prayer Model for Empowering Prayer

God, I feel inadequate in my prayers. I open myself to your power. Empower me to be an effective channel for healing. Fill me with your love that my prayers may have the energy necessary for blessing others. I accept the role of priest as I seek to bring your power into the life of the world. Amen.

HOW PENNY'S PRAYERS HEALED HER HUSBAND

One morning a desperate woman named Penny phoned me concerning her husband, Lewis. He was in the advanced stages of heart disease, having been too ill for two years to leave his home except to see his physician. As they entered my church study that morning, it was obvious that Lewis was sullen and withdrawn, unwilling to cooperate. Penny knew about spiritual healing and had heard of me. She was filled with hope. Because of Lewis' negative attitude, I felt private prayer was not going to work with the reluctant Lewis, so I invited them to our weekly healing service.

Lewis arrived with Penny and their son. They actually carried Lewis into the chapel. That first evening Penny told their story, openly crying by the time she finished. The woman next to her held her hand. Later, two men helped Lewis come to the front for healing. The four healers at the front welcomed Lewis and Penny with hugs. Lewis sat on a folding chair and we invited Penny to join us in touch-healing and prayer. Afterwards we embraced them again. Before they left, I suggested that Penny pray aloud with her husband twice daily, placing her hands on the front and back of his chest while offering a simple prayer for healing.

The next week, to my surprise, Lewis movingly shared his own history, a painful story of declining health, early retirement and despair. We all wept with him. The following week we beheld a miracle! Lewis walked in unassisted, his wife glowing with joy. In reverence, Penny shared with us the miracles unfolding in their lives. When she prayed with Lewis, her hands now tingled. They both felt the heat radiating into Lewis from Penny's hands. They both glowed with love and faith. Day by day, she was seeing Lewis' health visibly improve.

The next week they both joyfully described having three couples over for dinner, the first time in three years that Lewis' health had permitted such a strenuous event. The following week, Lewis entered the chapel, strutting like a young man and radiating vitality. While Penny sat contentedly, Lewis enthusiastically told of going to their parish's St. Patrick's Day dance and dancing all evening, mostly vigorous polkas. We all joined them in rejoicing. In a subsequent visit to his cardiologist, Lewis was diagnosed as free of heart disease. God had healed Lewis in body, mind and spirit.

What can we learn from this story? It shouts for all who would hear that a loving spouse and a small group of compassionate people, gathered for love and prayer, can bring God's healing, even to a reluctant healee. Caring was evident as each person heard the pain and responded with spiritual compassion.

Penny and Lewis had earlier heard other people sharing their pain (naming their fear). They had seen the acceptance and the loving responses throughout the group. They had heard others share their good news of personal healings. They came to experience a miracle readiness -- a burning hope that God would heal. Penny's prayers each morning and evening had at first been brief. Then with experience and growing excitement, her prayers lengthened to a half-hour at a time. She knew that God was using her as a channel for healing, and she eagerly accepted this role.

If this account of love, caring and immense compassion accomplishes anything, I hope it empowers people with a sense of their own potential. The good news is that everyone and anyone with compassion has direct access to the love of God and his power to heal. Simply claim the right and the power which God has granted each human being to be a holy channel for healing through prayer. Anyone who cares deeply about himself or others can pray effectively for healing. *You, yourself, can act as a priest in bringing the power of God into the life of the world.*

Chapter Ten

Science Clarifies Religious Beliefs

"A new principle is an inexhaustible source of new views." ...Vauvenargues

"The Deity possesses all the positive attributes of the universe, yet more strictly it does not, for it transcends them all." ...Dionysius, the Pseudo-Areopagite*

"An examination of the reports of religious experience discloses two psychological characteristics: (1) a new zest that adds itself like a gift to life; and (2) assurance of safety and a temper of peace, and in relation to others, a preponderance of loving affection." ...William James*

Life energies research data and the practice of touch-healing prayer provide a revolutionary new understanding and foundation for religious beliefs and practice. *They supply rational explanation for what have always been considered religious mysteries, answering many of the questions about religion that people begin asking in childhood and that may remain unanswered throughout a lifetime.* They provide new reasons for participating in a religious community. They can be the basis for genuine understanding and cooperation between religions. As with any new understanding, they may give birth to new theological thought. They may also spur religious revival.

This new understanding is not for everyone. My own Wesleyan Christian tradition accepts knowledge about God that comes from scriptures, tradition, experience and reason (which includes science). This tradition accepts science and experience as valued means for knowing about God. Yet, even those persons whose beliefs are based solely upon sacred scriptures will find insight into the Word through the knowledge and processes described here.

RATIONALLY KNOWING GOD

In the Western religious traditions, understanding of the nature of God is based upon sacred scriptures and religious dogma. These essentially appeal to the spiritual mind by saying, *"Accept the spiritual truth of these scriptures and dogmas and you will find the basis for your religious beliefs, practices and salvation."*

The increasingly rational mind of modern humanity rejects the spiritual truth of scriptures and dogma. The rational mind can neither enter the necessary spiritual mind, based in a state of awareness, nor respect it. Thus, the rational mind is forced to reject sacred scriptures and religious dogmas. This has produced today's secular individual, family, community and society.

Life energies research data and the practice of touch-healing prayer can convince the rational mind that God exists. They also tell the rational mind about the nature of God and God's actions. With this new understanding, the rational mind is able to look at existing religious beliefs and practices with new awareness and appreciation.

THE RATIONAL MIND VERSUS THE SPIRITUAL MIND

Previously we have explored the opposing worldviews of Aristotle versus Plato, of Newtonian medicine versus Einsteinian medicine, and of the thinking-sensing personality type versus the feeling-intuitive personality type.

The Rational Mind. Aristotle's philosophy, Newtonian medicine and the thinking-sensing personality type all view the world in practical terms. Everything that matters in the world can be physically measured and quantified through rational thought and logic. This is the rational mind and worldview. There is no place in the rational mind for a powerful God who interacts with humans and heals through prayer. The rational mind must reject the significance of God, prayer, healing, love, compassion and forgiveness. The rational mind emphasizes that science and reason are the only guides that people need.

The Spiritual Mind. Aristotle's philosophy, Einsteinian medicine, and the feeling-intuitive personality type all view the world as originating from the spiritual, with the human spiritual dimension being immensely significant. This is the spiritual mind and worldview. The spiritual mind views spiritual transformation or renewal as a crucial stage in normal human development. Without spiritual renewal, humans cannot reach their full potential or a higher level of evolvement. *You cannot transform the Earth until you have spiritually transformed humanity.*

The Clash. These two approaches to life have disagreed throughout human religious history. From a religious perspective the rational mind represents fallen and sinful humanity. The demonic can be defined as that which opposes God's acting in the world. Therefore, the rational mind represents the demonic in humanity.

FALLEN HUMANITY AND SPIRITUAL AWAKENING

God's image in the Original Creation. Most of the world's religions believe that in the ancient past humanity was spiritually awakened. In those days, humans had direct contact with God, were bathed in spiritual wisdom, lived joyously and responsibly, and possessed divine powers. Humanity was created in the image of God and was sacred.

Most religions preserve an account of the *"fall of humanity"* into its present state of spiritual unconsciousness. For Muslims, Christians and Jews, humanity's *"Fall"* is described in the story of Adam and Eve in the Garden of Eden, in Genesis 3.

The Veil. At that time, a veil (or cover) was placed over the Spirit in each human. Because of this veil, people could no longer find that sacred spark within themselves, the Spirit, that connects them to God. Humans were forced to solve their own problems, to discover for themselves what was right and wrong. Without God, their options were limited by their reliance upon reason and logic, the rational mind.

The world's religions, each in their own way, tell the story of how humanity could not survive by its own wisdom and power without divine transformation and awakening. Individuals lost their capacity for such higher feelings as love, compassion, forgiveness, honesty and integrity. Humanity fell into a life of selfishness and sexual immorality, hatred and betrayal, murder and war. When the rational mind rejected the awareness of God and unbelief became common, humanity lost the source of its moral grounding and began responding only to the stimuli of self-interest and physical sensation.

Finding God. The purpose of most religions is to provide the means for humans to reestablish a firsthand contact with God. Those who establish this contact are transformed and awakened. These awakened persons, through divine guidance and experience, help others to find God. Always, it has been awakened persons who have generated the world's sacred writings.

The Spiritual Viewpoint. From the viewpoint of the spiritually awakened/renewed mind, or the spiritual mind, the rational mind is severely limited in its abilities. Humans are both flesh and spirit. To be whole, the physical, mental and emotional qualities must be nourished by spiritual awareness. They need direct contact with God in order to fill all seven energy fields with life-giving information, wisdom and power. Look at the following chart of Brennan's model of the human energy fields cited in chapter five.

THE FUNCTION OF EACH HUMAN ENERGY FIELD

1. Physical functioning and sensation.
2. Emotional life and feelings.
3. Mental life and linear thinking.
4. Love and the emotion of love.
5. The divine and the power of the Word.
6. Divine love.
7. The higher mind of knowing and integrating the spiritual and physical make-up.

Brennan states: *"There are specific locations within our energy system for the sensations, emotions, thoughts, memories and other non-physical experiences."* The rational mind can only nurture and program the first three energy fields of physical functioning and sensation, emotional life and feelings, and mental life and linear thinking.

A Major Breakthrough. The rational mind has little input into the four outer energy fields dealing with love, divine power and the Word, divine love and the higher mind. Humanity, through various religions, has struggled for thousands of years to understand these spiritual qualities and how to achieve them. We are now in the midst of major breakthroughs. Research data and the practice of healing prayer provide the missing pieces of the spiritual puzzle.

THE SEARCH FOR GOD'S GUIDANCE AND POWER

God Chooses Moses. Because the rational mind failed ancient humanity, alternatives were needed. In the Western religious traditions, Moses had a peak religious experience at the burning bush when God chose him as a prophet, as described in the third chapter of Exodus. During this peak religious experience, Moses was filled with ecstasy, joy, bliss, peace and wholeness. These qualities are characteristics of the transformation and empowerment experiences of everyone who becomes spiritually awakened.

Rules for the Rational Mind. The spiritually awakened Moses, possessing direct contact with God, gave his people the Ten Commandments and the Law in order to lead them away from their destructive way of living. The Law is composed of rules of good behavior devised for the rational mind with suitable punishments for disobedience. These were substitutes for the guidance to be had from the awakened spiritual mind, which humanity was not yet able to understand. (This is the same failed approach practiced in today's America, where harsher laws and punishments are viewed as the only solution for a morally failing culture. The only practical solution lies in a spiritual awakening of individual Americans.)

Throughout subsequent centuries, awakened prophets arose who spoke of the spiritual qualities of love, compassion and forgiveness -- and of a future time when rational laws would no longer be necessary, for God's Spirit would dwell within human hearts and personally guide each individual.

Spirit's Action. In the Christian tradition, Jesus became the God-Man, the Savior, a spiritually awakened person who had direct access to God and all the powers of God. In the coming of the Holy Spirit at Pentecost, everyone touched by the New Word of God in Jesus and the power of the Holy Spirit, became spiritually awakened and connected to the spiritual body of Christ, the Church. The rational mind takes a quantum leap forward in human evolution when it becomes awakened. Spirit-filled people became transformed into New Persons. Each new Christian, baptized with the power of the Word and the Spirit, had direct contact with God and the divine power to heal and perform miracles.

From the viewpoint of life energies research and touch-healing prayer, Jesus provided the spiritual information (the Word) and, at Pentecost, God's Spirit empowered that information. Forming a powerful sacred group energy field, the waiting followers experienced inner transformation as the information carried by the living, acting sacred group energy field bathed them. Not only did they experience spiritual transformation, they were, as well, empowered with divine abilities.

The sacred energy connection bonding the participants to each other is known as the mystical Body of Christ, the Church. All Spirit-filled practicing Christians today remain united and empowered by this sacred group energy connection as members of the Church. This bond is strengthened by peak religious experiences and the awareness that this sacred energy connection exists. This sacred energy connection between believers must have been taught to the baptized as a part of the secret knowledge available only to the initiates -- the new members of the Church.

Spiritual Results. These spiritual minds were made whole. They were not only filled with the Spirit, but also with the Word of God. This gave them the ability to integrate spiritual love, compassion and forgiveness with rational morality, responsibility and integrity. In other words, all seven human energy fields were filled with the healthy information for which people had been starving. This information acted intelligently to make them fully alive and whole. Becoming inspired and creative through the actions of the Spirit, the new believers found that the power of their new spiritual mind permitted their rational abilities to blossom.

Until the fifth century, all Christians were awakened by God's presence. They were baptized only after their spiritual transformation. This baptism connected them to all other Christians through the sacred group energy field connection -- the mystical Body of Christ. They were then initiated -- given special knowledge -- into the mysteries of the faith. This nurtured further awakening. God lived in their healthy energy fields. They lived constantly in a state of peak religious experience, filled with ecstasy, joy, bliss, peace and wholeness. They invoked this inner spiritual power to overcome the fear and pain present in the rational world, and to fight the darkness with God's marvelous light -- a light that filled their minds.

The Rational Mind Barrier. By the fifth century, the peak religious experience and the awakened mind became suspect. The rational mind of church administrators began hindering peak religious experiences. The knowledge of faith was confined within the context of rational sacred scriptures, writings, doctrine and tradition. Peak religious experiences were no longer considered appropriate, and rationally structured information about God became endorsed by religious authorities.

We see this pattern unfolding repeatedly throughout the centuries. A great need for change and reform would arise, followed by a wave of spiritual renewal. The renewal occurred when a peak religious experience transformed and awakened a leader and his followers. Reforms in spiritual practice, theology, or social consciousness would follow, and then, in the guise of administering those reforms, the rationally-minded church administrators again would put the lid on the people's free experience of the actions of God. Consequently, a sense of personal connection with the energy of the sacred disappeared from church tradition.

Universal Experiences. Most of the world's religions originated from similar peak religious experiences and the resulting awakened leadership. Most religions emphasize the teaching that without God, humans struggle. Most religions have a history similar to Christianity, wherein rational administrators and dogmatic traditions first hindered and then suppressed the peak religious experience of God-awakened believers.

Organized religion is the most conservative institution in any culture as it seeks to conserve religious, moral and social traditions, making them resistant to change. Organized religions have not been able to break out of their traditional molds to respond to the immense social changes that have swept humanity over the past three generations. The problem is that most religious traditions represent the rational mind, which does not possess the intuitive genius of the spiritual mind.

An ongoing struggle continues between awakened spiritual minds and rational minds, between the thinking of Plato and Aristotle, between the thinking of Isaac Newton and Albert Einstein. The rational mind insists on leaving out both God and the spiritual journey, even within organized religion.

RELIGIOUS RESPONSES TO THE RATIONAL MIND

The world's religions were not unaffected by the dominance of the rational mind. A rational acceptance of information about God, originally acquired through ancient peak religious experiences, is now considered to be all the connection to the spiritual that a believer needs. The experience of divine transformation and awakening are no longer regarded as necessary. Believers are suspicious of peak religious experiences, which they view as too irrational, emotional and scary -- an untrustworthy roadmap.

Fundamentalism arose in all the world's religions as the rational mind went to religious extremes. Fundamentalism takes religious beliefs achieved through peak religious experiences and entombs them in dogma and doctrine. The rational mind sees its creation of a legalistic Law of God as the Absolute Truth about God. It is characterized by manipulation, control, fear, anger, a distrust of non-believers, the hatred of many enemies, self-righteousness, human pride and nationalism. Like the rational mind without God, religious fundamentalism is demonic -- enslaving believers, turning people against each other, and creating the conditions for war. Love, compassion, forgiveness, freedom, transformation and a bonding with all Creation are in short supply for religious fundamentalists. By their fruits you will know them.

Charismatic and Pentecostal believers usually combine the recognition of the peak religious experience with the fundamentalist rational mind. While rejoicing in the peak religious experience, they express their fear of it by confining group members to a rigid set of traditional and rational religious and moral beliefs. If the transformed and awakened do not conform to these beliefs, they are labeled satanic or evil, and are shunned or ejected. Within these boundaries, no divine creative-intuitive guidance for reform exists. The new wine of the Spirit is always poured into the old wineskins of tradition.

I experience a personal sadness in this analysis. I am a charismatic Christian who has been nurtured in the liberal theological tradition. I, like millions of others like myself, do not feel comfortable as a member of any Christian community.

Even today, our shifting religious climate has only caused the rational mind-set to become more stubborn in its resistance. The present inconsistencies shown by members of the world's religions are cause for the non-believing rational mind to rejoice. Rationalists can point to many religious believers whose behavior makes a mockery of their own stated religious beliefs. Even when rationalists accept the idea that God exists, they point to such deluded believers as proof of God's inability to act effectively or meaningfully in the world.

New Agers. The New Age Movement has grown because of the interest of those who wish to learn more about their intuitive abilities and apply them in worthwhile ways. Most New Agers place a high priority upon a spiritual

journey with God. Many New Agers reject traditional Judeo-Christian beliefs. Instead, they build their belief system -- their theology, their Word of
God -- upon many religious traditions and *"channeled"* or inspired contemporary intuitive religious truths.

Their theology represents the spiritual mind gone to irrational extremes,
just like the Christian Gnostics in the Early Church. New Agers place no
value on developing a systematic theology that is rationally consistent.

One glaring example is their inconsistency in combining unconditional
love with karma. Karma is the world's most legalistic religious concept. It
is based upon the belief that no sin can be forgiven during a person's current earthly lifetime. Adding to this inconsistency, New Agers reject the
concept of sin that is basic to all karmic beliefs. Unconditional love is directly contrary to karmic concepts. In another inconsistency, unconditional
love is only possible through the existence of forgiveness, which is rejected
by New Agers. New Age theologies are irrational and, thus, unbelievable.

New Agers also ignore religious history. The world's religious beliefs
and sacred writings were built upon previous religious tradition, religious
communities and the inspired wisdom that flowed from them. They did not
build upon a vacuum in religious knowledge. Inspiration is channeled and
either elevated or distorted by the human mind that produces it. Any future
original revelation of God will **not** flow from intuitive inspiration alone. It
must come from the highest state of consciousness -- peak first-hand experiences of God that transform and empower a person into a *pure* or divine
channel for humanity's next evolutionary step upward.

SUSPICION OF ANYTHING RELIGIOUS IS WIDESPREAD

Nothing prepared me for the complete rejection of the word *"religious."* As I
began talking about the *peak religious experience,* people generally wanted
me to change the word *"religious"* to something else. The general public
wanted me to call it a *"peak spiritual experience."* Church people wanted
me to call it a *"peak faith experience."* I was shocked with the negative
emotional connotations associated with the word *religious.*

All my life, I have defined *religious* as that which pertains to God. Thus,
the ancient and respected term, *peak religious experience,* means a peak
experience of God. My Webster's Dictionary defines *spiritual* as pertaining
to the spirit or soul, although it popularly does refer to a journey with God.
My dictionary defines *faith* as unquestioning belief in God or specific religious beliefs, although popularly, it, too, refers to a journey with God. However, neither of these two terms are appropriate substitutes for the word *religious* in this context.

I am on a *faith journey,* a *spiritual journey* and a *religious journey.* When
you or I have a peak experience of God, that is a *peak religious experience.*
But however academically uncomfortable I feel about it, I bow to the negative feelings associated with the word, *religious.* I will from this point onward refer to the peak religious experience as *"a peak experience of God."*

The Spiritual Journey. As a parish minister for thirty years, I have
found that less than ten percent of church members were interested in a
spiritual journey within the Church. I also discovered that most members
were on a spiritual journey of their own, outside of organized religion.

This trend has increased. Today, most people are on a spiritual journey with God. Most do not accept all of the orthodox beliefs of the Church. They are each building a set of religious beliefs on their own, borrowing from many faith and cultural traditions. Continuing this trend, only about twelve percent of Americans are actively pursuing this journey within organized religion. Most of the other eighty-eight percent are privately exploring their own personal spiritual journeys. They seek spiritual transformation, awakening and wholeness. PrayWell provides understanding and guidance for anyone on the spiritual journey.

THE PRESENT HUMAN CONDITION

The rational mind has had three hundred years to prove its worth as creator of the dominant thought pattern in Western civilization. It believes that adequate education, knowledge, government, laws, income, housing, food, medicine and technology can solve all human problems and usher in a Golden Age of peace with justice and happiness for all.

Those are all worthy social goals. But, knowledge does not and cannot transform humanity. Transformation occurs through peak experiences of God that produce spiritual evolution. The products of the rational mind have left us in the dark pit we find ourselves in today, the same dark pit of which the Adam and Eve account warned.

Even today, the rational mind believes it can solve all problems. Everyone in the United States is demanding solutions to increasing violence, to the disintegration of the family, to personal isolation and the lack of community. But laws and punishment alone cannot transform people.

We all want a kinder, gentler, more caring nation. The rational mind cannot provide the solutions. In this perspective, the truly evil element in the world, the real demonic power, is that which opposes God's acting in the world -- the rational mind.

Resolving the Crisis. Our society is breaking apart and needs to be put back together. How do we love, rather than hate? How do we care in our depersonalized world? How do we build values that enhance life? How do we build a sense of community? How do we stop the violence, nurture and heal dysfunctional families, and rehabilitate chemical abusers and criminals? How do we enable people to love, express compassion, forgive, and become emotionally whole?

The answer is so easy. By tending to the health of all seven human energy fields. By providing ample opportunities for peak experiences of God that transform and nurture people into wholeness. These experiences lift people to a higher ground of human awareness and evolution. To do this requires joining with others in prayer.

HEALING PRAYER AND THE PEAK EXPERIENCE OF GOD

Here is where the importance of prayer enters the picture. Healing prayer produces peak experiences of God that can spiritually transform and awaken people. When I practice touch-healing prayer, I am consistently aware of an inner bliss. *Bliss* is defined as spiritual joy or great happiness. This experience of bliss makes healing encounters the happiest moments of my life.

Accompanying this bliss, this spiritual joy, are other emotions. There is always a sense of peace -- of an inner calmness or serenity. There is always a sense of heartfelt love -- of a joyous, generous, shared love. There is always a sense of holiness -- of a breathtaking and inspiring awareness of God. There is always a sense of connectedness with all life -- of a oneness with a larger whole. One is no longer tied to the boundaries of the physical world. There is no awareness of the physical body, emotions and thoughts.

These are the qualities of all peak experiences of God. No other human activity comes near to producing the bliss, peace, joy, holiness and connectedness of the peak experience of God. I have a strong suspicion that a natural yearning for peak experiences of God accounts for the large crowds at faith-healing services. This experience of holy bliss draws people to the charismatic movement and to Pentecostal churches, to daily prayer and to the search for spiritual renewal. *One peak experience of God can drive one to search for a life-time for a means of recapturing that initial bliss with God.*

EXPLORING THE PEAK EXPERIENCE OF GOD

Peak experiences of God are a normal and necessary part of any spiritual journey. But, the peak experience of God's Spirit does not transform and awaken the consciousness without possessing a consistent set of religious beliefs -- a meaningful theology. This set of religious beliefs is called God's Word.

A person can meditate, contemplate, visualize and pray for twelve hours a day forever without achieving transformation and awakening. God's Word must be present for these to happen. You can have a wonderful sense of ecstasy, joy, bliss, peace and wholeness, but without the knowledge of the divine Word, there is no spiritual transformation.

In this setting, peak experiences of God are just a wonderful sensual experience. They are a far better experiences than alcohol or other mind-altering drugs, but afterwards, they leave you just as far from God. Your energy fields temporarily light up and then dim again with no transformation. You end up unchanged.

In addition, one person alone may not produce enough divine power to ignite transformation. The power of God in prayer is the square of the number of people praying. That is a primary reason why people gather together for religious rituals. In doing so, they form a sacred group energy field that bathes everyone in God's Word and Spirit.

I am not saying that one cannot have a peak experience of God alone. Millions of people do. As will be shared later, I had a peak experience of God while alone during a health crisis that regenerated a diseased organ of my body. It took place following six weeks of daily meditative prayer. I have had hundreds of such experiences spanning my life. I have no way of knowing how many others have had similar experiences.

I had an advantage. I had already been transformed and awakened during a peak religious experience at age ten when I became a Christian. I had been bathed in the Spirit and the Word for almost thirty-years within the Christian community when this peak experience of God, and the subsequent healing, occurred. I was connected to the mystical Body of Christ. The Spirit and the Word already lived within me. I am aware of them as I write these sentences.

There is another side to this. The Word, alone, has little power to transform. God's Spirit makes the Word come alive. Yet, often the Spirit is contained in the Word. This is the primary reason that Christians distribute the Bible -- the Word for all Christians. Millions have been transformed and awakened by reading the Bible. One can read the Bible with the rational mind to learn information. The information, the Word, can also awaken the spiritual mind.

I never know when this will happen for me. While reading the Bible for information, unexpectedly the Spirit moves within me. A peak experience of God then overwhelms me and tears of joy will stream down my cheeks. Christ may be there with me, speaking personally to me.

God's Spirit causes religious information to take on a life of its own. It empowers religious beliefs so they can become encoded into the seven human energy fields. Without valid religious beliefs, peak experiences of God cannot transform and empower.

Most religions teach that God's Spirit transforms the believer into the revealed image of God, the Word, and, then, empowers that same believer with divine abilities. Most religions focus on these two essentials, the Word of God and the power of God's Spirit. You cannot succeed on your spiritual journey without these two elements.

PEAK EXPERIENCES AT THE MENNINGER CLINIC

During the past three years, accumulated scientific evidence indicates that any time a person is able to achieve a peak state of consciousness, personal transformation and empowerment can occur. Using biofeedback, you can learn to enter the low theta brain-wave state of four to eight frequencies per second. At that point, you get into a state of consciousness where you can move up and go into a state of revelry -- a peak state of pleasure, of ecstasy, joy, bliss, peace and happiness. This state is called the autogenic shift. At this point, you are operating at the back of the head in the left cortex or the left occipital lobe of the brain.

Elmer Green, PhD, who set up the Psychophysiology Lab at the Menninger Clinic in Topeka, Kansas in 1964, reports that through biofeedback a Westerner can attain the mystic state of the Tibetan or Hindu yogi in two to three days. The body, emotions and thoughts are quieted as you enter the unconscious, upper four levels of consciousness. This is known as self-mastery.[1]

In this state, you are at the *"white light"* level of the peak experience of God. In Zen Buddhism, this is known as the True Self. In Christian mysticism, this is known as the Christ Level. In Tibet, they call this place the Jewel in the Lotus. The Sufis and the Kaballa, and in fact, all religions talk about this level of consciousness.

At this consciousness level, you can focus your intentions downward for the transformation of the body, emotions and thoughts. When alcoholics get up to this theta state, they can turn their attention downwards to the hypothalamus and are able to rewire the hypothalamus so that they no longer want to drink. This has been done with six thousand alcoholic subjects at the Menninger Clinic.

During the peak experience of God, the Word and the Spirit, working together, begin to automatically transform the believer into the qualities of the revealed image of God through the hypothalamus area of the brain. Along with transformation can come ongoing empowerment with spiritual abilities, such as prophecy and healing. You have an experience of Heaven and bring it back to earth with you. *You must be personally transformed before you can begin transforming the world.*

COMMON ELEMENTS OF RELIGIOUS EXPERIENCES

An enduring or perennial spiritual wisdom runs through all the world's religions. This comes from mystics -- those who encounter God at the highest levels. A beneficial peak experience of God contains an awareness of ecstasy, joy, bliss, peace and wholeness. This experience includes an awe and wonder of God and a oneness with God, the Creator and Sustainer. It begins a transformation that includes spiritual love, compassion, forgiveness, the need to serve others, a sense of inner freedom and sacredness and a connectedness with other believers. At the highest levels it results in a oneness or connectedness with all humanity and everything that God has created.

Discernment. If your peak experience of God contains the opposite elements of any of these qualities, be careful. Either your religious beliefs (Word) are faulty, or you are tapping into your own baser self, or you are being influenced by the destructive religious beliefs of others. Being able to determine the beneficial qualities of any religious experience is known as discernment.

THE HUMAN INFLUENCE IN RELIGIOUS EXPERIENCES

From healing research data and experience, we know human intentions and expectations affect the results. In touch-healing, a depressed or cynical healer or pray-er may cause an illness to become worse. The transmitted energy is not at a healing frequency when the pray-er is feeling anger, hatred, resentment or inadequacy. Such prayers can harm others.

Voodoo magic can be used to heal or to harm. The results are based upon the intentions and the Word used by the practitioner. All religious rituals are a form of magic. All religious rituals invoke a spiritual power or entity to act and to have an effect in our physical universe. Prayer is a form of ritual magic.

Any prayer that seeks to harm another person is a form of harmful or black magic. When you are seeking the destruction of an enemy through prayer, this is black magic. When Christians do this, it is not spiritual warfare. It remains black magic -- an evil.

When you are convinced that a critically ill person is going to die, do not pray for their healing. The energy of your prayers will contain your negative beliefs and hasten a death that might not have occurred without your negative energy.

Human Influence. The human mind has a powerful influence upon the Spirit's actions. Everyone agrees that there is one Divine Spirit for all humanity. In the exploration of group energy fields, <u>PrayWell</u> has repeatedly noted that all groups form energy fields and the information present within those energy fields is produced by the intentions, attitudes, emotions, thoughts, beliefs and actions of those participating in the group energy field.

Limits of Healing Energy. A healing group energy field is not the best setting for transformation and awakening. That is not the intention of the information in the energy. The intention is to produce healing results in the three inner energy fields: physical, mental and emotional. The healing energy lacks some of the qualities necessary for spiritual transformation. In most such healing services, I sense a powerful energy and peace. Sometimes an element of love is present, but it is rare to sense ecstasy, joy and bliss.

The Spirit Alone. My observation is that God's Spirit, when left alone, is religiously and morally neutral. God's Spirit (subtle energy or life energy) fills the universe. Left on its own and independent of humanity, the Spirit does possess information that acts to create and sustain life. Its energy is the source of life for all living organisms as it quietly acts to sustain and restore energy fields.

The Living Word. When you have been spiritually transformed and awakened, then the Spirit acts within you according to the Word that is now living within you. However, there seem to be exceptions to this. Noah, Moses, Ezekiel and Isaiah appear to have been called by God to service in order to declare a new Word. The Christian-persecuting Saul appears to have been possessed by Christ because God needed him to be an evangelist and missionary. At times, the purposeful Word takes us over, producing transformation without free will. This is known as predestination or divine destiny.

Satanism. In the case of Satanism, the Spirit of God is being called upon to do evil. I believe this is due to the evil Word used in the intentions and rituals of the participants. They are invoking evil to happen through ritual magic. Being itself essentially neutral, the Spirit empowers the content of *any and all* religious beliefs.

Identical Results. The end results of religious transformation and awakening are identical in most religions. In the limited contacts I have had with awakened people of other faith traditions, I have sensed no difference between their energy field information and my own. I sense love, peace, joy and acceptance. I feel comfortable with my brothers and sisters of other faith traditions. The perennial wisdom of the mystics is present in the awakened of all faith traditions.

I have also sensed the energy of Satanists and black magicians in which I have been aware of information at great variance with the perennial wisdom. On those occasions, a discordant shiver of fear has passed through me and I have needed to disconnect from them.

Spirit Possession. Like attracts like. If we are not filled with God's Spirit, being empty, we are susceptible to being filled with other spirits (energy forms). The rational mind is more susceptible to addictive-compulsive-obsessive behaviors. We can be filled with the spirit of obsessive, compulsive and addictive behaviors -- chemical dependencies, obesity, materialism, consumerism and sexual deviancy. We can be filled with the spirit of greed, jealousy or envy. We can be filled with spirits of illness. We can be filled with the spirits of hatred, violence, coldness and cruelty. These often begin with small ventures into one of these areas that attract negative energy forms that slowly possess and eventually completely dominate and enslave. Our best protection is through being filled with God's Word and Spirit. Some spirit energy forms are so resistant to leaving their hosts that only a ritual of exorcism works to expel them.

The rational mind does have access to God. The rational mind can be filled with God's Spirit through a person's life-style. Moral actions based upon love, compassion, forgiveness, caring service, and peace-making, can fill one with God's Spirit. Becoming close to nature opens spiritual awareness. The fine arts -- music, visual arts and literature -- can produce spiritually transforming experiences without the mention or awareness of God. All these work to repair all seven human energy fields.

The birth of each of my daughters was a joyous and satisfying experience. But for my wife, Dana, it was an even more powerful experience. Following the birth of each child, I observed Dana in the midst of a peak experience of God, her face glowing with bliss and ecstasy -- in awe of the sacred miracle of birth.

A RATIONAL "WORD OF GOD"

Every prayer would be answered if God's healing energy flowed freely and purely through us. Unfortunately, as the healing energy passes through us, we change its quality. Our feelings, thoughts, attitudes and beliefs alter the purity, frequency, and intentions of the healing energy. They program it.

One major factor we can attempt to control is our religious beliefs. If we don't know what we believe about God, our prayers tend to be tentative and to lack power. Consistent and clear beliefs about God also produce a purer quality of healing energy. These beliefs become God's Word, programming the energy of our Therapeutic Prayers.

You already hold religious beliefs, some of which may sabotage your Therapeutic Prayer intentions. Here, PrayWell seeks to provide you with religious beliefs based upon life energies research and the practice of healing prayer. Perhaps we need only one belief -- that God's love and healing power are ever present and available to you, the pray-er. Yet, we must be careful not to hold other beliefs that dilute or negate our pure intention of expressing love.

Life energies research and the practice of healing prayer provide us with rational knowledge about God. From this, we can build a rational theology -- a set of religious beliefs, or the Word of God for prayer. Here is a rational creed -- God's Word for prayer.

A RATIONAL CREED -- GOD'S WORD FOR PRAYER

I believe in God, who created the physical universe and continues to sustain it. God is always present, seeking to provide the optimum conditions for all life.

I believe that God reveals the divine nature through the physical creation, through first-hand experiences of God that provide knowledge, wisdom, revelation, transformation and empowerment, through the life energy that fills the universe, and through the process of science and reason. Through intuitive-creative guidance, God personally provides us with direction and purpose.

I believe that God is the source of all love, joy, peace, awe, ecstasy, compassion, caring, goodness, wholeness, renewal, unity, and justice.

I believe that God created us in the divine image, meaning that we are, like God, intelligent, creative, energy bodies who are eternal, and thus, will always exist.

I believe that we are connected to each other and to everything that exists through God's information-bearing, intelligently-acting energy that pervades the universe.

I believe that God calls all humanity to be co-creators and co-sustainers of our universe. God transforms and empowers us for this purpose through peak experiences of God and in our acts of love, creativity, justice-seeking, prayer and religious ritual. Through these, we become priests, bringing the power of God into the life of the world.

I believe that prayer is the primary means by which God is able to restore purpose, order, love and goodness to the universe, replacing chaos and evil with divine good and purpose.

I believe that through prayer we accumulate, attune and transmit the divine life force or healing energy, as we bring the power of God into the life of the world. Life energy renews the human energy fields, working like a cosmic antibiotic to produce physical, emotional, mental, spiritual and interpersonal health and happiness. Life energy can heal any disease.

I believe that God wills every person to be healthy and whole. Any failure to achieve this is due to human ignorance and interference.

I believe that God calls us to live in peaceful community with all humanity, through love, unity, respect and cooperation. These act to produce understanding, forgiveness and reconciliation, cooperation and support, justice and responsibility, and true wholeness.

I believe that God transforms and empowers us to live on a higher ground of spiritual wisdom based upon the divine Word. Through prayer, God unites human beings in energy-laden sacred group energy fields that bathe everyone with the Word. The Word, empowered by the Spirit, connects, transforms, and empowers individuals, couples, families, friends, communities and nations, encoding the Word into their energy fields and producing wholeness. Sacred group energy fields also hold the power to restore every other portion of God's creation.

I believe God is consistent in all these qualities because God's basic nature is to nurture the optimum conditions for life and abundant living.

RATIONAL REASONS FOR RELIGIOUS BELIEFS

What does the data of life energies research and the practice of healing prayer teach us about the rational reasons for religious beliefs and practice? These articles expand our faith understanding.

The Soul and Spirit. Achieving contact with the soul and the Spirit is the central purpose of all religions. I feel inadequate in defining the soul and the Spirit. I want, nevertheless, to share my understanding with you.

The soul consists of all the information present in the seven human energy fields. The soul is the energy blueprint for not only the physical body, but also for our thoughts, memories, personality, emotions and spirituality. The soul is our identity, our personality, our *spiritual body.* The soul, minus the first energy field, the physical energy field, is eternal and survives the death of the physical body.

The purpose of the soul is to grow and evolve into a higher awareness. This is achieved through spiritual and moral transformation in which the Word of God and the Spirit bathe the soul with new life. This is a process occurring throughout one's life. Transformation fills one with love and the need to live a selfless life devoted to serving others.

Transformation also unmasks a person's Spirit, which bathes the soul with God's power from within. This is the purpose of all religions; to help people get into contact with the Spirit. The Spirit resides within every soul. It is the free gift of God's presence in every person. It is one's core of life energy. It is hidden from our awareness and most often lies dormant until freed through transformation and awakening. It is like a three hundred watt light bulb covered by a shield that only permits ten watts of light life to glow until touched by God, who slowly removes the shield as awakening continues.

Only a few ever glow with the full three hundred watts. When they do, they become celebrated mystics who expand on God's works and the Word. The Spirit is the true self. As one's Spirit is unveiled, one's life is transformed, empowered and guided. Your Spirit is connected to God and, as such, is always perfect as it is.

God cannot touch our souls nor free our Spirits until we voluntarily open ourselves. Touch-healing confirms the reality of human free will. The healing energy cannot enter a person without permission, as we can shield our energy fields from all outside energies. In my own faith tradition, we ask people to invite Christ into their lives and verbally to accept Christ as the Lord of their lives.

Sin simply means to be separated from the Spirit -- to live a life veiled away from God. Barbara Ann Brennan[2] produced clairvoyant drawings on the effects of the specific damage caused to human energy fields by drugs, alcohol, anger, grief, etc. The accuracy of these drawings is proving itself over time as they provide effective working models for healing efforts. These drawings reveal that human energy fields may become polluted, darkened and unhealthy, producing the need for restoration. The drawings also display the enhancement of human energy fields produced by music, play and meditation.

In the practice of touch-healing, we know that drugs, alcohol, anger and grief hinder the ability of the human energy fields to be in contact with God.

We also know that Therapeutic Prayer restores the ability of people to experience God. Healing and salvation can occur through any action that repairs or transforms the human energy fields.

Salvation means that we have been transformed and awakened by the Word and the Spirit and have taken on the spiritual mind. The experience of the human condition is that our energy fields become distorted, weakened and crippled through life experiences. As the energy fields break down, we become physically ill, emotionally upset, mentally confused, interpersonally alienated and morally vulnerable. Salvation restores the energy fields.

We have sayings like, *"Christ makes all things new,"* and *"God created and he continues to recreate."* These saying become literally true at the moment of salvation. God *is* the life energy in its purest form. We become whole -- another term for salvation.

The quality of the human energy fields takes a quantum leap forward as one becomes a New Person as God's information-containing, living energy field is integrated into one's personal human energy fields. Taking on the *mind of Christ* means that the qualities of Christ have become encoded into the human energy fields.

Heaven. Acquiring *eternal life*, which must be done in this physical world, means that the human energy fields have become so transformed that they are able upon physical death to enter a specific afterlife sector like Heaven, because the quality of the human energy fields match the electromagnetic frequencies of the energy fields dimension of that sector.

Hell. Evil is an expression of chaos. Chaos occurs in the absence of the Word and the Spirit. When at death, the human energy fields are in a state of utter chaos, the soul enters the afterlife sector with the energy frequencies of chaos. This is what we call Hell, the spiritual dimension where utter chaos rules. Through prayer, God introduces order and purpose into chaos. Without God, utter chaos rules, enabling evil to live and to act.

Backsliding. Salvation occurred for me at the age of ten. That does not mean that I remained in that optimum state. For this to happen, I needed a continuous bathing in God's power through a variety of means. When that did not happen, I backslid. Remembering how wonderful full salvation is, I hungered for it. I wanted to be restored to full wholeness through God.

Spiritual renewal is soul development as one seeks to renew all seven human energy fields. An individual's beliefs, thoughts, attitudes, worship, meditation, prayer and loving actions all help transform the human energy fields. Each energy field vibrates at a different frequency. Clinical evidence suggests that these frequencies change with spiritual growth.

It is likely that we already have the scientific capability to measure these frequencies. With application, we will be able to determine the frequencies of the various levels of wholeness. This will enable us to quantify levels of health and spiritual maturity, and lead to simple ways of determining the truth of persons and situations. Hypocrites will no longer be able hide behind masks of respectability. We will be able to stop lie detector and psychological testing, instead choosing quality workers, spouses and friends according to the compatible frequencies of their energy fields.

The practice of touch-healing prayer began opening my thinking in this whole area. While praying for wholeness in body, mind and spirit, I sensed God's healing energy being transmitted to the healee's spiritual body (human energy fields). I noticed that even when healing did not occur, the healee often experienced the presence of God's love, joy and peace for about two days. It sometimes imparted the information through changes in thoughts, emotions, attitudes and beliefs. I realized that, in the proper context, prayers for healing produce a salvation experience. But religious knowledge is necessary for this to occur. The healing energy's presence made the existing religious knowledge, the Word, come alive in the healee for a brief time.

Religious rituals empower the Word and the Spirit. Gathering believers together in ritual, bathes everyone in the resulting sacred group energy field. This intelligent-acting information works over time to unite, transform, awaken and empower believers.

During the ritual of **Christian baptism**, God's Spirit is intentionally transferred by touch to the recipient. God then begins living within the recipient's energy fields. For a time, the energy fields of the baptized glow with and are protected by God's energy. Of course, God is literally present in all religious ritual. I, myself, have witnessed countless physical, emotional, mental and interpersonal healings occur during baptism, confirmation, communion and ordination.

Wedding rituals form an energy-bonding uniting the bride and groom into a spiritual, emotional and physical oneness as *"the two become one."* From that time on a cord of divine energy continues to unite them, unless it is broken. This created unity may make some spouses feel smothered.

One of the reasons that separation and divorce are so painful is because divine energy, the tie that binds, still exists. A prayer ritual can sever this cord, ending much emotional anguish. Such a prayer ritual is provided in Part Four. Love among family members and friends produce similar energy bonding/uniting. Casual sexual contacts can also produce such ties.

Grief is deepened by two energy factors. First, we miss the presence of the deceased one's energy field. Second, we may continue to be linked through the energy cord that binds. Touch-healing prayer can restore wholeness to grieving energy fields.

The Word's Significance in Healing. The Word of God must be present in every healing encounter. The Word comes from the qualities present in the energy of the healer's mind, soul, intentions and energy fields. In healing, the content of the Word of God involves many qualities. The Word of God for the healer involves such qualities as love, acceptance, faith, hope, compassion, expectancy, trust, confidence. Thankfully, in therapeutic spoken prayer made by caring loved ones, people of all religions naturally express the Word of God for wholeness and renewal.

Best Expressions. The Word of God is primarily expressed by all religions in the printed Word and the spoken Word. PrayWell is an expression of the printed Word. The therapeutic prayers in the practical applications of Parts Two, Three and Four are expressions of the spoken Word. The Spirit empowers both the printed and spoken Word. Without the Word, the Spirit does not act powerfully nor significantly.

Ineffective Idealism. There can be no spiritual development without the Word. Meditation, contemplation and visualization possess no spiritual power unless the participant is aware of the Word of God. In the absence of the Word, a person can feel peaceful and centered, but without any significant transformation or empowerment occurring.

Deep Belief. Religious commitment or deeply held religious beliefs (the Word) further empower God's Spirit. So, no matter what rituals are being used, the Word must be clearly expressed. If you want God's Spirit to act powerfully in a sacred group energy field, it helps to have all participants sharing common, deeply held, religious beliefs.

The Spirit in Groups. Any time two or more people gather together they form a group energy field. Healing encounters, couples, families, classrooms, work places, communities and nations all form group energy fields. If you wish health and happiness in any of these settings, then Therapeutic Prayers should to employed by every participant, expressing the Word for that situation, to empower the actions of God's Spirit. A sacred group energy field will then be formed that bathes everyone, transforming and empowering them.

A SCIENTIFIC SOURCE FOR LIFE ENERGY

Physicist John Zimmerman,[3] founder and president of Bio-Electro-Magnetics of Reno, Nevada, proposes a rational source for life energy. Dr. Zimmerman suggests that the source of life energy is our planet, Earth. Earth resonates with the Schumann Frequencies that exit with the Earth-ionosphere resonant cavity at seven to eight hertz. He asks, *"Is it not within the realm of possibility that some people can perceive the seven to eight hertz brain-wave frequency of the Earth?"*

Zimmerman's theory is that healers have either the innate or trained capacity to detect the weak variations of the earth's electromagnetic fields, the Schumann Frequencies. He suggests that the healing frequency varies, as do the Schumann Frequencies, with the time of day, month and year and the phases of the moon. The Schumann Frequencies vary from plus or minus 7.83 hertz. That variation appears to be identical to that of the healing frequency. Attuning for healing occurs by matching human brain-waves with the varied frequencies of Earth.

It is also necessary for the healer's respiration rate either consciously or subconsciously to adjust itself to become an exact sub-harmonic of the ongoing Schumann Frequency to facilitate the brain-wave synchronization. Normal respiration is about twelve breaths per minute.

If the Schumann Frequency is 7.8 hertz, the healer would need enough control to breathe exactly 0.195 breaths per second, the equivalent of 11.7 breaths per minute. This would give a Schumann Frequency and respiration rate of exactly 40 (7.8 divided by 0.195). The healer must then transmit this frequency to the brain of the healee, producing synchronized brain-waves.

Dr. Robert Beck, nuclear physicist, confirmed Zimmerman's theory. Beck found that during healing encounters, the healer's brain waves became both frequency- and phase-synchronized with the Schumann waves.

"That means the healer's brain waves pulse not only at the same frequency but also at the same time as the earth's Schumann waves. It could be assumed that healers are able to take energy from the magnetic field of the earth for the healing of patients. This process is called field coupling."[A] It is clear that what healers call "grounding into the earth" is the action of linking up with the magnetic field of earth, both in frequency and phase.

Dr. Edgar Wilson[5] proved that Israeli healer David Joffee impressed his brain-wave pattern upon a healee in order to produce healing. The healee must voluntarily allow this entraining to occur.

Dr. John Zimmerman went a step further. He found that once healers have linked up with the Schumann frequencies, the right and left hemispheres of their brains become balanced with each other and show a 7.8 to 8 hertz alpha rhythm.[6] In touch-healing, it has been shown that patients' brain waves also go into alpha and are phased-synchronized with the healers', as well as right-left balanced. The healer has linked the client with the earth's magnetic field pulses and has thereby tapped into a tremendous energy source for healing.[7]

Scientists possess evidence that life energy permeates not only our planet but our whole planetary system and our galaxy, as well. Earth as a single energized planetary body may be energetically linked to all physical matter in our solar system, producing an information-bearing, intelligently-acting energy field that encompasses our whole solar system. Our solar system may be similarly linked to the systems of other stars. Or, our solar system may be unique in possessing life energy -- the basis for all life.

Other scientists are exploring life energy as a new energy source capable of replacing nuclear power. Is life energy the fifth minor force scientists are looking for to balance their equations about the nature of the universe?

This discussion raises theological questions. Is the peak experience of God due to attunement with the Schumann Frequencies? Is Earth a living, breathing, information-bearing, intelligently-acting entity attuned to bring optimum life and spiritual wisdom to all of her inhabitants?

SACRED GROUP ENERGY FIELDS IN RELIGIOUS HISTORY

I have always considered the miracles of the Bible to be quite literally true. I have also chuckled at the attempts of biblical scholars to explain away miracles as symbolic stories or of scientists to explain specific miraculous events rationally. The existence of powerfully acting sacred group energy fields provides all the credibility needed for miracles.

How did Jesus calm a stormy sea? Storms are filled with energy and all he needed to do was to change the energy patterns and the storm and waves could be calmed. The energy released by a group in prayer can produce similar results.

The two most astounding group events in the Bible involve the Exodus and Pentecost. Here is a scientific energy field explanation.

The Parting of the Red Sea. The Bible indicates that both Moses and Aaron possessed immense spiritual abilities. They were obviously ENFJs. (See chapter eight.) They were group catalysts, attuners and psi sensitives.

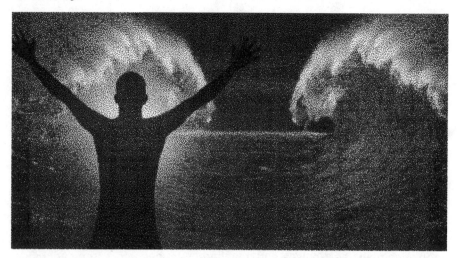

Figure 8. *Moses parting the Red Sea by focusing the immense energy of the sacred group energy field created by the fear and aspirations of the fleeing Hebrew people. A prayer-induced planetary group energy field would produce the most powerful man-made creative force ever known.*

With the ability of their personality types, their divine destiny and the sacred group energy field created by the high emotional and spiritual energies of two hundred thousand Hebrews fleeing before the advancing Egyptian army, parting the waters of the Red Sea would have been possible. They possessed the skills and forty billion energy units of prayer power. With this, they created two energy barriers as solid as poured concrete, damming the waters so they could walk across the sea bed. When all had passed, the energy barriers were withdrawn, trapping the pursuing Egyptian army. Read the story (Exodus 14:10-15:18). Moses' actions match this description.

Pentecost as a God-Empowered Group Energy Field. The Resurrected Christ told the disciples to wait in Jerusalem for the Holy Spirit to bring them power (Acts 1). At Pentecost, fifty days later, that power of the Holy Spirit swept over them (Acts 2). They were told to wait, to stay together, to expect God's power. They did all this in the context of Jesus' ministry, his teachings, the drama of the Passion and the post-Resurrection appearances. For the disciples, these events all formed a powerful drama of God's revelation to them. This is the revealed image of God and the Word of God for Christians.

The beliefs of those who awaited Pentecost are important. Those beliefs are the contents of God's revelation of the Word to the Disciples. God is love. God heals. God transforms and awakens. God in Jesus overcomes the world. God resurrects. God empowers. These are a part of the content of their revealed image of God. When the Holy Spirit came with power at Pentecost, it was in the context of that belief system, the Word of God as known in Jesus. The Disciples and others, gathered in expectation of the Pentecost, helped create the enormous sacred group energy field by their memories, thoughts and anticipations. This preparation was necessary for the Holy Spirit's actions on Pentecost.

God acts apart from humanity to shape human history. God's revelations are always filtered through the person and personality of a human being, through an Abraham, Isaac or Jacob, a Moses, or a Jeremiah or Isaiah. God also acts through groups of persons gathered together, as on Pentecost or in religious ritual. Their intentions, and the information in individual energy fields, creates a sacred group energy field that we have always thought of as God, acting alone and independent of persons.

God's power at Pentecost was like a nuclear explosion. Tongues of fire from the Holy Spirit -- God's living, intelligently-acting energy -- encompassed the waiting crowd. Thousands were gathered. They all knew the revelation of God in Jesus, their revealed image of God. The power of God and this new revelation of God's love -- the Word -- interacted. The energy fields of those gathered were encoded with this combination.

God's power in the Spirit enabled the believers to fit all the pieces of the new revelation together so that it made sense. Three thousand believers were transformed and empowered by baptism that day. That is nine million units of prayer power plus the power of the Word and the Holy Spirit. The power of Pentecost, placed in the human energy fields of each believer as their revealed image of God, was passed on powerfully by touch and by energy fields throughout the next four centuries of preaching, conversion, miracle-making and healing that dominated and then overwhelmed the cultures it touched. In the Fifth Century, the rationally-minded church administrators deadened the connection to the Holy Spirit. They continue to do this today.

Understanding this, a planetary Pentecost-type explosion of re-creation and transformation could happen if humanity had a new, universal revealed image of God exciting to everyone. Just imagine using the mass media to unite five billion people in common prayer for renewal. The energy created would be 25,000,000,000,000,000,000 units of prayer power. Theoretically, this could transform every person on earth to optimum health and life. It could bring about the ecological restoration of the planet Earth's oceans, air, ozone layer and forests, ushering in a Golden Age of peace with justice for all life. It is a vision that you can promote by pioneering experiments as explained later in PrayWell.

GOD'S LOVE IS UNIVERSAL

Parts of the Christian revealed image of God may also be present in persons who are not believers or church members or who are of other religions. Christians do not have an exclusive patent on the divine quality known as love. Most religions believe in the importance of love. The Christian revealed image of God's quality of compassionate love can be found in most persons at some level. In the Christian context, when the Word and the Holy Spirit come alive and produce salvation in a person, it does transform him into a person who shines with God's love.

This all sounds good on paper, yet it is quite complex. It may take a lifetime to integrate love into responsible expressions in the other energy fields. Compassionate love appears to have strong genetic and hormonal elements. New medical evidence indicates that the natural nurturing qualities of women are both genetic and hormonal. Compassionate love may be more rooted in innate personality traits than religious belief, with salvation only amplifying personality traits.

An individual's personality traits may be highly regarded in one religion while being seen as negative by another. American Christians hold in high regard the personality traits of persons who are warm, friendly, loving, generous and outgoing. We say these are *Christian* traits and the qualities necessary for sainthood, when in fact their source may be due more to the genetics of the personality traits and cultural expectations of American Christians. An American who is the reserved, introverted, thinking personality type may be out of place within a Christian community, yet feel right at home in another religion like Hinduism.

All of this is important for our understanding of group energy fields. A group energy field is created by the contents of individual human energy fields; all the mental, emotional, moral and spiritual qualities present in each of the individual human energy fields combine in the group energy field focused upon a specific goal or event.

There is one God of all creation. He is the God of Jews and Christians, of Hindus and Muslims and of all other religions. There is one God who reveals his true nature to all cultures and peoples. The qualities of God as Creator and Sustainer are known in all religions. In all religions, God transforms, empowers and heals. These attributes are known in every community and religion.

In a like manner, healers throughout the world emanate a healing energy at identical frequencies. The healing effects of all healers are identical. Being in contact with God and being compassionate are common factors of healers in all cultures. These universal qualities promote health and wholeness.

HEALTH RELATED TO RELIGIOUS PARTICIPATION

With this background understanding, it comes as no surprise that two 1992 studies linked religious participation to better health. Purdue University medical sociologist Kenneth F. Ferraro, reporting in the *Journal for the Scientific Study of Religion,* concluded that those who practice their faith regularly are healthier than those who don't. In his study of 1,473 people randomly selected nationwide, those who practiced their religion through prayer, religious services and religious study were more than twice as healthy as those who don't. Nine percent in the non-practicing group reported poor health in comparison to only four percent in the religion practicing group. Those associated with mainline denominations such as Episcopalians, Presbyterians, Methodists, Lutherans and Roman Catholic had better health than Jehovah's Witnesses, Mormons, Christian Scientists and some Baptists.

In *Psychological Reports*, William Oleckno, professor of community health, and Michael J. Blacconiere of Hines Veterans Administration Hospital, found religious commitment to be strongly related to wellness, non-use of tobacco, alcohol and drugs, and use of seat belts among 1,077 Northern Illinois University students. This correlation was directly related to the frequency of attendance at religious services.

Chapter Eleven

Evidence for the Existence of God

"Every man takes the limits of his own vision for the limits of the world." ...Arthur Schopenhauer

"Religious experiences should be evaluated in terms of their philosophical reasonableness and moral helpfulness." ...William James*

"God intended that his unity be reflected by unity of life, and that unity requires that prayer be an essential part of life." ...Olive Wyon*

Humanity has always yearned for evidence that God exists. Throughout the centuries, philosophers have attempted to prove the existence of God through reason, based upon what was known about the physical universe. No philosophical arguments have ever been convincing to me. The only branch of philosophy popular today is metaphysics, which seeks to explain the nature of the universe through intuitive means, like channeled information. No metaphysical explanation has been convincing for me. Only a subjective knowing of God through religious experience, beliefs and commitments had provided me with any certainty. That is how I became convinced of God's existence. Let us take a look at my own subjective knowing of God.

As a youth, I was rooted and grounded in Christ and the Church. This included infant baptism, an early conversion experience, Christian education classes, confirmation, singing in the church choir and leadership in the youth group. Then, as a nineteen year-old engineering student, I took a step backward. Despite my having had many peak experiences of God, God had become remote to me, like someone I had dreamed of in the distant past. I was no longer being bathed by God's presence in the Church. My despair became intense. I yearned for some enormous proof that God existed. I now realize this was *"the dark night of my soul."*

Then came the evening when I found myself on the roof of the dormitory in the midst of a monstrous thunderstorm. The winds howled and the rain pelted me. Deafening thunder roared in my ears and great bolts of lightning tore at my eyes. I found myself filled with an enormous rage. I stood soaking wet and shook my fist at the sky in defiance, shouting a challenge, *"God, if you are out there, then strike me dead with a bolt of lightning! Then, at least, I will know that you exist!"*

I had had an urgent hunger to hear God speak or, at least, show some evidences of his presence in the universe. God had manifested himself to biblical characters in ancient days. Why didn't God show himself vividly to his people today? I would squirm uncomfortably while singing the hymn stanza, *"I ask no dream, no prophet ecstasies, no sudden rending of the* veil of clay, no angel visitant, no opening skies; but take the dimness of my soul away." Those words were contrary to everything I wanted to experience. I yearned for visions, for prophetic ecstasies, and to see or hear God firsthand.

During the ensuing years, my hunger for God did not diminish. My theological education provided me with a meaningful Word. Worship and the Christian community bathed me in the Word and the Spirit. I did draw closer to God. I found satisfaction in donning the mantle of priesthood and serving as a parish pastor. I felt God's Spirit dwelling quietly within me. I had a few peak experiences of God whose effects were brief. In the midst of this, I desired more than anything else to see God at work in a more evidential way. I wanted an ongoing "rending of the veil of clay" -- to see the ancient evidences of a God who reveals himself with words and performs miracles. Then God responded to my yearnings by playing his little joke upon me.

Here I was, a well-educated clergyman starting on my path to professional success. I did not believe that God heals. I had even denounced any such possibility from the pulpit. Then, while praying with a dying man, I had a peak experience of God, in the midst of which I felt an energy descend upon my head and shoulders, and flow down my arm and into the dying man's hand. This resulted in the man's complete healing during our five-minute prayer. The healings continued and a sense of excitement accompanied each healing encounter. Along with this came frustration. What do I do with this newly discovered ability in a church and society that, not only do not believe in healing prayer, but ridicule and shun those who practice it? Who ever heard of an intellectual liberal Christian who practices touch-healing prayer? I think God is still laughing at my dilemma.

I eventually realized that God had given me the divine experiences for which I had so deeply yearned. It was a side-effect of touch-healing prayer -- consistently repeatable peak experiences of God. I was shocked by the dawning realization that healing encounters fulfilled my previous yearnings for God. Exploring this phenomenon has kept me fascinated for more than a quarter of a century. Each healing encounter has placed me, and still places me, in a state of spiritual ecstasy. "O Joy that never lets me go; my heart is forever filled with You!" That is subjective certainty about God's existence.

YOUR POSSIBLE DIFFICULTIES WITH GOD

I have summarized my own personal faith journey to inspire you. You may have your own doubts about the existence of God as you use PrayWell. That may be more of an issue for you than the question of the truth of healing prayer. Is there really a God who responds to my prayers? Church rituals, deep love, altruistic service and prayer are all effective means by which God's presence can enter our lives. As you practice self-healing or touch-healing, you will develop a wonderful awareness of God's presence. That is a given. As you learn to practice spoken prayer with loved ones, you and your whole family will be filled and constantly bathed with God's renewing and sustaining presence. Until then, you may be filled with doubts about the existence of God.

THE ISSUES

Aside from assuring people who need a scientific argument for the existence of God, what other issues are involved? The issues are many.

Public Attitudes. I seek to remove the sense of secrecy and shame that surrounds the practice of prayer. Although surveys report that ninety-nine percent of Americans have prayed, most people prayer secretly, hiding this activity as if with a great sense of shame. It is socially forbidden to pray aloud outside of a religious setting. Those who do so can count on being shunned or rebuked or regarded as a bit weird. If the existence of God can be proven as a scientific fact, this shame and secrecy will diminish.

The Use of Therapeutic Prayer. If the existence of God becomes accepted as a fact, then prayer may be released from its exclusive religious connections. Religiously neutral prayers may carry few of the negative public implications of religious prayers. Most personal prayers are not connected to organized religion, because most personal prayers are practiced during personal crisis to express caring. As explained in chapter two, the caring prayers of all humanity take on a universal form and purpose that transcend religious beliefs. Because of their caring nature, these prayers are more therapeutic at their core than religious. The day may come when a person praying with someone in public can say to onlookers, *"This is Therapeutic Prayer that I am offering to express my caring and to bring God's energy into the life of this person."* To which onlookers will respond with a smile and a nod of social approval.

The World's Religions. Most religions envision their own particular religious beliefs spreading throughout the earth to bring their version of the kingdom of God to all humanity. Historically, such idealistic but aggressive religious visions have always divided people and often produced religious suspicion, persecutions and wars. In today's world, the political Cold War may be succeeded by religious wars. We are ominously moving towards huge rivalries between religions that could suddenly propel us in the direction of a world war. These religious rivalries also involve national and ethnic pride, competition and aggression. PrayWell intends to build bridges of understanding and respect between diverse religious groups. With awareness of Therapeutic Prayer and its implications may come a recognition of common goals among diverse religions, enabling leaders of differing religions to work together toward peace with justice for all peoples.

Helping Religions. This new awareness will help, not hinder, organized religion. It will make people feel far more comfortable with religious rituals and far more understanding of religious beliefs. For the first time, many people will understand the *why* of religions, the connection of religious beliefs and ritual to everyday reality and benefits.

Community Issues. The use of Therapeutic Prayer in public settings as an expression of public caring will be readily understood in most communities. It eliminates partisan religious concerns. The energy released by prayer programs divine purpose and order into chaos, violence and rage. PrayWell's promotion of therapeutic group energy fields formed to bring the restoring energy of God into public gatherings and communities will be applauded by most people. Without being able to voice it, many people have sensed that God's presence in the community is therapeutic.

Legal Issues. The need to separate public practices from formal religious ties at high school graduation exercises was acknowledged by the United States Supreme Court, even as I am writing this. A student may offer such a prayer, but not an ordained clergyperson representing any religion. The Court is thus setting a legal precedent for acceptance of caring community prayers or Therapeutic Prayer. Therapeutic Prayer changes the legal context of public prayer.

My layman's understanding of the present legal perceptions of the United States Supreme Court is that any prayer offered in a public education setting is perceived as an example of the state's promoting religious beliefs, and is, therefore, illegal. There are three bases for a new argument to change this legal stance.

First, it is necessary to distinguish between Therapeutic Prayer and religious prayer.

Second, it must be proven to the Court that the existence of God is no longer a religious issue, but a scientific fact. This would void previous legal decisions banning religiously neutral public school prayers. The beliefs of atheists would be proven to be scientifically untrue, opening the door to acknowledging God's presence in the public classroom. Then, Therapeutic Prayers in the public schools can be used for the therapeutic purpose of nurturing students and not for the promotion of an organized religion's beliefs.

Third, if the Court would not accept the scientific proof of God's existence, the Court could acknowledge the scientific existence of a life force or energy whose properties are clearly defined and can be used for bringing wholeness to students in the public classroom, and to their parents as well.

The Court's acceptance of any of these approaches would change the face of America. It would enable parents, teachers and students at a particular school to bathe students and families in therapeutic group energy fields that produce physical, emotional, mental and interpersonal health. This would restore educational integrity to the classroom while healing all participants of anger, fear, despair, painful memories, drug abuse, alcoholism, crime and violence.

This may sound like pie-in-the-sky dreaming. We already possess personal awareness of the power of prayer to transform hardened criminals who are *"born again"* spiritually. We already have evidence that adding the power of God in prayer to drug and alcohol treatment works with Alcoholics Anonymous and other treatment programs.

The juvenile justice system already acknowledges the therapeutic power of church attendance for delinquents. The experimental evidence indicates that the power of prayer is the square of the number in the group participating. In a school of five hundred students, the students, teachers and parents would generate over twenty million prayer energy units of therapeutic love bathing everyone.

SCIENTIFIC PROOF OF THE EXISTENCE OF GOD

We possess almost as much objective data about the qualities of healing energy as we do about another energy source, electricity. This data provides objective proof that the concept of God is not only a religious belief to be found in personal experience, but also a scientifically measurable truth of the universe. Thus, God is like such other proven facts of the universe as the sun, ultraviolet rays, electricity, and atomic energy. Just as we use these energy resources to improve the quality of life, the use of individual and group Therapeutic Prayer to improve the quality of life is objectively justifiable.

All religions believe that there is a Supreme Being, God, who is the creator and sustainer of the physical universe. In this same context, they all believe that God transforms believers into the revealed sacred image of God, and then enhances believers with divine power. Finally, all religions believe that God uses believers as vehicles for divine healing, which results in positive effects, proving God's creative, sustaining attributes. The science of life energies confirms all these religious beliefs as scientific fact. The fact is God is now a scientific truth of the universe. This proof is not based upon philosophy or metaphysics. It is based upon hard scientific evidence. The scientific data indicates that life energy produces the effects attributed to God by all religions.

1. SCIENTIFIC EVIDENCE THAT LIFE ENERGY HEALS VERIFIES THE RELIGIOUS BELIEF THAT GOD HEALS

A. Dr. Bernard Grad's classic 1957 Wounded Mice Experiment[1] provided the first evidence that the human transmission of life energy produces a clinically measurable healing effect. This experiment was replicated by Dr. Remi Cadoret and G.I. Paul at the University of Manitoba.[2]

B. In 1990, Daniel J. Benor's statistical evaluation of one hundred thirty-one controlled trials on cells, enzymes, yeasts, bacteria, plants, mice and humans demonstrated a positive effect of human transmitted life energy in the fifty-six trials, with a statistical analysis at a significance level of $p<.01$.[3]

C. In human clinical studies, Daniel P. Wirth[4] demonstrated the effects of human, non-contact, transmitted life energy, with the statistical results indicating significant healing with $p <.01$.

Conclusion. *All religions believe that God heals, and scientific studies verify that life energies have a healing effect on living organisms. All religions believe that God heals through prayer and some of the scientific studies used praying humans who transmitted a life energy that heals. It appears that "God" and "life energy" are interchangeable words. Life energy is an aspect of God.*

2. LIFE ENERGY POSSESSES MOST OF THE ATTRIBUTES OF GOD

A. Life energy transmitted by fourteen different healers caused a significant variation in the pattern of an infra-red absorption spectra of water placed in sealed vials during a 1986 study.[5]   Both life energy and God have an effect on the physical world.

B. Life energy transmitted by human hands to bottled water caused barley seeds to grow statistically faster than did normal bottled water.[6]   Holy water and healing spas are religiously considered to be filled with God's presence.

C. Life energy transmitted by human hands to cotton and wool produced healing results in mice identical to the touch of humans.[7]   Holy relics, including the clothes of the saints, are attributed with healing power.

D. Life energy was transmitted by human hands to surgical gauze that was applied as a wound dressing, resulting in a faster rate of healing.[8]   Similar to "C" above.

E. Regardless of their religious beliefs, all world-class healers display an identical brain-wave frequency during their healing attempts.[9]   There is a universal biological basis for all healing abilities that transcends religious differences.

F. Regardless of their religious beliefs, all healers possess an identical brain-wave frequency at all times.[10]   Again, there is a universal biological basis for all healing abilities that transcends religious differences.

G. Life energy can be photographed with infra-red film showing the energy emerging from the palms and finger pads of a healer's hands.[11]   All religions believe the power of God is passed through the hands.

H. Life energy from a world-class healer's hands immersed in water causes water protons to emit an 8 hertz frequency.[12]   This is consistent with all healers having identical brain-wave frequencies and identical healing frequencies.

I. A 5.xxx frequency induced cancer in radiated mice within forty-eight hours.[13]   Some human-transmitted energy produces negative effects as we saw with Grad's study of depressed patients.[14]   and Solvin's test of a scoffing volunteer healer.[15]   All religions believe that there are dark or evil forces in the world. Every force possesses a specific frequency. (I do not give the exact frequency for cancer out of fear that someone might use this knowledge as a weapon of destruction.)

J. When the mice were radiated with an eight hertz frequency, their tumors were healed within forty-eight hours.[16]   They were radiated with the life energy or God's healing frequency.

K. Life energy is information-laden and acts intelligently to restore health, an observation made by Grad. All religions believe the presence of God's Spirit provides knowledge and acts intelligently to make all things new.

L. Life energy produces the optimum state of health for life, according to a study using water-soaked beans that had been prayed for.[17]   God restores and makes all things new.

N. Life energy increases the amount of oxygen in the blood by up to twelve percent.[18] God heals.

O. Life energy is extremely stable. According to Grad's research, the power level of life energy in bottled water does not diminish during two years of storage, nor does it leak out to contaminate adjacent bottles. Only sunlight and heat at over the boiling temperature of water will de-stabilize healing energy. These qualities are the same in life energy-charged cotton or wool cloth.

Religiously viewed, the healing energy acts like religious holy relics and holy places that maintain their level of power century after century. Subjectively sensed, God's religious presence has qualities identical to those subjectively sensed in healing energy.

P. Life energy dissipates when imparted to living organisms, with the evidence present in a blade of rye grass growing more rapidly due to absent-prayer.[19] Religiously, humans must have ongoing contact with God to remain faithful because God's power is used up as it heals, transforms and empowers people.

Conclusion. *All religions believe that God heals, and scientific studies verify that life energy has a healing effect on living organisms. All religions believe that God heals through prayer, and some of the scientific studies used praying humans who transmitted a life energy that heals. It appears that "God" and "life energy" are interchangeable words. Life energy is an aspect of God.*

3. HUMAN ENERGY FIELDS REFLECT HUMAN HEALTH

A. Ramesh Chouhan's research data in chapter five shows that cancer, arthritis and pregnancy can be diagnosed through changes in the human energy field before the symptoms can be detected by other medical methods. Religions believe the soul reflects the wholeness of humans.

B. The Chouhan-Weston Clinical Studies indicate that the normal human energy field changes color and size during the transmission of life energy in touch-healing prayer, going from blue to white and becoming about twice as large. This is consistent with the white halos around the heads of those filled with God's presence in religious paintings. This is consistent with the pure white light perceived within the mind during peak experiences of God. This is consistent with white universally being regarded as the color of holy purity.

C. The Chouhan-Weston Clinical Studies indicate that the common cold, chronic back pain and cervical cancer all respond well to life energy transmitted by touch-healing prayer. All religions believe God heals.

Conclusion. *These factors are consistent with religious beliefs.*

SUMMARY ARGUMENT

During twenty-eight years of practicing healing, I have always considered God to be the source of the power and energy that I sensed. During the healing encounter, I am strongly aware of the presence of God. I have no doubt that healing research data proves the existence of God.

On the other hand, a troubling issue has not been satisfactorily resolved. World-class healers are born with the healing ability. Their brain-waves and energy fields are at all times attuned to the life energy frequency. As Bernard Grad points out, most healers used in clinical studies do not pray and some do not consider God to be the source of life energy.

From experience, most healers believe the life energy is empowered by such factors as love, concern and intention. I have already listed the many factors that trigger my own healing flow. I again quote the Bible, *"God is love, and he who abides in love abides in God, and God abides in him"* (I John 4:16b). In the Christian faith, love is considered to be the most powerful force in the universe. *"Faith, hope and love abide, but the greatest of these is love"* (I Corinthians 13:13). If God is the source of all love, then God is empowering the healing of all who love the hurting.

For legal purposes, I am willing to stipulate an alternative to God. Science has proven the existence of a life energy. If it does not come from God, then the life energy can be used at any time, even in public schools, in prayer for therapeutic purposes.

GOD IS LIFE

In my public practice of healing, I ask my clients what name they would like me to use for God during our Therapeutic Prayer. No matter what name I use in addressing God, I always sense the God of my Christian faith. Christ dwells within me, providing the context for my prayer power. When I mentioned God to one client, she painfully winced at that name. *"Then, what name would you like me to use?"* I asked.

She responded, *"Life."* I prayed with her, using the word Life. We had a wonderfully transformative healing experience. "Life" is not such a bad term for God. After all, God is the Source of all Life. I could open a Therapeutic Prayer with, *"O Life, the source of our being; grant this woman healing. Fill her with Life and restore her. Thank you. Amen."*

Chapter Twelve

The Significance of Spoken Prayer

"We should take care not to make the intellect our god; it has, of course, powerful miracles, but no personality." ...Albert Einstein

"We should establish in ourselves a sense of the Presence of God by continually talking to him." ...Brother Lawrence*

"The prayer of a righteous man has great power in its effect." ...James 5:16b

The significance of the use of prayer in the healing encounter has been downgraded to the point of extinction except in organized religion. I know of no healing technique that even mentions prayer. Healers usually belittle any suggestion that they pray. I, myself, remain convinced of the value of healing prayer.

When I work in silent group healing, the introduction of spoken prayer dramatically increases the group's energy and success. For that reason, spoken prayer has always been heartily welcomed by those with whom I share it, for the focus and power it brings to the group effort. Regardless of the attitude of healers, prayer remains the primary means by which most of humanity seeks God's presence, power and wholeness.

THERESA'S DRAMATIC HEALING THROUGH SOAKING PRAYER

As you read the following account of Theresa's healing, the scientific working model for healing prayer provides you with a practical understanding of this dramatic healing encounter. Francis MacNutt, one of the world's most knowledgeable healers, relates Theresa's story in one of his books[1] when writing about the intensive healing process known as *"soaking prayer."* This incident took place at a Roman Catholic retreat for priests in the Diocese of Sonson, Rionegro, Columbia in February 1975.

On the evening of the first day of the retreat, a group of nuns and laywomen sought Father MacNutt's assistance for Theresa, a nineteen-year-old woman whose withered right leg was six inches shorter than her left leg and twisted at an angle. This was the result of stepping on a sharp object in a swamp at the age of five. The untreated infection had entered her bones and developed into osteomyelitis, an inflammation of the bone.

The women had been praying all day with Theresa. Father MacNutt joined them in prayer. The eight-person group *"soaked"* Theresa in prayer that evening, each taking turns touching Theresa's leg. The day's earlier prayers had produced an inch of new leg growth. After two hours of gentle evening prayer, her leg grew another inch. The following day, a two-hour session resulted in another inch of leg growth.

During this soaking prayer process, the leg began straightening, scar tissue healed, shrunken toes grew and a deformed foot reshaped to normal. When they finished their soaking prayer at the end of the week, her right leg was only one-half inch shorter than the left. The leg bone and foot were normal. Theresa's healing is not unique. It is a clear textbook example of soaking, touch-healing prayer.

HOW DEPENDABLE IS SPOKEN PRAYER?

Spoken prayer is one of the most powerful spiritual tools known to humanity. It is a more powerful spiritual tool than thought, meditation, visualization, centering and silent prayer. It has historically proven its power as the basis for religious ritual. The spoken word is the best way for humans to communicate and draw closer. The spoken word in prayer can draw upon the wisdom of sacred writings, the Word of God. The spoken word is the basis of divine power in all religious ritual and is superior to thought, meditation, visualization, centering and silent prayer because of this.

Think about it. If you were given time to inspire one hundred people gathered for religious purposes, what one method would you use? Standing and thinking -- silent meditation -- inner visualization -- inner centering -- silent prayer -- or using the spoken word? The spoken word transmits energy that is information-bearing and acts intelligently. God's power is expressed more effectively and consistently through the spoken word than through any silent activity taking part in the brain alone.

A personal quality essential for enhanced healing skills is the ability to utilize spoken prayer. This is a controversial statement. The use of prayer has been considered to be religiously partisan, and thus controversial. But PrayWell has overcome this concern through the use of Therapeutic Prayers to express simple caring. These prayers are religiously neutral.

Because prayer has become so identified with religion, those who are hostile to religion may resist including prayer while using a healing technique. In fact, many of those who do not use prayer in healing may be unable to do so. They may simply not be skilled in spoken prayer.

My insistence upon the importance of spoken prayer is usually perceived as unfair. Few people presently possess this ability. Spoken prayer is a specialized form of communication with its own unique style and language. One survey verified that only one couple in a hundred has ever prayed aloud for the needs of a spouse. We have privatized prayer, even within the family setting. Yet, spoken prayer is also the key for two or more persons to achieve spiritual unity and create a sacred group energy field.

Most people have had no opportunity to learn this skill. In order to learn, you need a teacher or coach, just as you would if you were trying to learn to play a musical instrument or a sport. You can learn to pray aloud competently and confidently within a few weeks, as you will see. Throughout PrayWell, prayer models are provided to assist your efforts. The principles of PrayWell can be employed in conjunction with silent prayer, inner centering, the intention to transmit healing energy or just the intention to offer healing. But remember, it is spoken prayer that normally enhances the power of the healing encounter.

EIGHTEEN REASONS FOR USING SPOKEN PRAYER

1. Spoken forces the pray-er to focus intentionally upon what s/he is thinking and doing.

2. Spoken prayer establishes an emotional and spiritual link between pray-er and healee, or a sense of unity among those gathered.

3. A spoken prayer can express acceptance and compassion.

4. Spoken prayer uses the voice, the frequencies of which possess healing power.

5. Spoken prayer uses words whose meaning programs and empowers healing energy.

6. Spoken prayer can express a theology of God's love and healing. This expresses the pray-ers intentions and is God's Word for the prayer.

7. Spoken prayer can affirm the healee's life journey including, his/her hurts, fears and struggles, his/her faith, hope and trust, and the sacredness of his/her life.

8. Spoken prayer can acknowledge and accept brokenness, forgiveness, reconciliation and renewal.

9. Spoken prayer is the most reliable means for attuning the pray-er to both God and the healee so that all are united as one, enhancing the effectiveness of the healing energy.

10. Spoken prayer can command healing in God's name.

11. Spoken prayer can fixate the desired healing results.

12. Spoken prayer can thank God for the healing that is taking place.

13. Spoken prayer can praise God, from whom all blessings flow.

14. Spoken prayer enhances the significance of healing touch.

15. Spoken prayer has historically been the most powerful medium for channeling God's power and miracles.

16. Spoken prayer is the best means for building spirituality, and for increasing an awareness of God's spiritual presence in family, groups, community, and nation.

17. Spoken prayer is the best means for creating healing group energy fields.

18. Spoken prayer produces a sense of God's presence, love, joy, peace and unity among all those who use it. This is one of the most consistently blissful experiences known to humanity, resulting in a yearning for more. Our hearts are restless until they find their peace in God, and spoken prayer provides a direct path to that peace.

SOME CULTURES AND RELIGIONS DO NOT USE PRAYER

Some Asian cultures do not utilize prayer. Chinese are skilled in using *Wu Chi,* an Ineffable Life Energy. In Taoism, it is known as the *Tao* -- the Way or the Voice.

There is little or no religious overtone in traditional Chinese philosophy regarding Ineffable Life Energy. Taoism says that the *Tao* existed before Heaven and Earth, carried out the process of creation and exists within all things and life forms.

According to traditional Chinese medicine, the sun, moon and stars radiate energy toward the Earth in a pattern that varies in ten ways, according to their relative positions during the year. The Earth changes its energy state with twelve different annual patterns, effecting all life. Therefore, the state of energy and blood flow in the human body is subject to influences of the Ten Energy Interferences from Heaven and the Twelve Energy Changes from Earth.

The quality and nature of the Ineffable (meaning inexpressible, or too sacred to be spoken) Universal Life Energy in the human being is called the spirit. The spirit of each human being exists in the universe like a droplet of water in the vast ocean of universal life energy. When the human body is formed, the power of spirit is housed in the organs, where it directs and energizes various psychological and physiological functions. The one who tunes his or her spirit with the Universe can live long in health.[2]

Chinese use *Chi* to balance the life energy throughout the body for health and longevity. To do so, they utilize techniques such as herbology, massage, acupuncture (inserting needles in the energy meridians) and t'ai chi (a martial art} -- complex cultural techniques that can take a lifetime to master.

In conversations with a few Chinese citizens, I have found a complete indifference to both God and prayer. Their way of utilizing Ineffable Life Energy works.

In a similar way, Western healers with the psychic ability to see and to manipulate the human energy fields for health, see no reason for using prayer. Their way of utilizing life energy works. *For the rest of us, praying is an easily learned skill for utilizing God's power or life energy. It, too, works.*

THE ABILITY TO PRAY FORCEFULLY

Personal prayer styles tend to be passive. Healing prayer takes on a different and far more forceful style. This is true because in healing prayer one is acting to bring the power of God into human lives. The power of God's light and love is battling with the forces of chaos, which is made known through evil and darkness. This is not a time for being timid or passive. You are using God's power to overcome the evils of physical illness, destructive emotions and alienated relationships. Though the basic tool is love, that battle demands a forceful style.

Most people are not familiar with the forceful style of healing prayer. When they attempt to make the necessary transition into the healing prayer style, they tend to retain the passive personal style. They remain uncomfortable with forceful prayers. This discomfort goes beyond accustomed style.

Traditionally, most people have viewed prayer as involving expressions of appreciation and the making of requests. In other words, their prayer content has always involved thanking God and asking God for specific blessings. As channels for God's power, we need not ask. The healing power is always present and available. In healing, we are called to use that power forcefully. People who are new at praying are uncomfortable with this new style of forceful prayer. To the experienced healer, most people's personal prayer comes through as wishy-washy.

Here are some examples. One style of prayer pleads, *"God, if it is your will...?"* It is assumed by most persons that we do not know the will of God for a specific person's illness. However, God created and wishes his power be used to recreate and make people well. We do not doubt that God wishes everyone to receive appropriate medical care. If healing prayer is seen as a constructive way to bring healing, then we can express this caring in a forceful way through our prayers.

Another way of praying humbly requests healing from God. *"God, I ask you to please heal Bill."* This style assumes that God is like a great heavenly computer granting some requests for healing while denying others. The scientific evidence suggests a different approach, one that recognizes that we are partners with God during the practice of healing prayer. When we unite with God for healing prayer, it inevitably results in an unlimited supply of healing energy moving through us to the person for whom we are praying.

This brings us to the forceful style of healing prayer. This involves a blessing or a command for wellness. Most religious traditions offer similar ritual blessings in a commanding style. It is usually called a blessing, but the form in which it is stated is a command in God's name.

In my own Christian tradition, in baptism we forcefully say, *"John Smith, be baptized...."* In joining the Church, we forcefully state, *"John Smith, be confirmed as a faithful member...."* In benedictions, we forcefully bless, *"The power of God be present with you...."* Believers feel comfortable with each of these styles. In a similar context, to pray forcefully, *"God, use me as a channel for healing," "God, I open myself to being a channel for healing," "God, heal John," "In God's name, be healed,"* or *"In God's name, I command the spirit of illness to depart,"* makes sense.

The ongoing resistance to offering a blessing or a command for healing comes from the reluctance of most persons to accept the concept and the role of priesthood. Anytime we pray effectively, we are acting as a priest, bringing the power of God into the life of the world. The only way that God can act to bring about healing is when a person is willing to become a channel for God's healing flow. Therefore, in healing prayer, as transmitters of God's healing power, we must forcefully command, *"In the name of God, be healed."*

NAMING THE ILLNESS IN PRAYER

Fear and denial are common responses to the medical diagnosis of an illness. A century ago, the names of certain illnesses were never orally expressed, except in a hushed, secretive whisper. Cancer was one of those illnesses whose name created shame and terror among loved ones.

Not naming the illness is an expression of fear. It gives an illness far more power than when the condition is unveiled. Medical and mental health professionals have made great progress in diminishing the fear of illness through encouraging people to name the illness, talk about it and become knowledgeable about its nature and treatment. Clinical studies reveal that a person has a better chance of coping with an illness and marshaling his own healing resources to fight for his life when the illness is named.

By naming an illness in prayer, we are removing fear as we acknowledge its presence. We are also offering the faith and hope that there is a power in the universe that is greater than disease; that is the power of God to heal. This enables people to transcend their fear.

NAMING THE EMOTIONS

In enabling people to cope with a crisis, it is crucial to deal with emotions. This is also true of spoken healing prayer. During prayer, naming the emotions of everyone involved expresses compassion, creates emotional empathy and oneness between pray-er and prayee, and empowers and attunes the healing energy. To avoid the emotions, as though this will cause them to go away, is faulty magical thinking.

CONFESSION AND FORGIVENESS IN PRAYER

Confession and forgiveness are essential for inner wholeness and the full acceptance and use of the healing energy. Confession means to admit or to acknowledge one's own inner state of being, including personal responsibility and accountability. Anger, anxiety, resentment and fear are often directed at oneself or others through blaming. These emotions diminish healing power. Confession and forgiveness during prayer are a means of letting go of these emotions. Doing so acknowledges one's responsibility for one's own emotions, thoughts and actions. Confession and forgiveness affirm one's control over one's life. They clarify thinking and reality. They empower one to cope with the crisis. Accountability assumes personal responsibility for our own role in the crisis, thus bringing one a sense of power over one's destiny.

Confession is performed in full awareness that all persons are imperfect and can learn and grow from their mistakes. It is a way of becoming totally honest and aware of oneself. In the process of self-awareness one may experience a sense of guilt, unworthiness and stupidity. Becoming aware of our mistakes is one way of making contact with our own true spiritual nature and with God. Confession cleanses and renews the human energy fields so they can become healthy.

Forgiveness serves a similar function. The stress emotions of anger, hatred, fear, guilt, and personal inadequacy separate persons from an awareness of human community, spirituality, God and wholeness. These emotions, disrupting the balance of the emotional energy field that effects the other human energy fields, help to cause and to maintain illness. They raise barriers to the reception and utilization of healing energy.

Emotions are also emitted as information and as a force by the human energy fields. They affect other people who come into contact with them. When negative emotions are held onto in a family setting, they act like a poison on the energy fields of all concerned. So refusing to forgive hurts not only oneself but detrimentally effects one's loved ones.

These are the reasons that confession and forgiveness are often included in healing prayer. Once confession and forgiveness have accomplished their purposes, reconciliation occurs. From reconciliation, mutually supportive love naturally flows.

THE NEED TO VOLUNTEER PRAYER

It is rare for anyone to request a prayer, especially a prayer for healing. Any clergyperson knows that requests for prayer in the hospital, home, crisis or counseling setting are rare. For the non-clergy to receive such a request would be even rarer. On the other hand, when prayer is appropriately offered, it is overwhelmingly accepted with deep appreciation -- unless it is a healing prayer!

You may be cautious about offering healing prayer for several reasons:

1. You may be waiting to be asked (which rarely happens).
2. You may feel inadequate to be used as a channel for healing.
3. You may feel awkward about doing something you have never done before.
4. You may lack the necessary skills.
5. You may fear rejection.
6. You may be embittered because your previous successful efforts have not been acknowledged and appreciated.

Healing prayer remains a gift of love that must be offered without thought of a return -- a generous gift offered with the intention to heal.

Without this understanding, you are likely to give up, for any of the above-mentioned reasons. For example, one healer became irritated with a dear friend, vowing never again to offer her healing. During four distinct health crises, he had volunteered healing to her, resulting in the alleviation of the symptoms in her painfully arthritic knees, an arthritic shoulder, and hip and knee damage incurred in a fall. During the current health crisis, she had told him, *"I do not think your previous efforts were the reason I was healed."* This produced his *"never again"* vow.

Like many others, this woman had great difficulty acknowledging the source of her previous healing results, so in order to allow herself to receive further assistance, she was impelled to make the above denial, an illogical move produced by the limitations of her conventional belief system.

This type of response is maddening to most healers, and is likely to continue to be an inhibiting factor for all those who offer healing prayer. Practitioners of healing must realize that, while their process is an effective and practical means for caring about people, it is different from others in that one's successful efforts may seldom be satisfactorily acknowledged, let alone appreciated.

Whether volunteered or requested, here are some guidelines for offering spoken prayer.

1. Begin the transaction in a private place. Most will welcome your offer if it is made in private.
2. Offer the prayer privately. People are often uncomfortable about praying in public, although there are exceptions. Clergy can acceptably offer prayer in many group settings. Prayer can also be offered by a family member within a family setting or by a friend among a group of close friends.
3. Ask, *"May I pray with you?"* Never ask *"May I pray for you?"* Many people will experience the latter request as demeaning.
4. Approach people as equals. Never imply that you have a better link to God or goodness than someone else.
5. Do not fear offering an unexpected prayer for healing. Such unexpected opportunities often produce rewarding results, even with someone you have just met.

AWARENESS OF OTHER SPIRITUAL CONTACTS

When one prays, are all spiritual contacts with God? If you are like me, you have personally known only the presence of God in prayer. Yet, throughout the centuries, people have reported contact with angels, saints, departed loved ones, spirit helpers, and evil or demonic spirits. In addition, dozens of parishioners have shared with me their stories of healing through spirit helpers. The stories usually follow similar lines.

After viewing me with trust and receiving assurance of confidentiality, parishioners have shared many experiences of spirit helpers. Extremely ill and lying in bed at night, the individual awakens and sees a ghostly figure at the foot of the bed, often accompanied by an inner message that the illness is being healed. Some report a voice assuring them of healing. People have variously identified this ghostly figure as a sacred person like Jesus, as an angel, a deceased loved one or an unknown being.

What is the role played by spirit beings in supporting our daily living? While serving an inner-city parish, I was confronted by armed and dangerous people a dozen times. During each encounter, I felt safe. I experienced an inner peace; my inner sense of time increased several times as the outer world went into slow motion; and I sensed a holy presence. This resulted each time in a mysterious resolution of the danger. I have never clearly understood what happened.

The explanation I gave myself at the time was that my guardian angel had intervened. But the concept of guardian angels is inaccurate. That is a concept popularized by movies. Rather than angels, I believe that it was spirit guides, persons from the Company of Heaven, that rescued me. Angels have never lived as physical persons, and rarely participate in human affairs. Spirit guides are human energies from the heavenly realms who continue to assist those of us on the earth plane after they have made their own transition into the spiritual dimension.

Scriptures describe people reporting contact with sacred figures from the spiritual realm like angels and spirit guides. Much of the spiritual healing movement believes and reports that persons other than God assist them in healing. In the three nations where spiritual healing is most practiced -- England, Brazil and the Philippines -- most healers state that their healing is empowered by spirit guides from the other side. Healers in Canada, Mexico and the United States produce similar witness. We need to be open to the possibility of our access to spirit helpers, such as the saints in the Roman Catholic, Orthodox and other traditions. If you have such an experience, honestly explore it and draw your own conclusions.

THE ROLE OF FAITH AND BELIEF IN HEALING

Of all the issues surrounding healing prayer, the importance of faith and belief during the healing encounter has been the most troubling for me. The public overwhelmingly believes that one must have great faith in God in order to be healed. This has been hammered into our minds by one television faith-healer after another. This belief, this requirement about faith, has then been repeatedly stated by the public to the extent that it has unfortunately become *"a Law of Divine Healing."*

Nothing antagonizes people more than my questioning the truth of this belief, but nothing hampers healing efforts more than this belief. This belief causes countless people to feel that God cannot heal them because they do not have enough *faith,* whatever that might mean. For, in many minds, faith implies being perfect before God. Few people view themselves to be godly enough, good enough, worthy enough or faithful enough to be healed. Consequently, this belief has become the major obstacle hindering healing results.

In a similar manner, this belief has also become the major obstacle to people practicing touch-healing prayer. They do not view themselves to be godly enough, good enough, worthy enough or faithful enough to offer touch-healing prayer. *The truth is that the only qualification for offering healing prayer is a loving concern. The only qualifications for being healed are the desire to become well and a trust in healing prayer.*

What is the true role of faith and belief in healing? I am not sure. I am still learning. I do know a little. There is no evidence that a pure faith in God alone produces any healing results. This type of faith can be used as a denial of the seriousness of one's condition. However, the certain belief that one cannot be healed, for whatever reasons, greatly hampers healing efforts. And a sense of personal inadequacy for the task hampers the practice and effectiveness of healing prayer.

My dilemma as an author, researcher and practitioner lies within myself. I grew up in the Christian Church. Since early childhood, I have been a believer. I have always prayed and felt God's presence during prayer. I have always felt close to God. His presence has always lived within me, transforming, guiding and sustaining me.

In addition, I am an optimist, an idealist, a dreamer. I believe that all things are possible. I have known many peak experiences of God. I have always believed in divine miracles. I have observed and participated in many encounters that could be considered to be divine miracles. Therefore, I would have to consider myself to be one who lives with a firm faith in God. That is also my handicap in addressing the issues of faith and belief in healing. My handicap is in not understanding what is going on within people who have not shared a similar faith journey. It is from this perspective that we will explore the role of faith and belief in healing.

Before doing that, we must focus on the real issue -- the effects that faith has on human energy fields. People voluntarily or involuntary exert control over their own energy fields during the healing encounter. Anything that blocks the entrance of life energy into the human energy fields, blocks any healing possibilities. The blocking of life energy occurs when a shield is raised against it.

University of California in Los Angeles (UCLA) researcher Thelma Moss photographed the fingertip energy fields of student volunteers using Kirlian photography. The resulting energy pictures reveal fascinating evidence of human energy fields interacting. In one study, Dr. Moss asked a male and a female student to place their fingertips beside each other to study the interaction.

While they waited, the man had found the woman to be attractive and had been flirting with her. The woman's response was one of irritation and rejection. Given this setting, the first Kirlian photograph showed the man's energy field reaching out towards the woman's, while the woman's energy field actually pulled back from the man's in rejection. This showed a negative interaction of energy fields with the unwillingness of the woman to have the man's energy field touching her's.

In the second Kirlian photograph, taken several weeks later, the man and woman had begun dating and the woman was now returning the man's affection. The photograph shows the couple's energy fields reaching out towards each other and merging. Out of affection, they had voluntarily opened their energy fields to each other. This experiment suggests the way energy fields interact.

What blocks the acceptance of life energy during the healing encounter? Whatever blocks the life energy from entering one's energy fields, blocks healing results. Here are my educated guesses. People block the healing energy during an encounter:

1. When they possess negative feelings like anger, hatred, fear and a sense of inadequacy,
2. When they possess total disbelief, distrust, distaste and suspicion,
3. When they are filled with chemical substances that block the life energy,
4. When for any reason they place a blocking shield around their energy fields,
5. When they do not voluntarily open their energy fields to the life energy.

Using these reference points, we can examine the issue of faith and belief in healing. Let's first explore the belief that one must have faith in order to be healed. For me, faith in this context means a faith that one will be healed. Faith has also meant believing in what a particular faith-healing evangelist says. Both these images need to be rejected. *Faith is a factor in healing but only if one takes some action on the basis of faith.*

Dr. Herbert Benson's research indicates that having faith that one's actions will produce healing, works. This is a result of the placebo effect. This includes faith in a physician, a medication, a medical procedure, a healer, a healing process, prayer, meditation, a special diet or exercise. This type of faith opens one's energy fields and can restore them to heath.

This type of faith is identical to that expressed by Dr. Bernie Siegel's *"exceptional cancer patients,"* who recover from terminal cancer because they have faith that a change in lifestyle will make them well. In each instance, faith is a belief that one will get well through a specific type of action or practice. This type of faith can reprogram the body's energy field into the perfect blueprint, and elevate the level of life energies.

In another context, faith can be defined as "a trust in." In this context, a trust in the person offering healing is faith. A trust that healing prayer works is also faith. This type of faith opens one's energy fields to the healing flow, a crucial factor.

Belief that a specific healing approach works is important. Filipino healers report the need to spend extra time with foreign clients in order to deal with their belief systems. They must persuade clients that their healing activity causes no harm and actually works. Most persons either do not believe in healing or are uncomfortable with the healing styles being practiced. These are barriers to the healing process because they block the flow of healing energy.

Another factor more important than faith in the healing encounter is the attuning of the healing energy. Attuning is simply accomplished through compassion and relationship: a oneness between the healer, the healee and God. My observation is that perfectly attuned healing energy opens up all energy fields to the healing flow.

I think that often the issue of faith is a tiresome excuse for why the healer failed in his or her efforts to produce healing. Rather than looking within himself, the healer blames the ill for not getting well. I am not comfortable with this. As a professional healer, I have a responsibility to my client to use any number of techniques to open the energy fields. These techniques include building relationship and trust, explaining the scientific data, caring for them and opening their fields with my hands.

This brings us to the beliefs of the pray-er. I see the beliefs of the pray-er as far more significant factors than the beliefs of the healee. The pray-er needs to believe in the sacredness of each person, in a God who heals and in himself as a channel for healing. It helps when the healee trusts or believes that this particular person can be a channel for healing. Yet, experience has taught me that skeptical healees are more likely to be healed than believers. It is rare for cynics to be healed. Assurance that the healing process is taking place is a part of belief.

If an ill person believes he is not going to get better or is going to die, that belief will likely negate any effects of prayer. God's healing love energy intelligently produces healing but it also respects free will. Any inner programming or script about the course of the illness is an important factor.

We may soon learn more about the role of belief. The physical energy field can now be recorded, using low-light one lux videocameras in bioelectrography. I can now record the interaction of the healer and healee to show what occurs in the energy fields of both persons before, during and after the healing session. We can also measure the frequencies of the energies emitted by all parties that will form a new picture of the frequencies of illness and of attuned healing energy. These hold the hope of clarifying the role of faith and belief during the healing encounter.

BARRIERS TO THE USE OF PRAYERS FOR HEALING

We have seen that the capacity for prayer to produce physical healing traditionally has been one for which the general public has shown little understanding or support. Yet, public surveys report that the vast majority of people pray. During a medical crisis, it could be expected that most of those pray-ers would offer a prayer for physical healing. Thus, a majority of human beings have prayed for a physical healing.

With such actions affirming the belief in the power of God to heal, it would be logical to conclude that the public believes in healing prayer. The public, however, claims not to believe. Here we encounter one of the great social mysteries of our day, and your number one barrier to effectiveness in healing prayer. People tend to believe that prayer heals only under certain limited circumstances, specifically, during a medical emergency.

During a life-threatening medical emergency, most persons will pray. Fearing the death of a loved one, they become ready for a miracle, any kind of miracle that will work. This miracle-readiness, which involves faith and hope, all but disappears after the medical emergency is resolved. If a healing miracle should occur while they pray in a state of miracle-readiness, few persons will talk about it afterwards, even privately with loved ones.

Once the medical emergency has passed, the survivor's loved ones, no longer in a state of extreme fear, seldom continue their prayers. If the ill one continues to live with a chronic or life-threatening illness, like heart disease, cancer or stroke, diabetes or emphysema, their loved ones tend to stop praying for healing.

I think that people are unable to make the connection between their prayers for God to rescue a loved one during a medical emergency and healing prayer. They did not observe that what they had offered was actually healing prayer. They had merely prayed for God to rescue a loved one. Therefore, they could not take the next step by continuing their healing prayers afterwards.

THE ILL MAINTAIN A STATE OF MIRACLE-READINESS

Usually, only the one who is ill maintains the needed state of miracle-readiness in which prayers for healing remain an affective option. Following the initial medical crisis, the ill continue to live in a condition of fear. This may produce the *survival response*, a state of faith, hope, and miracle-readiness based upon the belief that God will heal them. It is for such individuals that Part Two of PrayWell is designed. Part Two is addressed to anyone who holds an urgent desire to get well again, and who wants to take charge of his/her own journey back to health using prayer as the major tool.

In time, more and more individuals will discover the efficacy of healing prayer, as each undergoes his own form of crisis and is forced to override previous limiting beliefs. Until then, pray-ers must continue to prepare themselves to meet the suspicion and hostility of those who have not yet learned to think for themselves.

Even today, upon learning that I practice healing prayers with the ill, the majority of those I meet register strong emotions of anger, fear, suspicion, shame, embarrassment and rejection. You, too, must be prepared to face public opposition to your plans to pray for healing or self-healing.

The first barrier, therefore, to your pursuit of prayer as a healing technique is public opinion, as seen above.

The second barrier to your resolve involves your potential resistance to setting aside your present understanding and adapting to a new perspective based upon objective research findings. Some of these findings may contradict what you have believed. You will be traveling on unfamiliar ground. The research data is designed to provide a new roadmap for your own self-healing. The results will be the most convincing evidence of their own truth that you will need.

A third barrier -- and probably the greatest of all -- may be your belief that others are far more qualified than you to offer prayers for healing. The truth is that all persons have the inborn potential to produce effective prayer results. Much of this barrier arises from the human inability to accept the role of a priest who acts for God. As a pray-er, you are acting as a priest, bringing the power of God into the life of the world. Throughout history, humans have struggled with this identity of priesthood. Be aware that serving in the priestly role of pray-er has nothing to do with your goodness, worthiness, religiousness, age, education or any other status. It is based solely upon your personal willingness to be used by God to express love and caring for yourself and others through prayer.

A fourth barrier is your lack of knowledge and experience in prayer. PrayWell offers complete details, including prayer models, to help you feel comfortable and competent in your prayers. You may feel awkward at first. Most new endeavors require a clumsy learning period of practice in order to learn and become competent.

A fifth barrier is your image of how God works. Since earliest times, people have sensed that there was a power in the universe greater than themselves, the power they called God. That awareness of God is known as *"spirituality."* In other words, humanity has always possessed a spiritual nature or awareness. This sensing of God has always led to religious beliefs, an attempt to explain the universe in terms of how God works and to tell humanity how to live life with God.

PrayWell makes the religious statement that God created and continues to create, to recreate and to make all things new. But in human affairs, God does not do this magically. God seldom intervenes in human affairs unless people ask for help. Much of the creative power of God at work is due to the actions of people who pray. *The whole field of spiritual healing is united in the belief that a human being inevitably serves as the bridge between God and the healing results.* Prayer is a significant means by which God continues to create and to make all things new.

A sixth barrier involves belief. Doubt about the healing process is almost universal. The inner question is always *"Is anything really happening?"* We all want something dramatic and immediate as a sign of what is quietly occurring within. Healing prayer remains a process that takes place over a period of time. Believe in the process. Through prayer, God is helping people get well.

A pleasant surprise awaits you. As you journey on your path of prayer for wholeness, you will be blessed far beyond what you had ever hoped. The powerful presence of God makes prayer encounters joyous and rewarding moments. Much of humanity is longing for both personal wholeness and spirituality. PrayWell uses prayer to provide a path that leads to both. This book is committed to fulfilling your deepest spiritual yearnings. In the midst of this prayer journey, you will come to a deeper appreciation of the psalmist who declared, *"Our hearts are restless until they find their peace in God."*

Chapter Thirteen

The Unexpected Side-Effects of Prayer

"The attempt to define all mystical, transcendental, and ecstatic experiences, which do not fit in with the categories of consensus reality, as psychotic is conceptually limiting and comes from timidity which is not seemly for the honest open-minded explorer." ...John Lilly

"A man may be a heretic in the truth; and if he believes things, only on the authority of others without other reason, then though his belief be true, yet the very truth he holds becomes heresy." ...John Milton

"Discernment arising from disciplined practice is necessary for continually recognizing the movement of God's Spirit." ... John Woolman*

Throughout history, humanity has been sidetracked in its spiritual explorations by the unexpected side-effects of peak experiences of God, prayer and meditation. Even today, these side-effects are labeled by many as dangerous and evil, and therefore, unacceptable. The labeling continues, along with the hysteria and fear that accompany it. The unexpected side-effects of prayer are just as misunderstood as spiritual healing. This is tragic because it makes people afraid to continue on the spiritual journey.

What are these unexpected side-effects of prayer? They are an enhanced awareness and intuition. Enhanced awareness has enabled me to be more creative and purposeful. It has been a part of my prayer healing encounters for many years, enabling me to *feel* the emotions of others and tend to their needs. It is this enhancing of awareness that frightens many people.

The pursuit of any spiritual journey increases intuitive abilities. The Therapeutic Prayers for health and renewal in <u>PrayWell</u> work because of the enhanced intuitive abilities present in prayer. No book on healing prayer tells the whole story unless it explores enhanced intuitive abilities.

Most world-class healers employ a variety of intuitive abilities during the healing encounter. In chapter eight, healers were described as having the gifts of clairvoyance and telepathy and they are to some degree *"sensitives,"* able to see energy fields. I identified four healing abilities necessary for effective healing in groups and healing services. These abilities enable the healer to act as a group-catalyst, energy-attuner, healer-sensitive or energy-enabler. Intuitive abilities must be used for restoring and maintaining healthy human energy fields. Understanding and accepting these natural human intuitive abilities is invaluable for the prayer journey, healing and renewal.

PRAYER AND INTUITIVE ABILITIES

Prayer has always increased intuitive abilities. In my own case, intuitive abilities inspired this book. Intuitive abilities once led me on a confirmed out-of-body experience while sleeping. Intuitive abilities enabled me to hear encouraging words from a deceased parishioner. Intuitive abilities often guide me to people who are hurting. I have learned to telephone people when a name pops into my mind for no apparent reason. Each time I discovered a person in crisis. My car has been guided to the homes of hurting parishioners, or to a hospital. Christians call this the spiritual gift of knowledge. Parapsychologists would call it telepathic attuning. Why have such experiences been called evil or satanic in origin or purpose? The awakening of intuitive abilities like these in religious groups has caused whole congregations to back off from spiritual practices out of a sense of fear, shame and evil.

My mother has always possessed intuitive abilities. Recently, she sensed that her brother had just died in Las Vegas. A few hours later, her sister-in-law phoned to tell her that Foy had died, and at the very moment that my mother had intuitively sensed it. Was my mother's premonition in any way evil?

INTUITIVE ABILITIES EMERGE IN PRAYER GROUPS

Persons in every prayer group I have led experience enhanced intuitive abilities. A scientist began having dreams which solved research problems. A woman had a spontaneous out-of-body experience. Another woman reported vivid encounters with her deceased mother during meditation. A man had a deeply moving religious experience in which he had a conversation with Jesus and received a blessing of his life's journey. It was his first meaningful encounter with God, and it spiritually transformed him. A physician reported a new intuitive diagnostic awareness with his patients.

All these people reported that their experiences were astounding, rewarding and welcome. Most of these experiences addressed practical concerns of the individual. Some dealt with subconscious information. Some centered on expanded consciousness. While a few respond with fear, most people remain curious and eagerly explore their enlarged awareness. One woman developed two unwanted abilities overnight. In what parapsychologists call *distant viewing,* Mary was able to see her husband at work in his office ten miles away, knowing what he was doing and saying. At times, she had similar knowledge of her children living in a city fifty miles away. The second ability would be helpful in a gambling casino. It, too, could be called *distant viewing* or *mental telepathy* or the religious *gift of knowledge.* While playing cards, Mary effortlessly knew the exact cards that each player held. Along with these new abilities, Mary experienced unusual awareness during healing encounters. Mary's overall response was one of fear and anger. She vowed that she would never pray again because it was too scary.

OTHER WORDS FOR INTUITIVE ABILITIES

Intuitive abilities have many names. According to their names, intuitive abilities are accepted or rejected, good or evil, blessings or curses. The

Christian Church calls intuitive abilities either spiritual gifts or evil deviations. Social scientists study these abilities and label them paranormal, extrasensory perception or psi. The public calls these experiences psychic or psi. Are they all the same phenomena under different labels? We will be exploring this question throughout this chapter.

INTUITIVE ABILITIES IN HISTORY

When the sixteenth century Christian monk Martin Luther struggled through his faith journey and read his Bible, coming up with the revolutionary concepts for the Protestant Reformation, he did not figure it out in his mind, using reason. He dreamed his ninety-five theses. That was intuitive ability.

When the noted eighteenth century Swedish scientist Emmanuel Swedenborg had a vision (remote viewing) of his home city burning while he was hundreds of miles away from it, that was an example of an intuitive ability, clairvoyance -- a clear vision from a physical distance.

Twentieth century mathematician Albert Einstein did not reason through his many theories. The theories and equations came to his mind while he was sleeping or walking. He spent years seeking to prove his theories rationally, producing the mathematical basis for his equations. Einstein was an intuitive genius, not a reasoning genius. He had a clear vision of a revolutionary new intuitive means for describing reality. His intuitive ability supplied the basis for Quantum Mechanics and a new Platonic view of reality.

THE NATURE OF INTUITIVE REALITY

Chapter three discussed the two different views of reality described by Aristotle and Plato. Aristotle insisted that only what can be known by the five physical senses is real. Plato defended intuitive knowing and the spiritual nature of the universe, stating that the physical universe is a by-product of the spiritual reality/universe.

Episcopal priest Morton Kelsey has written a dozen scholarly books explaining spiritual reality. His contention is that physical reality is just the projected small tip of a wedge of human awareness. Most of that wedge extends into the infinite spiritual universe of God, heaven, the Company of Heaven, spirits, dreams, revelation, extrasensory perception, etc. The five physical senses give only a limited consciousness or awareness of reality. The miraculous events in the Bible could not have happened if there were only this physical reality. All religions require access to another dimension, the spiritual dimension wherein dwells God. Intuitive abilities and spiritual gifts cannot exist in a purely physical three-dimensional universe. Without the intuitive-creative-feeling process, there is no access to God.

Religious historian John Rossner carries this argument a step further by stating that we live in a multidimensional universe. Albert Einstein and quantum physics state that there are an infinite number of parallel universes, each existing at a different frequency from our Earth, and each a variation of our Earth universe. Access to these other universes is possible through what is known as the Einstein/Rosen Bridge.

The existence of invisible human energy fields, existing at seven different frequencies, provides a scientific basis for the understanding of quantum physics and intuitive abilities. As we attune our brains to specific frequencies, we can actually see these seven human energy fields. As we attune our brain for specific frequencies, we can experience any of the intuitive abilities that operate on those frequencies. When, through loving concern, we attune to the healing frequency of 7.83 hertz, we are at the intuitive frequency that heals. Perhaps at 7.7 hertz we can bend spoons with our minds. Perhaps attuning to a 6.45 hertz frequency gives us the ability to see into the future. Perhaps attuning to a 6.375 frequency can put us in touch with a parallel Earth universe.

INTUITIVE ABILITIES AS THE BASIS FOR SAINTHOOD

Sainthood is conferred by the Roman Catholic Church upon those who have exhibited spiritual and psychic abilities. An analysis of each of the twenty-five hundred thirty-two Roman Catholic saints from the four-volume Butler's Lives of the Saints, shows that some form of psi was mentioned for six hundred seventy-six saints or twenty-nine percent. These included three hundred ten saints known for their miracles, fifty-five saints with extrasensory perception, thirty-one cases of clairvoyance (knowledge of events through pictures in the mind), twenty cases of discernment of spirits (the ability to read consciences) and twelve cases of prophecy (precognition or knowing the future).

While alive, most of these saints were viewed with suspicion. Many were condemned by their church superiors during their lifetime. Throughout history, humanity has responded to enhanced intuitive abilities with the same distrust it has shown to spiritual healing. Perhaps that is why the Roman Catholic Church waits one hundred years after a gifted Christian's death before making the decision to bestow sainthood.

REMOVING THE MYSTERY FROM SPIRITUAL GIFTS

Six of the spiritual gifts are referred to in almost fifty percent of all New Testament verses. Without these spiritual gifts, there would be no Christianity and no religions anywhere on earth. Enhanced intuitive abilities must be present for any religious revelation, healing or miracles. Today, established churches either ignore the biblically documented spiritual gifts, dismiss them, deny them, view them as divisive, fear them or label them as evil. Just as spiritual healing does not fit into today's worldview, neither do the other spiritual gifts.

Most of today's churches focus on beliefs about God and seek a believer's mental agreement to those beliefs. This is followed by a commitment to living a life of love, morality and service. This approach is backwards. Historically, ancient people experienced God and then formed theological statements to explain their experiences. When religions deny the existence of the spiritual reality by placing power only in the five physical senses, they prevent the action of the mystical power of God, and the religious experiences accompanying mystical awareness.

Today's religions ignore divine visions, the current evidences of the afterlife, communication with the Company of Heaven, near-death experiences, out-of-body experiences, premonitions, precognition, extrasensory perception and spiritual healing. Yet, these ancient, biblically reported intuitive abilities still thrive among humans throughout our planet.

PEOPLE STILL EXPRESS INTUITIVE ABILITIES

Sociologist Father Andrew Greeley concluded a poll in 1974 for the University of Chicago's National Opinion Research Center. Sixty-three million Americans have claimed personal experiences of one or more psychic or supernatural events (closeness to a powerful force that seemed to lift them out of themselves). Thirty-four percent reported having had contact with the dead.

The United States National Institute of Mental Health at the Centre for Studies in Suicide Prevention, Los Angeles, published a study revealing that forty-four percent of those sampled were convinced that they had had several experiences of post-mortem contact with the dead. Twenty-five percent of these persons indicated that the dead person actually visited them or was seen at a seance, while more than sixty percent of the incidents involved a dream.

In 1980, a Canadian national poll conducted by a sociologist at the University of Lethbridge in Alberta revealed that twenty-two percent of all Canadians are sure that extrasensory perception abilities exist, with an additional forty-seven percent believing that such abilities exist, for a total of sixty-nine percent either being sure of or believing in extrasensory perception. Sixty-three percent say they believe in life after death. Forty-four percent of those who are very religious believe communication with the dead is possible, with thirty-six percent of those *"not very religious"* saying communication with the dead is possible.

Is the Christian Church perceived as being important in the exploration of these phenomena? Most people believed that science, not organized religion, is the place where future answers concerning these spiritual mysteries are to be sought. The same poll indicated that only twenty-eight percent of Canada's nominal Christians are regular churchgoers and that of these, only fifty-five percent still believe in the *'supernatural'* dimensions of their faith, as expressed in such traditional doctrines as the divinity of Christ and life after death.

WHAT IS THE CHURCH'S RESPONSE TO THIS DATA?

The Church's response to this data has been either silence or condemnation. Who is going to answer questions about intuitive experiences? Will the clergy continue to ignore them? Will the clergy and psychiatrists continue to label the psychically gifted as mentally ill or troublemakers? Do we label people who have intuitive experiences as evil, as satanic, as filled with evil spirits? Do we insist that anyone having a premonition or receiving assurances from a deceased spouse is deluded, misguided or evil? Do we continue to take the wonder of God out of people's lives so that they no longer believe he exists, so that the churches lie empty? Will we deny any acceptable place for God and intuitive experiences among church members?

Organized religion in America can only blame itself for the existence of New Agers -- those who are exploring and practicing the human intuitive dimensions. When an American has an intuitive experience such as a premonition, distant viewing or an awareness of future events, there are few places within organized religion that support such exploration and understanding. Many of the most intuitive-creative-feeling type of people have participated in aspects of the New Age because there is no other interest group that accepts them.

THE PHYSICS OF CONSCIOUSNESS

In November, 1977 at Reykjavik, Iceland, a group of international scientists gathered for what became known as the Iceland Conference to present the results of experimental and theoretical research on the physics of consciousness. The scientists presented papers on distant viewing (seeing events with the mind from a distance), precognition (viewing the future), teleportation (moving an object from an enclosure with the mind), the mind's ability to collapse the wave-function of matter, and the ability of children to bend metal by the use of the mind. Five of the papers were collected in a book, The Iceland Papers, edited by Andrija Puharich.

The results of five years of research conducted by Harold E. Puthoff and Russell Targ at the Stanford Research Institute were presented under the title, *"Direct Perception of Remote Geographical Locations."* The ability to perform *remote sensing* was brought to their attention by Ingo Swann, an individual who has the ability to perceive, and describe by word or drawing, distant scenes and activities blocked from ordinary perception. While in an enclosed room, Swann can describe or draw scenes of events that are happening many miles away. In over seventy laboratory experiments involving work with more than a dozen test subjects, the ability for remote sensing was scientifically validated. Today, this is known as "remote viewing."

John B. Hasted of Birkbeck College, University of London, described his experiments on paranormal metal-bending with children, in which he showed that he was dealing with real, controllable psychokinetic phenomena. Psychokinesis deals with the ability to affect or move material objects through the use of the mind. Hasted used sophisticated scientific tools that could quantify the forces involved in psychokinesis. He applied statistical and theoretical mathematics to explain the data.

DEFINING BASIC INTUITIVE ABILITIES

Dr. Hal Banks, a consciousness researcher, has written a book, An Introduction To Psychic Studies, that I have found to be an excellent source for defining the following intuitive terms:

1. **Parapsychology** is the branch of science dealing with ESP and psychokinesis. ESP stands for *"extrasensory perception,"* which includes telepathy, clairvoyance and precognition.

2. **Psychokinesis,** or PK, involves the power of the mind over matter. Gifted subjects can do both ESP and PK, which suggests a linkage or unity between various psychic abilities. They may be a part of a single system. Psychokinesis can affect the roll of the dice. It is strongly suspected that psychokinesis is involved in certain spiritual healing phenomena. Filipino healers appear to use PK as they dematerialize human tissue.

Levitation is included in PK. Levitation means to raise a physical object, like a pin, by using the mind. Levitation has also been associated with deeply spiritual or loving persons who are capable of rising into the air. Poltergeist manifestations are another form of PK, involving the moving of objects in a house. This has often been related to the actions of ghosts but in recent years it has been associated with the PK ability of adolescents with a focus ability.

3. **Telepathy** occurs when mind communicates with mind. It is frequently associated with crisis situations having a strong emotional content involving loved ones, and may occur during the healing encounter.

4. **Clairvoyance** is the awareness of some objective event or object without the use of the five physical senses. Dr. Banks lists four subdivisions of clairvoyance. The first is *"x-ray clairvoyance,"* which is the ability to see into sealed envelopes, closed spaces, boxes, books and rooms. This is also a part of what is known as *"psychometry."*

Second is *"medical clairvoyance,"* the ability to see within the human body and its mechanisms, and to diagnose disease. I have met three clairvoyant diagnosticians whose accuracy in diagnosing disease is excellent.

Third, *"traveling clairvoyance"* is the ability to change one's perception and to travel with the mind, and to describe a distant scene (*"distant sensing"* or *"remote viewing"*).

In the fourth, *"platform clairvoyance,"* one is able to see or perceive discarnate (not in the physical body) personalities. A clairvoyant working with a group can bring messages from spirit folk. This is also known as *"mediumship."*

5. **Clairaudience** means *"clear-hearing"* or receiving information through hearing it, like listening to spirits or God. Some healers are guided by the clairaudient ability.

6. **Psychometry** is a form of clairvoyance involving the ability to gain information through sensing the information in the energy of a person by touching an object the person owns or wears. Psychometry is also known as *"soul measurement"* or *"object-reading."*

Psychometry can be applied to archeological objects, personal jewelry, or religious objects. It can be use in sensing the energy of a photograph in a sealed envelope, or what has happened in a room. Individuals with this ability can read the past or present by touching or being near a physical object. It has been a valuable tool to criminology in tracking evidence or finding a lost child or a body. Many world-class healers use psychometry to read the energy fields of a client.

7. **Precognition** is a means of predicting the future. It is the knowledge through ESP of some future event. A historic example is Abraham Lincoln's precognitive dream in which he foresaw his own assassination and funeral. Healers sometimes have awareness of a person's future state of health. *"Retrocognition"* is knowledge of a past event acquired intuitively.

8. **Mediums and Mediumship.** A medium is a link between the living and the physically dead who are now alive in the afterlife. A medium is also known as a *"sensitive,"* and is one who has unusual awareness. Psychical researchers prefer the word *"sensitive,"* which does not imply afterlife survival. Spiritualists state that all healers are mediums as they bring the power of God into the life of the ill.

History is filled with experiences of mediumship. Two striking evidences of mediumship occur in the Bible. In I Samuel 28:7-25, King Saul seeks advice from a great deceased leader of Israel, the priest Samuel. King Saul goes to the medium of Endor who materializes Samuel. The troubled Samuel is told he and his sons will die in a battle the next day. In the New Testament, the Transfiguration of Jesus is a prime example of mediumship. With Jesus acting as a medium, Peter, James and John are able to see the manifested presence of the Old Testament heroes Moses and Elijah (Matthew 17).

There are two broad classes of mediumship. There is *"mental mediumship,"* which includes such phenomena as clairvoyance, clairaudience, precognition, psychometry, automatic writing, trance and telepathy. Then there is *"physical mediumship,"* which includes psychokinesis, levitation, apports, materialization, psychic photography, table-tilting, raps, direct voice and psychic lights. Any contact we have with the spirit world, including contact with God, is considered by some to be mediumship. In this perspective a medium is one who serves as a link between the world of spirit and this physical world. With a large proportion of Americans having claimed contact with deceased loved ones, each of these at such times was a link with the spirit world, and thus, momentarily a medium.

A COMPARISON OF PSI, PSYCHIC AND SPIRITUAL GIFTS

Christianity has always separated the paranormal knowing of parapsychology and psychic studies from the spiritual knowing of things religious, as seen in the spiritual gifts. The evidence points to the fact that they are all manifestations of the same phenomenon. When the paranormal gift is used within a religious community, it is often awakened and empowered by God's presence in the sacred energy field of that religious community. Once awakened, the paranormal gift often becomes actively alive within the context of a believer's faith in God, the content of one's religious beliefs and the depth of one's spiritual development.

For many centuries, humanity has been negative in its attitude towards parapsychology and psychic studies. Therefore, we have come to separate the church-sanctioned paranormal knowing in religion from the paranormal knowing of parapsychology and the psychic. This artificial separation needs to be bridged if only for the sake of intellectual integrity. The benefits of a deeper understanding will be productive for everyone. The following table attempts to match the wordings of the three categories of intuitive knowing.

A Comparison of Terms for Intuitive Abilities

Parapsychology	Psychic	Spiritual
Precognition	Prediction	Prophecy
Telepathy	Telepathy	Knowledge
Clairvoyance	Clairvoyance	Divine Vision
Clairvoyance	Channeling	Revelation
Clairvoyance	Mediumship	Mediumship
Clairaudience	Clairaudience	Voice of God
Guidance Dream	Psychic Dream	Divine Vision
Guidance Dream	Discernment	Spiritual Discernment
Paranormal healing	Psychic Healing	Spiritual Healing

DISCERNING THE BENEFITS OF RELIGIOUS RITUAL

Institutional Christianity does its best to separate paranormal and psychic phenomena from religious history. Christianity is untiring in its denial of paranormal and psychic phenomena. Time and again, the Church asserts, *"This is a religious phenomenon, not a psychic phenomenon."* Objective studies show there is no difference between psychic and religious phenomena. Are there evil psychic phenomena? Yes. We call them black magic because they are empowered by evil and demonic spirits. Are there evil religions? Yes. One form is Satanism, the personification of evil spiritual thought. Anytime a church spreads hatred and violence, it expresses evil.

It is so easy to condemn non-religious psychic phenomena or the beliefs of other religions merely because they differ from our own understanding. In the Sermon on the Mount, Jesus offered advice on discerning between religious beliefs. Jesus stated, *"Beware of false prophets, who come to you in sheep's clothing but inwardly are ravenous wolves. You will know them by their fruits.... So, every sound tree bears good fruit, but the bad tree bears evil fruit. A sound tree does not bear evil fruit, nor can a bad tree bear good fruit....Thus you will know them by their fruits" (John 7:16-19).*

Enhanced intuitive abilities or psychic abilities are the basis for all religious miracles. We discern the merits of any religious group, religious miracle or enhanced intuitive ability by their fruits. Do they produce goodness, love, responsibility, peace, justice and interpersonal harmony? Do they effectively empower people by enhancing their health, happiness and spirituality? Do they consistently help people? Using results as an evaluation tool may prove that there are groups within every religion that produce evil outcomes or consequences.

Religious rituals empower believers in every religion. My studies indicate that all religious rituals are magic rituals, or ritual magic. In Christianity, baptism, communion, confirmation, ordination, weddings, and prayers are all forms of ritual magic. Each uses ritual words designed to bring the power of God into human lives. Each produces similar fruits, bringing God's power into the human energy field to act in intelligent, loving, transforming, empowering ways.

Years ago, I was at a meeting where I angered a practitioner of black magic. I abruptly left his group and went home. Knowing how vindictive he was, I knew I was about to be cursed by a black magic ritual. Being an expert in magic rituals, I knew I could be harmed, so I sought a defense. I used Christian ritual magic to surround my home in a protective bubble of love while sending the whole black magic group Christ's love and peace. I slept the night in confidence, knowing that any magical curse directed toward me would be reversed and affect the perpetrators instead.

The next morning, I received a phone call from a woman in that group warning me that a spell had been cast upon me that would make me ill. An hour later, another woman phoned to tell me that the black magician had spent the night ill with a high fever, stomach cramps, vomiting and diarrhea. I could simply state that I had prayed for God to protect me. I had. But, I had done more than that. I had used a prayer ritual, or ritual magic, invoking Christ as the source of the power. The black magician had invoked demons to empower his ritual magic. Both the source and the purpose of my rituals represented goodness. The source, the intent and the results of his ritual were evil. We both used ritual magic, a morally neutral technique.

INTUITIVE ABILITIES ARE A GIFT TO ALL HUMANITY

In the box seen above, A Comparison of Terms for Intuitive Abilities, we compared the universal gifts that are the heritage of all humanity. The common element uniting all the world's religions is not just that we all worship the same God. Uniting all religions is the universal human experience of God and his spiritual universe through revelation, vision, prophecy, guidance, the afterlife, healing and communication with the spirit world.

The ability to act as a channel for healing exists in every culture and religion. Any person who loves another person with compassion and oneness can offer that person God's healing love energy. Since channels for healing exist outside of Christianity, the Church's exclusive claim for Christ as healer through the spiritual gifts is not objectively valid.

This is a necessary shift in thinking -- a demythologizing of how the Holy Spirit is at work in our lives. It is also an empowering concept. It implies that any religion that upholds God's love as the source of creation, wholeness and new life is valid in its teachings. This concept can lay new beginnings for all humanity. These approaches promise new life for the world's religions. They also lay the foundations for interfaith understanding, tolerance, respect and cooperation. They raise hope that the Golden Age of peace with justice may soon become reality for all humanity. This hope is rooted in the power of Therapeutic Prayers to restore and make all things new.

CAUTIONS FOR THE SPIRITUAL JOURNEY

Is there anything immoral or evil about intuitive experiences? In the Middle Ages, Christians meditating in monasteries had similar experiences. Their leaders discouraged them, telling them to focus only upon their religious purpose, experiencing God. Today, the same advice is given. When practicing prayer, meditation, or contemplation, a few people experience "bad trips." Vulgar, immoral or sacrilegious data may appear. This is usually attributed to outside evil forces and influences. In rare instances, this is true. Experts in the field provide another explanation. This material is produced by one's own subconscious mind.

Our subconscious minds may be filled with pain, fear, anger, hurt, shame and guilt, which become uncovered by the awareness awakened in spiritual practices. In rare instances you may come upon spirit entities, some of whom may wish to possess you. Subconscious and conscious forces can empower such beings. Panic and terror are the worst responses. Be aware that you do have control of your own mind. If problems persist, seek professional help. Those actively involved with traditional religious practices are protected by the presence of God's spirit, a sacred presence in the human energy fields. Spirit possession exists. But prayer, meditation and contemplation are far safer than walking, bicycling, or riding in an automobile as far as injury and death are concerned. I have heard of no one who has been physically harmed by spiritual endeavors. On the other hand, expanded inner awareness can be an exciting and rewarding journey.

Some caution is warranted. Those with unresolved painful or guilty memories will eventually confront these during the long-term practice of meditation or prayer. In such circumstances, a competent person must guide them. Passive and suggestive people lacking in ego-strength also need a guide. Persons with psychiatric histories of schizophrenia, mania, depression, paranoia, multiple personality and borderline personality should refrain from meditation, except under the guidance of a mental health professional. This is also true of persons on mood-altering prescription drugs and those with drug dependencies. The main danger comes from the fact that whatever is present within the mind of a person is expanded and empowered.

Criminals, abusers of others, and manipulators will have expanded access to both the higher self and the lower self. Possession by evil entities also becomes more probable for them and for those who have studied and believe in Satanism. Believe in Satanism and your beliefs will become powerful forces with a life of their own that controls you, beginning within the spiritual state and continuing when you return to a normal state of consciousness. Beware when any inner voice commands or suggests that you do something morally wrong, or sounds manipulative or ignorant. Don't obey it! It is probable that many serial killers and rapists are not just demonstrating uncontrollable compulsive behavior. Their statements to the media are consistent with what we know of possession by evil or demonic spirits. The use of the ritual magic of exorcism may be effective in eliminating their destructive compulsions.

Those actively involved with traditional religious practices are partially protected by God's spirit, a sacred presence in the human energy field. All persons need to take the precaution of using rituals to protect themselves from evil or random spiritual forces while in a spiritual state. Just addressing God provides protection.

Most cases of possession involve earth-bound spirits who are looking for vulnerable persons through whose minds and bodies they can continue an earthly existence. Earth-bound spirits belong to deceased persons who could not or would not leave this earth dimension following physical death. Some psychotherapists think that some chemical addictions are connected to the presence of earth-bound spirits that invade the bodies of vulnerable persons in order to continue practicing their addictions. Earth-bound spirits often leave when they are made aware of their circumstances and their destructive effects upon their hosts.

Familiar spirits, evil spirits, and demons do exist on their own, separate from the subconscious mind. Depossession may be required for resistant earth-bound spirits and for rare cases of evil, familiar, and demon spirits. This requires the team efforts of a clairvoyant and a healer or a knowledgeable priestly intercessor. Instances of possession as a direct result of meditation and prayer would be unusual. Possession is more likely to occur in a group setting, due to the powerful forces generated by group energy fields, or because of an individual's involvement with evil activities or persons.

THE GOLDEN RULE in the World's Great Religions

CHRISTIANITY: *"Whatever you wish that men would do to you, do so to them."*

JUDAISM: *"What is hurtful to yourself, do not to your fellow man."*

ISLAM: *"No one of you is a believer until he loves for his brother what he loves for himself."*

HINDUISM: *"Do not to others, which if done to you, would cause you pain."*

BUDDHISM: *"In five ways should a clansman minister to his friends and familiars -- by generosity, courtesy and benevolence, by treating them as he treats himself, and by being as good as his word."*

JAINISM: *"In happiness and suffering, in joy and grief, we should regard all creatures as we regard ourselves."*

ZOROASTRIANISM: *"That nature only is good when it shall not do to another whatever is not good for its own self."*

TAOISM: *"Regard your neighbor's gain as your own gain and regard your neighbor's loss as your own loss."*

CONFUCIANISM: *"Do not to others what you would not they should do to you."*

SIKHISM: *"As you do for yourself, so do for others. Then shall you become a partner in heaven."*

Copyright permission courtesy of Marcus Bach

Chapter Fourteen

Protecting Yourself from People Fatigue

"Every great discovery contains an irrational element or a creative intuition." ...Karl Popper

"As exemplified in Jesus Christ, love is the most durable power in the world." ...Martin Luther King, Jr.*

"...if we love one another, God abides in us and his love is perfected in us." ...John 4:12

For years, it affected me. Counseling sessions often exhausted me, especially with persons who were depressed, angry, anxious or fearful. When I walked down the hospital corridor of a cancer ward, I could feel myself being drained. An hour's trip through a crowded shopping mall left me exhausted.

Millions share my former plight, constant fatigue. People sensitive to the needs of others often pay a price, a sense of being drained of energy. Many of those affected are professional caregivers. A clinical psychologist once told me an eight-hour day with clients left him with no energy resources to share with his family. He felt this played a role in his divorce.

Teachers, nurses, doctors, counselors, clergy, social workers and salespersons have all shared the vocational problem of becoming drained day after day. Some eventually burn out and take early retirement. Others may be victims of Chronic Fatigue Syndrome, a condition that limits the lives of millions of Americans.

These people possess few hints about the source of their exhaustion. If the symptoms get too severe, they consult their physician, seeking the cause. Usually a physician suggests learning how to cope with stress. But, no matter what they do, the fatigue persists. What's causing this?

A dozen years ago, I came to the conclusion that mental effort, stress and physical health could not account for my fatigue. My energy could be restored by a good night's sleep or spending a day at home. It was spending time with certain people that seemed to cause my fatigue. I concluded that those people were somehow draining my energy.

ENERGY VAMPIRES

Then I heard a new term, *"energy vampire."* With that phrase, all the pieces of the puzzle began to fit together. As I counseled troubled persons, I came to sense that their energy fields were exhausting me. When I entered a hospital patient ward, the patients were draining me in some unknown way. Large crowds were somehow wiping me out. I was a victim of energy vampires.

When I studied life energies research, I found evidence that my earlier conclusions had a scientific basis. The radiations of human energy fields are not imprisoned by the outer skin of the physical body. They project constantly outwards, often to a radius of twenty-five feet, mingling and interacting with the environment.

All energy contains information that can influence human energy fields. Concern has been expressed about the effects of the various man-made electromagnetic frequencies bombarding us from high-power lines, computer terminals, microwave ovens, etc. Of equal or greater effect may be the energy interactions we have with other people.

Ambrose Worrall observed that life energy, like electricity, flows from a strong source of energy to a weaker source. People who cannot produce enough energy for their own needs are forced to steal it from other sources.

From clinical data we know that healers transmit an energy that transforms and brings health to others. In chapter seven, we discovered that group energy fields bathe their participants in information that acts intelligently according to that information. Group energy fields can influence people to love or to riot. Individual energy fields affect us as much as group fields.

EXAMPLES OF INDIVIDUAL ENERGY FIELD INTERACTIONS

Depressed People Drain. Many who work with depressed persons report large energy drains. A depressed person's energy field works in the same way as what astronomers call a *"black hole"* in space. A black hole absorbs all the energy around it but is never saturated. A depressed person's energy field seems to operate in a similar fashion. It absorbs all the energy around it but is seemingly not energized by it. The energy disappears as if going down a whirlpool-like drain into another dimension, or as if it is leaking through holes in a ruptured human energy field. Depressed persons are the worst type of energy vampires. Their enormous need for energy can only be satisfied by draining the energy from other people's energy fields.

Cancer Patients Drain. People with cancer display similar characteristics. The research data of life energy scientists suggest cancer cells develop energy fields independent of the physical body's energy fields. The energy field of cancer cells competes with the body's own energy system for energy. It seems to absorb the energy around it to reinforce its own cell strength. The patient is then forced to draw life energy from his environment, including from other people.

Energy Field Pollution. Evidence exists for human *energy field pollution.* When energy fields interact, one field can leave information -- mental, emotional, physical or spiritual -- which influences the energy field of another. If this is unwanted information, it is influencing and polluting another person's energy field. The energy fields of those persons who are angry, resentful, fearful, and feeling inadequate, contaminate the fields of others. Polluted energy fields coat you with foreign negative feelings and thoughts that short-circuit a normal flow and balance. This causes fatigue until the pollution is either removed or diluted by time. *This is a theoretical working model for energy field contamination.*

Energy Field Pollution and Illness. Researchers have been studying the role of the emotions in the onset of physical illness. This is mind-body work on the role of a patient's internal mental and emotional processes in the onset of disease. Unresolved anger has been linked to the onset of a number of diseases. All of these mind-body studies have only examined the emotions of the person who is ill. None has taken into account the negative emotions present in the patient's environment. Could living in a hostile emotional environment prove to be a primary link to disease?

My own observations in a hostile work environment suggest such a linkage. Energy field interactions provide the mechanism. Twenty-five years ago, as I began a ministry in the inner city, urban riots broke out in the neighborhood I was serving. In the aftermath of this violence, immense hostility and distrust arose between white and black residents of the community. Being a white professional in the midst of the black community, I became an available target for black hostility. I received weekly death threats from neighborhood residents for more than a year and was surrounded with hostility daily for almost five years.

Two other white clergymen shared a similar hostile environment. The first, Earl, suffered a heart attack a year before I left. I asked to leave that neighborhood because the stress had already produced hemorrhoids in myself. Eighteen months later, I had a heart attack from clogged coronary arteries. While recovering, I phoned my second clergy friend in that neighborhood, Bob, suggesting he leave that hostile environment *"because it might damage your health."* A year later, Bob suffered a heart attack.

Yes, our heart attacks were stress-related. But it was not the anger within us that corroded our coronary arteries. It was not self-generated anger. It was the anger directed at us by others, as an energy, that filled our energy fields with poisonous venom. I suggest that researchers examine the emotional environment that patients live in when exploring the mind-body connection. Medical treatment could include using touch-healing techniques that remove the negative emotions from the heart chakra.

Interpersonal Energy Interactions. An angry person sends angry energy field emanations with extreme power. Some recipients may cower in fear. When one person intimidates the other, it is not just the force of words or a conditioned response. The intimidated person cringes because of an invisible interaction of energy fields allowing the intimidation to occur. Any defense must not only involve assertiveness training, but a means of protecting one's own energy fields from attack

Energy Intimidates Family Members. I have counseled many wives who are routinely intimidated by their husbands. No matter how the wife attempts to cope -- even with assertiveness training -- she is always fighting a losing battle. Her irritated or angry husband dominates every encounter; his projected energy field always overwhelms hers.

Knowing this, dominated spouses can learn to marshal the resources needed to become equals in such energy field power struggles. Do not choose projecting anger as your weapon of defense. This escalates the anger and leads to violence. You form a group energy field during this interaction that quadruples the power of your individual emotions.

Any defense involves either blocking off the other person's access to your energy field with a shield or projecting an energy filled with compassionate love that neutralizes the anger, as acid is neutralized by an alkaline substance. The best psychological defense is verbally acknowledging the anger of the angry person. Example: *"I sense that you are angry."*

Loving Interactions. The sharing of positive emotions is the upside of energy field interactions. Huggers sense this. Family members share their love and peace with each other, forming a life-giving group energy field which others can easily sense.

Lovers know the passionate energy of their human energy fields merging into sensations of heat, tingling and pleasure. Lovers never lose their physical passion when they learn to merge their energy fields through Asian and Hindu energy field merging techniques.

One can feel the emotional warmth emanating from the rooms of a home where there is love, joy and peace. One can also feel fear, anger, or an emotional void, in the home of a dysfunctional marriage or family.

Caution is needed here. Yes, we can sometimes sense the information of another's human energy field. Note the word *sometimes.* Sometimes we may be attributing our own inner state or expectations to the other person. When you are sensing anger or fear in another, what does that mean? Is the person angry with you, with himself, someone else, or the whole world? Is the anger ongoing or temporary? Either way, what do you do with that information?

We need to be aware of both the temporary and long-term states of the human energy fields. When you are with a therapeutic personality or a healer, you will usually sense an atmosphere of peace and love. This is the 7.83 hertz frequency emitted by the healer's energy fields. Those persons may not feel its influence themselves, but others around them will. It is difficult to leave the presence of such persons because of the beneficial effects of their energy fields.

If you spend considerable time with a family member, friend or fellow worker, you are susceptible to what is going on within them, and they, to you. A fellow worker is despondent because his spouse has left him. How does that affect you? In your household, a family member is physically ill or emotionally troubled. How does his or her impaired energy field affect you? Do the energy fields of others have short- or long-term effects upon yours? If each disease has a unique frequency, can the interaction of energy fields increase the likelihood of your contracting the illness? If so, how long must a contact be sustained for it to have a permanent or harmful effect?

Feeling-Thinking Interaction. The love between two persons is transmitted in the information shared by their merged energy fields. Persons who lack this awareness are socially and interpersonally handicapped. When a feeling type of *"people-person"* expresses feelings to a thinking, logical type of person, the thinking type is usually unaware of the feelings expressed in the energy field. The thinking type tends to be blind to the feeling levels of energy and unable to pick up emotional information or cues from energy fields. Unable to sense the energy of feelings, the thinking type is labeled *unfeeling.* This is true, if he is unable to sense feelings in energy fields.

Minority Abilities. People who hold a minority status in any culture tend to be capable of picking up the feeling-information projected in human energy fields by the majority culture. It is a useful skill that is necessary for survival in a suspicious and sometimes hostile environment. Black Americans have told me that they have a sixth sense -- a survival trait, an intuitive ability -- telling them when someone holds prejudiced feelings towards them. Existence of human energy fields that are bearers of information accounts for this survival trait.

Group Negotiations. Information present and discernible in human energy fields explains many things. When any two individuals or groups are negotiating their differences, the interaction of their energy fields plays a major role in the results. Whether it is two different factions, races, cultures, nations, or management versus labor, beneficial results are more likely to occur when their interacting energy fields are taken into account.

A Promising Future. I can envision a future where a growing awareness of human energy field interactions plays a major role. If we can learn to sense the sacredness and humanity in the energy fields of every person, then the entire human race will learn to treat all persons with dignity and fairness. If those who inflict cruelty upon others begin sensing the pain, anguish, and hurt they are causing, this will slowly begin to transform them into more compassionate persons.

DR. SHAFICA KARAGULLA'S RESEARCH

I discovered energy field interactions through observation and life energies data. A neuropsychiatrist put together a similar picture. Dr. Shafica Karagulla's fascinating findings on eight years of research in the field of what she calls Higher Sense Perception are reported in her 1967 book, Breakthrough To Creativity.

Sensitives. Her research used *"sensitives"* (clairvoyants) some of whom could see into and through the human body. Their diagnoses of states of health and illness correlated accurately with medical findings. Other sensitives could see energy exchanges among individuals in a group and describe what happens when people experience the energy pull of human *"sappers"* (energy vampires). We now focus on the latter.

Interpenetrating Energy Fields. Dr. Karagulla states that some of the sensitives with whom she worked described interpenetrating fields of energy surrounding the human body. Three fields are *seen* and unified with each other. One is the physical energy field closely related to the body. Then there is the emotional energy field extending from twelve to eighteen inches from the body. Finally, extending two feet or more from the physical body is the mental energy field.

Emotional Persons. *Sensitives* observe that certain activities, ideas and experiences seem to increase the inflow of energy into the field of a given individual. Coming into the presence of a well-beloved person intensely brightens all three fields. Some people's energy fields are brightened by interesting intellectual conversation. The emotionally focused person likes to stir up emotional scenes around him that tend to cause those in his group to appear depleted and low in energy.

Many sensitives say we live and move in a vast and immense ocean of energy. People use varying means for taking in different types of energy. Emotions like grief or self-centeredness appear to diminish greatly the individual's access to this energy supply.

Within a group, there is often a stimulating exchange of energies between and among individuals, described as bright lines of energy connecting two people who may be across the room from each other, such as husband and wife.

Performers. When an actor is performing before an audience, the actor's emotional field seems to glow, expand and extend outward until the emotional field of the audience blends with the vastly extended field of the performer. A unified group emotional field is maintained for the duration of the performance. When the performer is unable to create this unified field, his performance is rated poorly. This may be similar to the exceptional ability of a healer to mold individuals into a strong healing group energy field.

A Charismatic Personality. We say that a person who can hold a group spellbound has a charismatic personality. How true that statement is! His/her charisma or energy field envelops the group, forms a group energy field and influences all participants.

KARIGULLA'S ENERGY SAPPERS

Dr. Karigulla's research data on *"sappers"* as described by sensitives is similar to my experience covered earlier in this chapter. Certain persons, having a closed-in energy field, seem unable to pick up their needed energy from the surrounding ocean of energy. It appears they take their energy *pre-digested* from people in their immediate vicinity. Sappers are usually self-centered individuals. Victims of the sapper's energy draining effects find that they feel a need to leave the presence of the sapper.

The sapper pulls the energy from whatever is a person's weakest energy vortex; it could be from a weakened heart vortex or throat vortex, or from wherever resistance is weakest. Some appear to use their voices, others, their eyes, to drain the energy of those around them. Sappers may be found among socially passive observers at a party or gathering.

Sensitives describe the sapper as having a wide opening in the solar plexus area. From the edges of this opening, streamers or tentacles appear to shoot out and hook into the energy fields of a person who is close, in order to steal his energy. Sappers who use their voices or eyes do not have to be close to drain others.

All who may benefit from the information provided by this pioneer researcher owe their thanks to Shafica Karagulla. Her contributions to this field are invaluable.

THINKING TYPES ARE IMMUNE TO ENERGY DRAINERS

People interact with the personal energy fields of others in varying ways. Some may have a natural immunity to both energy vampires and energy polluters. They were born with or have acquired a shielding that protects their energy field. This immunity may come from either their innate personality type, an act of will or a state of consciousness.

In terms of the Myers-Briggs Type Indicator, thinking types are likely to have this immunity, an immunity that makes them appear to be insensitive to the feelings of others. The truth is that they are unaware of the energy fields of others and to the emotional content of those fields. Sensing types

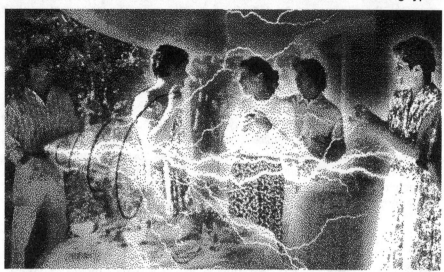

Figure 9. *Energy interchanges always occur in group settings. Quiet observant people may acquire an energy high in such gatherings as they unknowingly steal energy from others, acting as sappers.*

may also possess various forms of immunity. Introverts may be immune until they open themselves to others.

Using this theory, the person most immune would be the thinking-introverted-sensing type personality. Such personality types may have difficulty receiving healing energy. They also may not understand this chapter nor find it helpful, except for self-understanding.

FEELING TYPES MOST VULNERABLE TO DRAINERS

Other personality types may have far fewer natural defenses to the energy fields of others. The feeling type may be the most open to harm from other energy fields, with the extroversion and intuitive traits adding to the problem. The extrovert quickly exchanges energy with others. The intuitive person is often too unaware of what s/he is sensing to create a defense. The profile of a healer provides evidence that healers display all three of these traits, making them extremely vulnerable to energy vampires and polluters.

People in the caring professions often exhibit one or more of these traits that give them a natural ability to care for people. When they have compassion for another human being and reach out in a caring way, they risk having their energy fields drained and polluted by the very people they are seeking to help. This happens any time one is empathetic. Because the energy of love is so powerful, the one possible defense would be to be sure to project love when entering into a compassionate and empathetic link with another.

School teachers may find themselves so badly drained by their daily contact with students that they spend their free time simply sitting in a stupor of fatigue. Once teachers learn to protect their energy fields from drainage, their lives can be transformed into ones of satisfaction, rather than weariness. Anyone whose vocation involves continued contact with people may experience *"people fatigue."*

Feeling types are the most vulnerable. They are badly disturbed by arguments because of the resulting energy field interactions. During periods of alienation between members of a household, feeling types are vulnerable to the negative feelings of those from whom they are emotionally separated. Members of a household may project their negative feelings like anger, anxiety and fear, even while sleeping.

Feeling types will have found these concepts to be helpful. They will identify with the theoretical model that has just been presented because it fits their personal experience. When they learn to protect and to cleanse their energy fields, their quality of life will be greatly enhanced.

PROTECTING ONE'S ENERGY FIELDS

There are several ways to protect one's energy field. The basic strategy involves erecting a protective covering or shield around one's own energy field. This can be done in one of several ways. The shield is put in place before entering a situation where negative feelings or energy drains may be present.

Always pray for God to protect you in what you are doing. A prayer I have found helpful says,

"God, please protect my energy field from being depleted or polluted by others. Surround me in your love and light. Let the method I am using be all I need."

Other options include the following, with the first three options providing protection for about an hour.

1. **Space Suit Protection.** Imagine donning a space suit that protects you, zipping it up to cover you completely. Say the above prayer.

2. **Protective Bubble.** Use a protective mental bubble. Entwine the straightened fingers of both hands with each other. Begin at the groin and, keeping your elbows slight bent, move your hands to behind your neck and then do the same as you move back down to your groin area. Say the above prayer.

3. **Filled with God.** Keep yourself filled with God's love and continually project it.

4. **Saran Wrap** protects you for six to eight hours. Take a piece of Saran Wrap (reportedly only Saran Wrap will do) about ten inches long. Stretch it both ways. Then place it over the area of your solar plexus (diaphragm), which is located between your rib cage and your navel. Se-

cure it in place with clothing. After six hours, restretch the Saran Wrap and put it back. The solar plexus is the primary energy center where energy drainage and pollution occur.

5. **Cross Limbs.** Crossing your arms with your hands around your sides protects your diaphragm's energy field. When sitting or lying, crossing your ankles provides similar protection.

6. **A Watch.** Wear a special watch on your left wrist that broadcasts an extremely low frequency wavelength in the seven to nine hertz range. This keeps one's energy field balanced and protects it from the frequencies on which negative energies are broadcast. Most health food stores can tell you where to order one. All these protective measures work for me. My energy levels remain constantly high. Yet there is a possibility that my belief in these methods provides protection through subconscious projection.

CLEANSING AND RECHARGING ONE'S ENERGY FIELD

When energy field pollution exhausts you, how do you cleanse and replenish your energy fields? Again there are several possibilities.

1. **Showering.** Taking a shower cleanses the energy field. This suggests that the best time to take a shower is after work or after an argument. Once the water cleanses the energy field, the gross fatigue will vanish and in time you will fully recharge yourself. Be aware that showering also makes one more vulnerable, washing away one's own energy field protection for an hour or more.

2. **Water on Wrists.** Some spiritualists believe that running cool water over both wrists is quicker and safer. They caution about showers making one's energy field more vulnerable, suggesting fewer showers. It might be prudent to avoid taking a shower an hour or two before going out in public.

3. **Water Rinsing.** Rinsing one's face and hands in water is a partial cleansing.

4. **Epsom Salts.** Bernard Grad suggests soaking one's feet in Epsom salts.

5. **Salt and Soda Bath.** Barbara Ann Brennan prescribes a twenty minute bath in a warm tub of one pound sea salt and one pound baking soda. She cautions that this may make you weak as it draws large quantities of energy out of the body, so be prepared to rest afterward to replenish yourself.

6. **Drinking Water.** Barbara Ann Brennan suggests drinking water to cleanse one's energy fields.

7. **Hand Cleansing/Recharging.** My favorite method for a quick cleansing and recharging during moments throughout the day is this. Hold your open hands palms up. Pray, *"God, use my hands to cleanse my energy field."* Then, beginning at the feet, move your hands all over your body in a scooping motion. Don't forget your head area. While doing this, periodically place the energy you are scraping off onto the floor. By patting your palms flat against the floor, you are releasing the energy you have removed into the Earth, which will purify and reuse it.

Then, to recharge (you can also do this after a shower), hold your open hands before you, palms up. Pray, *"God, use my hands as channels to recharge and balance my energy fields."* Using a straightened hand, palms towards the body and not touching the skin, move your hands over your entire energy field. I prefer about one inch from the skin. I often repeat the procedure further out at about four inches.

8. **Embrace.** You can embrace someone you love. Children and dogs are great for this.

9. **The Sun.** You can lie in the sun.

10. **A healer** can recharge you.

11. **Many other ways.** Recharging can also be done through deep breathing exercises, inhaling through the nose and exhaling through the mouth, self-relaxing techniques, meditation, reading poetry, listening to classical music, singing sacred songs, using prayer and contemplation, attending a religious service, strolling through a garden or walking through woods. Feel free to put your arms around a tree to draw energy.

A CAUTION

Some will feel uncomfortable with these exercises. A decade ago, my wife and I visited Massachusetts on vacation. After a day of sightseeing with old friends among large crowds, we pulled into a restaurant parking lot for dinner. I felt fatigued. After explaining what I was about to do, I practiced Hand Cleansing/Recharging beside the car, feeling refreshed afterwards. Our friends remained troubled by what I did. Out of concern, one advised, *"Walter, if you must, be more discreet."*

When people complain of undue fatigue, I have sought to help them protect and restore their energy fields, with mixed responses. Those who have experimented report good results. My reputation has suffered in the eyes of scoffers.

Discreetly experiment to see what works best for you. If you have a friend who is also seeking to protect, cleanse, and re-charge his or her energy fields, share what works with each other.

PRAYWELL

A GUIDE TO
SELF HEALING

RESOURCES FOR THOSE WHO STRUGGLE
WITH CHRONIC, LIFE LIMITING OR LIFE THREATENING
MEDICAL OR EMOTIONAL CONDITIONS

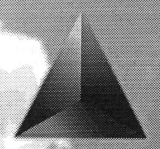

PART TWO

A PRAYER IN THE MIDST OF AN ILLNESS

God, I am puzzled by what has happened to me. My life has abruptly changed. My plans have been interrupted. My confidence has been shattered and my peace destroyed. I am angry. I am hurt. I am fightened. I am not sure I can face tomorrow, yet I really have no choice, for today is here and tomorrow comes. Who will deliver me from this endless nightmare? You, God? Are you my strength and my salvation?

I feel as if somehow I have failed. I feel guilty about being sick when I truly wish to be well. I am proud. I have always considered myself to be so competent and self-reliant and yet now I feel so helpless. Enable me to accept the loving care of those who love me. Hold me in your love. I seem to be dwelling more and more with you, God. You are becoming my strength and my salvation.

God, remove my anger, my hurt, my fear, my loss, my darkness, as I seek to dwell in you. Fill my soul with your transforming light. Hold me in your never-failing strong arms and never let me go! Yes! You have become my strength and my salvation!

I often feel sad. Will I ever run again with the breeze caressing my face? Will I ever dance again with vibrant life coursing through my veins? Will I ever laugh without a bitter edge? Will I ever sing with joy filling my soul? Will I ever be loved again because I am strong and whole? Lord God, please heal my inner being and fill me with your strength, with the love, joy and peace of your presence. For you, God, are my strength and my salvation.

God, I often ponder the death of my dreams. I have struggled and have grown. I have laughed and I have played. I have created and achieved. I have loved and known deep love. I have dreamed of many years down the road. I once thought earthly life was endless, but now I know that each earthly journey is limited. Open me to new dreams which will still yield happiness and fulfillment. Teach me the joys of this day. For you are my strength and my salvation!

God, assure me that my soul is eternal. Let me live in your love, that when this earthly journey ends, with trust, I will gladly rest in your everlasting arms -- free to grow and to become forever. I know that you are with me in life, in death and in life beyond death. For you are my strength and my salvation!

God, help me to see clearly through new eyes. Open me to the opportunities and joys still before me. You have enabled me to take control of my life. I choose to live each day fully and satisfyingly. I choose to live, to love, to care! I choose to live in your presence. Completely transform my inner being so that I am filled with love and light! Heal me in body, mind and spirit that I might become a blessing to myself and to others. I know that new life awaits me. For you are my strength and my salvation! Amen.

Written by Walter Weston in the midst of his own struggles with heart disease.

Chapter Fifteen

Healing the Emotional Issues of an Illness

"Sudden illness occasions the thought of life's variableness and of the soul's imminent danger in face of the body's death." ...John Donne

"We experience God in our lives as the will to love." ...Albert Schweitzer*

"There is no fear in love, for perfect love casts out fear." ...John 4:18a

---

From the moment you receive a frightening medical diagnosis, the emotional issues begin overshadowing the physical symptoms. You now feel trapped in an unreliable body with no way out. These emotional issues have the power to hinder or block the efforts of medical treatment and therapeutic prayer. It is crucial to give first priority to the emotional issues before tackling physical self-healing through prayer.

Facing an illness can be just as frightening as military combat. Combat soldiers become heroes while facing terror on the battlefield. Many of the ill face similar fears and dangers. We have all known people who should have been awarded a medal of valor for their courage in the midst of medical battles.

During a health crisis, the emotional issues are predictable. Others with a similar health problem will have comparable emotional responses. You are not only physically sick; you have been emotionally wounded. The ability to work through these emotions will determine your ability to cope with your illness.

PrayWell provides the emotional and spiritual resources you need to help you fight for your health and your life. This will enhance the results of both medical treatment and healing prayer. I have faced several major illnesses. The emotional issues I faced mirror yours in many ways. To provide you with insight for your own journey, here is my own story of woundedness and self-healing.

A PERSONAL TALE

In 1975, at the age of thirty-nine, I found my life rudely interrupted by a heart attack. It had all begun on a beautiful summer's day in Ohio, but the weather now no longer mattered. Even my personal and professional responsibilities had faded into the background. I was now entirely focused upon fighting for my life.

I spent three weeks in the hospital's coronary care unit. Before I was discharged, my doctor told me the medical truth. My heart muscle had been badly damaged. I would never work again. I would never move faster than a slow walk. When pressed, he admitted that he did not expect me to live through the year. As my wife drove me home, I sat immersed in emotional shock.

I had only been home a few hours when I saw my wife, Dana, pass by my doorway. I was immediately haunted by that brief glimpse. Her eyes were red from crying and her features were etched in anguish and fear. While I was a patient in coronary care, Dana had daily entered my hospital room cheerfully, wearing a big smile. As we visited, she would chatter lightly about family and work -- no serious talk. Yet, I had noted the strain in her face and the fear in her eyes. Now we were home together again. She, too, had just heard the doctor's grim prognosis. She, too, was experiencing emotional agony. My heart went out to her. After she passed my doorway, I called her name. She took time to become composed and then entered. I asked her to sit next to me and held her hand.

Sharing. I opened our conversation with, *"You have been very brave the past three weeks with your smiles and reassurances. I know how tough it has been on you. Your tears deeply move me. I feel good about being loved that much. I have been scared, too."* We both began crying; an emotional release of all the pent-up feelings we had been hiding from each other for weeks. After the tears were gone, we looked at each other with intense love, caring and spiritual compassion. We affirmed our common woundedness by talking about it. This was sealed with a hug and a kiss. We then joined hands and prayed aloud. It was one of the most deeply rewarding experiences of our marriage.

The honest sharing of our deepest fears and the support of a mutual love was life-transforming and empowering for both of us. Our individual isolation was gone. Traveling this journey together made the future bearable.

Weak and Vulnerable. The next morning I was left alone. Dana was at work and our three children were in school. For the first time since childhood, I was afraid of being alone. I felt weak and vulnerable. That first day's events only confirmed these feelings, as I attempted to take a walk. Following an extremely slow thirty-yard walk, the angina pain in my chest forced me to sit down for five minutes before I returned to the house, exhausted. That evening, during the excitement of watching an action-adventure on television, the angina pain returned. As I got into bed for the night, the coldness of the sheets again set off the pain. I knew these were signs that my heart muscles were screaming for more oxygen.

Shock Waves. As the days passed, one emotional shockwave after another hit me squarely as the significance of what was happening to me continued to sink in. I could not hide the truth from myself. As a parish pastor, I knew the reality of illness and dying. Besides fighting for physical survival, now came the lonely inner mental, emotional and spiritual battles that overshadowed most of my waking and sleeping hours.

My first emotion was anger. My life had been rudely and brutally interrupted; it was changed forever. My pride had been bruised purple. I was deeply disappointed about things that could now never be. I felt a moral indignation, an anger at my condition that led me to ask, *"Why me?"* Spiritual wisdom finally answered, *"Illness can come to anyone and has little to do with one's goodness, worthiness or lovability. God still loves you and wishes you to become whole."*

The major emotion was fear. How long did I have to live? What happens to me when I die? In my remaining time, how could I cope with the many changes and limitations that had so suddenly taken control and changed my life? Who would support my family? How much of a burden was I to loved ones? I feared dying and I feared living. At first, I buried the fear of dying. I denied my vulnerability and my frightening future.

Confronting the fear. I was forced to confront this fear as I lay fully awake in bed for hours, night after night. My heart attack had occurred while I was sleeping. Now I was afraid I might not awaken if I went to sleep. It took me ten days to understand that fear was causing my insomnia. I asked questions about my fears, knowing the answers would help conquer these fears. Had my life been worthwhile? Do I have any regrets? Are there things I want to do before I die? Do I really believe that death is but a transition into the spirit world of God? The answers, combined with prayer, brought me assurance and inner peace. My religious faith assured me that God was with me in life, in death, and in life beyond death.

I also had a sense of desperation. I felt panic at being trapped in an unreliable body. For the first time in my life, there was no way out -- no creative answer. A deep sadness came over me, robbing me of already diminished energy and lessening my ability to sleep, eat, be cheerful and have inner contentment. I recognized this as depression.

I soon made the decision to fight. I asked my sixteen-year-old daughter to drive me to the public library for the most recent books on heart disease. I spent a week learning all I could about my disease. I continued to follow my doctor's orders and took my medications. I also decided to utilize spiritual resources. I had participated in many prayer healings, but held little hope for my own physical healing. Medical experts had written that it was impossible for the heart muscle to regenerate. I was merely seeking God's presence for emotional and spiritual support.

I studied the books in my library on the subjects of prayer, meditation and wholeness. From these, I chose what I would include in my daily meditative prayer. These included scripture passages, sacred songs, meditation exercises, contemplation, visualizations of wholeness and prayer.

A Spiritual Journey. Even though I was a clergyperson, I had never before so immersed myself in the spiritual journey. The urgency of crisis motivated me. For the first time, I had no responsibilities and plenty of free time. Every morning I spent one to two hours in meditative prayer. My colleagues later chuckled, saying that it was far longer than needed. At the time, it seemed just right. If faced with a similar health crisis today, I would spend similar amounts of time. As I practiced daily meditative prayer, I was surprised by the inner transformation. The immense struggle within began to subside. I sensed God's love, joy and peace. I came to an inner knowing that God was with me. I lost my fear of living and my fear of dying. I no longer struggled. I just placed myself in God's care. I wrote this prayer to describe my journey. You might use it as a model for your desired healing.

A PRAYER IN THE MIDST OF ILLNESS

God, I am puzzled by what has happened to me. My life has abruptly changed. My plans have been interrupted. My confidence has been shattered and my peace destroyed. I am angry. I am hurt. I am frightened. I am not sure I can face tomorrow, yet I really have no choice, for today is here and tomorrow comes. Who will deliver me from this endless nightmare? You, God? Are you my strength and my salvation?

I feel as if somehow I have failed. I feel guilty about being sick when I truly wish to be well. I am proud. I have always considered myself to be so competent and self-reliant and yet now I feel so help-less. Enable me to accept the loving care of those who love me. Hold me in your love. I seem to be dwelling more and more with you, God. You are becoming my strength and my salvation.

God, remove my anger, my hurt, my fear, my loss, my darkness, as I seek to dwell in you. Fill my soul with your transforming light. Hold me in your never-failing strong arms and never let me go! Yes! You have become my strength and my salvation!

I often feel sad. Will I ever run again with the breeze caressing my face? Will I ever dance again with vibrant life coursing through my veins? Will I ever laugh without a bitter edge? Will I ever sing with joy filling my soul? Will I ever be loved again because I am strong and whole? Lord God, please heal my inner being and fill me with your strength, with the love, joy and peace of your presence. For you, God, are my strength and my salvation!

God, I often ponder the death of my dreams. I have struggled and have grown. I have laughed and I have played. I have created and achieved. I have loved and known deep love. I have dreamed of many years down the road. I once thought earthly life was endless, but now I know that each earthly journey is limited. Open me to new dreams that will still yield happiness and fulfillment. Teach me the joys of this day. For you are my strength and my salvation!

God, assure me that my soul is eternal. Let me live in your love, that when this earthly journey ends, with trust, I will gladly rest in your everlasting arms...free to grow and to become forever. I know that you are with me in life, in death and in life beyond death. For you are my strength and my salvation!

God, help me to see clearly through new eyes. Open me to the opportunities and joys still before me. You have enabled me to take control of my life. I choose to live each day fully and satisfyingly. I choose to live, to love, to care! I choose to live in your presence. Completely transform my inner being so that I am filled with love and light! Heal me in body, mind and spirit that I might become a blessing to myself and to others. I know that new life awaits me. For you are my strength and my salvation! Amen.

Renewal. Meditative prayer filled me with faith, hope and peace. I no longer feared death, and felt renewed joy in living. Every morning and evening I thanked God for this joyous day of life. I experienced the intensity of the beauty all about me. Tears came easily as appreciation for my family grew and I treasured the previous years of my life. A deep sense of self-worth was emerging.

A Physical Healing. Then in the sixth week of these spiritual disciplines another miracle occurred. My dead heart muscle was healed, regenerated. Here is that experience:

Lying on my bed in the midst of a healing meditation, I found myself filled with a sense of God's presence. First, I felt a marvelous peace descend upon me, followed quickly by immense love, and then great joy! I felt tears of happiness streaming down my cheeks. I became aware of a Holy Presence. Brilliant white light filled my mind. I was in holy ecstasy. (The term "holy" is a traditional term for what the sensed presence of God feels like.) My arms, which had been resting at my sides, were suddenly lifted by some unknown agent and my hands were placed upon my chest. I was immersed in immense holiness. God. The hands resting upon my chest grew painfully hot. I felt the heat penetrating my whole body.

This peak experience of God seemed to be endless. Time stood still. A part of my intellect asked, *"Am I being healed?"* When I arose, I felt whole.

Confirmation. A few weeks later, during my three-month checkup, an EKG showed my heart muscle to be completely normal. The amazed cardiologist checked it against the ones originally taken in the coronary care unit and said, *"This is impossible. Such a thing has never been reported in medical literature. You are a miracle patient!"* He did not want to hear my story and refused to write up the healing for a medical journal. *"No one would believe me,"* he said.

I do not want to give the impression that my health problems ended with this healing of the heart muscle. Each of three heart catheterizations over a two-year period showed another coronary artery was completely closed, but I had developed life-sustaining capillary bypass circulation. Ten weeks out of the coronary care units, I was walking two miles daily. Eight months later, with medication, I was able to resume playing volleyball and racquetball three times a week. I continued daily meditative prayer. By 1979, I no longer required any medication. I thought I was home free. In 1983, walking again produced angina pain. A fourth heart catheterization showed that the artery feeding my coronary arteries was ninety percent occluded, a normally lethal condition. Quadruple coronary bypass surgery followed. Since that time, I have led a normal life with neither physical limitations nor need of medication.

I believe my healing was made possible by any number of circumstances. I experienced the love and support of my family, which filled our home with God's presence (as the healing energy). Family and friends sent me their cards and prayers. Self-examination and the experience of being ill changed my thinking and perspective. As a former eighty-hour a week workaholic, I now realized the preciousness of my family and the importance of a personal life. I placed God, my family, and myself as my highest priorities, subsequently expending more energy and time with each.

A Changed Lifestyle. I intentionally changed my lifestyle to combat heart disease. I attempted to change my Type A Behavior -- a life of endless hurrying and accumulating achievements. I stopped to smell the roses, as the saying goes, and fell in love with the fragrance. I took control of my life and began doing what brought personal satisfaction and happiness. Daily I reserved time for myself, my family, walking, praying and playing. I followed a low-cholesterol diet. I stopped over-scheduling myself and no longer wore a watch. All of these components enabled meditative prayer to work its miracles of healing.

God's Role. I know that God's intention is always for perfect health. Why didn't God heal my coronary arteries? The generated healing energy may not have had time to make arterial plaque disappear but I did develop collateral circulation. I am thankful for the healings that took place. I am even grateful for the health crisis. It deepened my faith, changed my perspective, enriched my lifestyle, and increased my joy.

A Shared Experience. I share this story because it is not unique. Humanity is united by its common experience of physical and emotional suffering. Others in similar circumstances would struggle with similar issues. The spiritual healing of my heart muscle was a result of the spiritual technology described in PrayWell. This is based upon the evidence and experience that spiritual healing processes work for everyone. PrayWell adds to the faith and hope welling within the hearts of all humanity in the midst of crisis. It also deepens existing relationships with God and others. I also believe that my success in resolving emotional and interpersonal issues removed any barriers that might have blocked spiritual healing.

YOUR FIRST INNER BATTLES

The Battle of Crisis. The first inner battle is brought on by the crisis itself. Daily plans and responsibilities will probably need to be put on hold. Being acutely ill, hospitalized, or emotionally immobilized or receiving a fear-inducing diagnosis, all call for refocusing your energies solely upon yourself. Life will momentarily have to go on without your contributions. Others will pick up the slack! You are more important than any of your former responsibilities. Assert your determination to deal with your own immediate needs, because your survival depends upon it.

Perspective. Put your crisis in perspective. Most crises are accompanied by disruptions, pain, fear, confusion and a sense of helplessness. These are not pleasant experiences but they are normal human reactions. If you are reading this, you survived. Even in life-threatening medical emergencies, ninety-eight percent survive the immediate crisis.

A health crisis can eventually be recognized as a friend. It may be an early warning sign that can eventually enhance the quality of your life. It may indicate that your lifestyle needs change through diet, exercise, stress management or cessation of smoking, alcohol and drugs. It may mean that you need to make major changes in vocation or family life in order to fulfill the need for personal happiness and satisfaction. It may begin an inner search for what needs to be healed within you, like painful memories, emotional trauma, anger, fear or a sense of personal inadequacy.

A health crisis can become a maturing experience. It can change your outlook and values for the better. It can lead to the appreciation of the essentials of life. It can place everything in better perspective by changing priorities and focusing upon deepening your relationship with loved ones. It can lead to more compassion and caring for others. If one chooses, a crisis can lead to a closer relationship with God. One's spiritual resources are a major factor in emerging from the crisis as a stronger, wiser, more mature person.

The Battle with Fear. Fear is the reaction we deny most, but fear has a purpose. It warns us that something we regard highly is being threatened. In this case, it is life itself, as well as all that your life is focused upon. Admitting fear lessens it. As a first step, admit to yourself that you are fearful. Then, admit this inner anxiety to loved ones and medical professionals. This helps you handle difficult situations. If you are fearful, your loved ones are also likely to be fearful. Talking about your fear and sharing it with them strengthens everyone.

Concern about physical pain is a common fear. Pain also serves a purpose. It warns us that something in our life needs attention. Assurances that the pain is not life-threatening can lessen it. Fear of pain increases its intensity. Focusing on pain makes it worse. Loving and being loved, concentrating elsewhere, self-hypnosis and prayer all reduce the severity of physical pain.

Medical diagnosis and prognosis can be the greatest causes of fear and the attendant emotional shock. This is normal. To hear that you have a life-limiting, chronic, life-threatening, or terminal illness is usually terrifying. Again, sharing your reactions with loved ones gives courage and strength to everyone involved.

The fear of dying and the fear of living are tied together. Once one conquers the fear of death, both fears end. Exploring the fear of dying involves several questions. Do I have any regrets? If so, how do I make amends? Has my life been worthwhile? If not, what can I do now to make it worthwhile? Is there anything I deeply desire to do before dying? If so, can I still in some way accomplish it? Do I really believe in the afterlife at the deepest emotional and spiritual levels? What spiritual assurances do I need in order to believe?

A THERAPEUTIC PRAYER FOR COPING WITH FEAR

God, my life has changed abruptly. Nothing will ever be the same again. I am tense. I know that much of that tension is due to fear. I fear this illness. I fear for my health. I fear for my future. I fear the limitations that have been placed upon my life. I fear for my loved ones. I fear about money matters. I fear death. I fear fear. I am not sure I have the strength needed to handle my life as it is.

God, I know that fear is draining me of energy that could better be used for my healing. Rather than seeking to defeat the fear through my own strength, I let go of my fear, God. I place my fear in your hands. I release my fear to you, God. I place myself in your hands. I accept your strength and your salvation. Fill me with your love, your strength, your assurance, your peace. You are with me in life, in death, in life beyond death. Make me aware of my own sacred and eternal nature. Your power and presence course throughout me and dwell within me. Thank you, God. I rest in your care. Amen.

The Battle with Vulnerability. Illness can destroy one's sense of invulnerability, power, confidence and competency. We feel weak and helpless. We will probably struggle to maintain control over our lives. We may need to rely upon many others, but this need not lead to dependency. People need to maintain a sense of control over their lives. If possible, do not relinquish control over decisions affecting your life. All medical treatment legally requires consent. Do follow medical instructions on self-care. To do otherwise is a form of denial that your condition is serious. The condition itself may directly relate to your attitude.

Seek to maintain as much independence as your condition permits. Graciously accept the care of medical personnel and family. It is necessary and normal to be assisted during an illness. Never consider yourself to be a burden, unless others are doing things for you that you are capable of doing for yourself. To deny loved ones the opportunity to care for you is robbing them of the means for expressing their love for you. You are worth loving. Try to remain in as much control of your life as possible.

A THERAPEUTIC PRAYER FOR COPING WITH VULNERABILITY

God, I feel so weak and helpless. I place myself in the care of others, trusting in their loving motives. In doing so, I feel safe and secure. And yet, I ask for confidence. I am essentially the same person I have always been, although my life has been changed. Fill me with your peace as I seek to maintain control of my life. I choose life. I choose to live each day as fully as possible. Make me aware of the love shared with people around me, of the beauty of this day, of the hope that dwells eternally within my heart. Be my strength and my salvation, God. Amen.

The Battle with Change. Many illnesses require drastic changes in lifestyle. Your physical activities may be limited. You may need to give up responsibilities on the job or at home. Your income may be reduced. Dietary changes may be required. You may have to give up certain things that have been satisfying parts of your life. This produces a sense of loss, of grief. You will adjust to the changes if you are willing to work at it. Most of life's options for happiness still remain open. To try clinging to that which must be changed is normal. Common sense usually wins. Learn to let go of the past, live in the present, and enjoy what is possible now. Emphasize what you have left, not what you have lost.

A THERAPEUTIC PRAYER FOR COPING IN THE MIDST OF CHANGE

God, my life is dramatically changing. A new way of living and thinking is forcing its way upon me. I feel a sadness about things that will no longer be possible. It is scary at times. Yet, most of what I truly value in life is still available to me.

God, enable me to find happiness and satisfaction as my new lifestyle emerges. Let my complaints become a source of humor as I discover possibilities for joy and happiness. I place myself in your care. Please guide me as I place my trust in your strength and guid-

ance. **Fill me with your love and light, provide for my needs and protect me from all harm. Thank you. Amen.**

Seeking to Cope. As people attempt to live with a major medical condition, they may use five common strategies in coping. These are denial, anger, bargaining, depression, and acceptance. They were identified by Dr. Elizabeth Kubler-Ross as the stages undergone by the dying, but they also may apply to those dealing with any major medical condition. The emotional shock and the resulting five strategies for coping are obstacles that often permit the disease to win without a fight. They detour one from the more urgent task of combating the disease. Being aware of these strategies can lead to an earlier resolution of the crisis. Unfortunately, these five strategies are not planned. They are unrehearsed responses to danger.

The Value of Hope. Fortunately, there is a way to avoid these responses. That is the way based upon hope. To hope means that even though you have discovered this terrible medical condition in your body, a bearable and fulfilling future still lies ahead. When hope dies, the danger responses grow stronger and can rule a person.

Two groups promoting the efficacy of hope are the mind-body advocates and practitioners of spiritual healing. Both assert that the medical diagnosis and prognosis are not the final word; they are only statements about the limitations of medical science, not about the future of your health. Diseases resistant to medical treatment may respond to the alternative approaches of mental-emotional and spiritual resources. As Bernie Siegel states, *"There are no incurable diseases, only incurable people."* This is a basis for realistic hope.

The combined data on the mind-body effects and spiritual healing results indicate that many illnesses resistant to medical treatment will respond to other approaches. The responses vary from the complete alleviation of all symptoms to vast improvements that increase the quality of living. This produces joy and a sense of usefulness. Should you go through these processes and still die, you will by then be so transformed that death becomes an acceptable Final Healing. Death can come, not as an enemy to be feared, but as a peaceful transition into further growth and fulfillment. These thoughts are the basis for realistic hope.

A THERAPEUTIC PRAYER OF HOPE

God, fill me with hope. Make me believe that I can cope with all that is before me. Help me to make my life worthwhile. Strengthen my determination to maintain control over my life. Enable me use all the resources available for my healing. Open me to the healing flow of your presence and love.

I know that you want me to become whole and I trust that you will struggle with me in my efforts. I place my life in your care. Fill me with a living hope for today, tomorrow and forever. God, thank you for being with me in life, in death and in life beyond death. Amen.

FIVE REACTIONS TO A MEDICAL CRISIS

These reactions do not come in any specific order, though acceptance is usually last, if it comes at all. Several or all may be occurring at one time. The self-healing therapeutic prayers in this chapter are designed to heal these reactions.

Denial. Denial involves not hearing, not accepting and ignoring the medical condition, or having hope of a miraculous intervention. About to leave coronary care, I taped my doctor's twenty-minute explanation of my heart condition. Afterwards, I realized that I recalled only a small portion of the information. At the end of the first replay of the cassette, I still remembered only half of what I had heard. I came to realize this only after making a complete written transcript of the cassette. This was a *not hearing painful news* type of denial.

Recovering from a heart attack, Sam could not accept his medical condition, but he followed his doctor's medication orders. Both Sam and his wife chose to remain ignorant of information on heart disease and aftercare precautions. This response is caused by a fear of the illness. This is another form of denial. A few weeks later, during a second heart attack, their wrong responses led to more serious heart damage. If denial is practiced for too long, it prevents you from fighting for your life.

A male colleague, Bill, ignored the seriousness of his condition. In coronary care, Bill stated that his heart attack *"was all a big fuss over nothing."* Arriving home, Bill boasted that nothing was going to keep him down. He made no changes in his lifestyle. Two days later, a second heart attack brought death.

Melissa's diagnosis was cancer. Her response was a faith statement, *"God will not let me die."* She refused all medical treatment, saying that God had already healed her cancer. Nearing death, she was puzzled that God had not intervened. Her response, though encased in religious belief, was a form of denial.

No clinical evidence exists that a faith in God alone will relieve the symptoms of cancer. *Taking actions based upon faith does open opportunities for healing.* The health-giving actions include following the doctor's directions, learning all you can about your illness, resolving the emotional issues of your illness, exploring the mind-body connection and seeking self-healing through prayer and other spiritual resources.

These are some reasons for denial. Denial can be necessary. It is a normal human defense mechanism. A person can only handle so much fear. Denial allows the medical truth to sink in slowly as one becomes emotionally able to handle it, one bit at a time. Denial can hold one in a hypnotic-like state where one is unable to see reality, even when others try to force it upon us. The evidence is that we can do little to help a person work through her/his denial. All attempts at intervention will fail to produce the desired results. Forcing persons to accept their medical conditions can hasten the arrival of death.

Time after time, I have heard loved ones and physicians say, *"You must accept that you have terminal cancer and you will not recover."* This is cruel and untrue. A few have survived terminal cancer. This statement robs people of the power of hope, faith and belief. It writes a script that usually leads to earlier death.

One way of working through denial is by sharing your concerns with supportive loved ones or a wellness support group. What are your denials? What fears prompt them? What can you do to resolve those fears?

A THERAPEUTIC PRAYER IN THE MIDST OF DENIAL

God, I have always been so self-reliant and competent. I had thought of myself as being strong and secure. Now I know fear and helplessness. There is no easy way out. There is no quick fix. This new journey is difficult. As I seek to handle it, let the truth slowly sink in. Provide me with the hope that I can handle all that is before me. Enable me to make the changes I need to fight for my health and my life.

God, I need you now as never before. Strengthen my inner self with your presence and power. Assure me of your love. Fill me with your peace. Grant me wholeness in body, mind and spirit, for you are becoming my strength and my salvation. Amen.

Anger. Anger is always present, even when suppressed and denied. Anger is the direct response to the illness. It is the result of life being disrupted and endangered, of fear, of frustration, of moral indignation. Anger is seldom directed at the illness causing it. The anger is often inappropriately directed at family and friends, medical personnel, the hospital, God, religion and clergy. Anger can become a mindless rage that alienates caregivers, thereby further isolating the ill.

I was once the focus of the anger of a terminally ill cancer patient named Ida. Ida became hospitalized for the final four weeks of her life. At our first meeting, I permitted her to voice her anger. She initially expressed her rage towards God and then addressed her growing rage at me, a priest, a human representative of God. The last two weeks, she would shout her rage at me the moment she saw me. I would quietly stand beside her, placing my hand on her shoulder while offering a silent prayer. A few days before her death, Ida weakly beckoned me to her bedside and we talked. Ida was still angry but resignation now dominated. She said, *"I am sorry for how I have treated you. But you represent death. Now, help me to die."* I did. Ida died with an inner peace.

Expressed anger can serve as an opportunity to the listener. As you listen to an angry person, a statement like, *"You are really angry about your illness and what it is doing to you, aren't you?"* can give a person permission to talk about this emotion and fear. This helps heal anger. Some do not express anger because they are people-pleasers who feel expressions of anger are not nice, or show a lack of courage, faith, or maturity, or are denials of goodness or will result in rejection. When anger is not appropriately expressed, it can lead to depression and the inability to fight for your life.

Have you misplaced your anger on loved ones? Can you now begin focusing your anger upon your disease? If so, vocally express it. Are you angry with yourself for a destructive lifestyle that may have contributed to your illness? Express your anger appropriately and responsibly, forgive yourself and others, and then constructively use your energy in seeking happiness and personal fulfillment.

A THERAPEUTIC PRAYER FOR HANDLING ANGER

God, I have been feeling much anger lately. My medical condition has upset me. I am angry about being ill. My life has been rudely interrupted. It isn't fair! All the changes have made me irritable. This is a scary experience. I just want to blame someone for all the pain and change. I know the doctor wants the best for me. I know my loved ones have been trying to help me. I know that you, God, are not responsible for my illness. You want me to be healthy and whole.

If I give you half a chance, you'll offer me new life and provide an energy to help improve my health. So, forgive me, God, for being so angry with everyone. I am going to try to focus my anger upon my medical condition and concentrate upon what I can do to find happiness and satisfaction. I release my anger into your love, knowing that you can handle it. Help me to take charge of my life responsibly. Amen.

Bargaining. Bargaining is used to seek a way out. Bargaining is partially based upon guilt about being ill. It involves the belief that if I become a better person, I will somehow magically be blessed with health. Bargaining asks anyone we think has power -- God, the universe, the self, the family or a doctor -- for one more chance to become well in exchange for changing and leading a better life. It states, *"If you will let me become well, I will do this...."* This assumes that becoming well is related to moral goodness, religious commitment or a better lifestyle.

Bargaining is based upon magical thinking. It can increase our hope but it does not cure disease (on its own). If bargaining is based upon the realistic hope utilized by the mind-body movement or spiritual healing therapy, it will contribute to your health. Keeping bargains that involve following medical orders and other healthy life-styles does help. If you succeed in becoming a better person, it will certainly help you and your loved ones to be happier.

A BARGAINING THERAPEUTIC PRAYER

God, I would do almost anything to become well again. So, I want to bargain. I need to be realistic. From this moment on I intend to be a better person. I am going to love and appreciate my loved ones more. I am going to follow my doctor's orders.

I forgive everyone who has ever hurt me and, at this moment, let go of any hurts inflicted by others. I forgive myself for the hurts I have inflicted upon others and will seek to make amends. I forgive myself for the guilt I am feeling about being ill. I let go of my anger, my hurts and my fears. I will seek to create happiness and satisfaction within my life.

I will rely upon your healing power in my life. Please provide your healing flow through my prayers and the prayers of others. I accept your power into my life. Thank you. Amen.

Depression. Depression is a normal part of a health crisis. It is like the delayed shock syndrome of the combat soldier. A health crisis involves physical, emotional and mental shock. One's whole life has been changed. There is sadness and grief over the many losses. Unexpressed or unresolved anger can result in depression. Our sense of self-worth suffers. Of-ten, we see ourselves as useless burdens to both ourselves and others. Illness can deepen our sense of failure in life, resulting in feelings of guilt and a deeper sense of personal inadequacy.

Surgical recovery is often followed by short-term depression. Returning home from a hospital stay can produce depression as the stresses at home take their toll. The symptoms of depression are often delayed. We may do a marvelous job of coping with an illness only to find depression overwhelming us months after the initial crisis is over. Emotional and physical shock can traumatize the human energy fields that may become torn and unable to maintain needed energy levels. Following my heart attack and wonderful healing, I still experienced mild depression for a year. My symptoms included dulled emotions, limited energy and weight loss.

The symptoms of depression may also include an emotional flatness, too much or too little sleep, tasteless food, gaining or losing weight, lack of energy, being negative and pessimistic, expressing bitterness and a missing sense of appreciation for the care given by others. During depression, the brain tells convincing lies which distort reality. These lies paint everything in the most convincingly negative terms. Those who have been close to God usually that find their ability to sense God is severely diminished. A health care professional should be consulted when your depression is deep or accompanied by suicidal thoughts or destructive anger.

Most depression is self-limiting, disappearing as quickly and mysteriously as it began. Depression can be faced by accepting it as a normal human reaction to shock and loss, appropriately expressing your anger at the illness and taking responsibility for your own life. It is helpful to go through the motions of seeking happiness and satisfaction. Doing your best to love and care for those around you.

A THERAPEUTIC PRAYER IN THE MIDST OF DEPRESSION

God, life seems so bleak and useless right now. I do not have any energy and do not have much ambition. I am really feeling down. I feel down on myself and down on everyone around me. Even as I pray, I do not sense your presence. But I go through the motions, knowing that you are still with me. I know that I am sacred and precious but they are just words right now. I know that my life has been worthwhile, full of many wonderful people and experiences, much happiness and joy. But I feel little of this right now.

God, all I can do is affirm the goodness of life and try to hold on until the darkness is replaced by your light and love. Help me to spot

the lies that my depressed emotions are telling me. Life is good. I am good. You are good. My loved ones love me. Life will be beautiful again. Soon, I will see the beauty around me again. Soon, I will again know vitality and purpose, happiness and love. Until then, give me the strength and hope to survive this day.

Help me to smile and laugh, if even for a moment. Be my strength and salvation. I ask you to restore me and make me whole. Fill me with the Word and the Spirit that I might be recreated anew. I praise and thank you. Amen.

Acceptance. Acceptance of one's illness or possible death is not resignation. Acceptance emerges from the struggles surrounding one's condition and a growing maturity. I find acceptance can best be attained through the spiritual journey with God.

Following my heart attack, I did my best to deal with all the issues included in this chapter. These changed my perspective. Daily meditative prayer empowered my ability to accept my new situation. Over a period of weeks, my anxiety and fear diminished. They were replaced by an inner calm and serenity. I became closer to God and attained a sense of God's presence and love. The Word of God came alive and my religious beliefs were true and living in me. I lost my fear of living and my fear of dying. I accepted the limitations placed upon me by my illness. I trusted in God's care, no matter what happened. I never became passive. I was determined to fight for the highest possible quality of life. The inner battle was almost won. I came to accept and respect the new me. I was filled with hope. Yes, there is light and life at the end of the tunnel, whether in limited living or even death.

Many people report that acceptance was the first step in their journey back to wholeness. Acceptance permits focus and intention to come alive. I personally discovered that my health crisis was not all bad. It shook me out of my complacency. It enabled me to ground myself in what was truly essential in life -- personal satisfaction, loved ones and God.

An illness contains many positive messages, making it a friend in disguise. It may be a helpful warning message that one's life is focused upon the wrong priorities. If you do not change your life, you may grow sicker or suffer a series of illnesses until you do either change to life-giving priorities or die. We tend to resist change, especially that which is quickly and involuntarily forced upon us.

When I reached the acceptance stage, I knew that I had learned my lessons. I rejoiced in the new me that was emerging. It was far more satisfying than the old me. Acceptance is not resignation, passivity or depression. It is making peace with your situation. It is the result of conquering fear, coming to terms with anger and coping with despair.

A THERAPEUTIC PRAYER OF ACCEPTANCE

God, this is the most difficult struggle of my life. I do not want this illness. If I had a choice, I would be well. This is so unfair in many ways. I cannot escape this physical body of mine. I can see no way out. I am angry, frightened and indignant at what is happening to me. I am not sure I can adjust. Some days I live as if nothing has happened. On other days, reality hits me squarely and I hurt.

God, give me the strength and wisdom to accept what has happened to me and to alter my life accordingly. Enable me to see my life as worthwhile and meaningful. Help me to celebrate the joys that I have known and the fulfillment still before me. Help me to live each day as happily as possible and to awaken each morning with the words, *"Thank you God for another day."* Provide me with guidance on how to get my life together. Grant me your presence and peace. Thank you. Amen.

THE WONDERFUL RESULTS

This is one of the most important chapters in PrayWell. When you have worked through the devastating feelings and thoughts brought on by your illness, you have achieved a major victory. You now feel mentally and emotionally healthy. This frees you to use all available resources to cope. Think of this chapter as an ongoing resource. Read it again and again. Use the prayers regularly. Use this chapter along with the following chapters to find healing.

My own struggle with heart disease has been rewarding. My life is richer now. I have grown. I have matured. I am fully alive. I am happy. This is not to say that I would wish disease upon anyone. Perhaps the healthy do not need the lessons I learned. Health is a wonderful thing. As performer Mae West stated, *"Too much of a good thing is wonderful."*

LOVE in the World's Great Religions

CHRISTIANITY: *"Beloved, let us love one another; for love is of God, and he who loves is born of God. He who does not know love does not know God; for God is love."*

ISLAM: *"Love is this, that you should count yourself very little and God very great."*

HINDUISM: *"One can best worship the Lord through love."*

SHINTO: *"Love is the representative of the Lord."*

BUDDHISM: *"Let a man cultivate towards the whole world a heart of love."*

TAOISM: *"Heaven arms with love those it would not see destroyed."*

JUDAISM: *"...you shall love the Lord your God with all your heart, and with all your soul, and with all your might."*

SIKHISM: *"God will regenerate those in whose hearts there is love."*

BAHA'I: *"Love Me that I may love you. If you love Me not, My love can no wise reach you."*

ZOROASTRIANISM: *"Man is the beloved of the Lord and should love Him in return."*

CONFUCIANISM: *"To love all men is the greatest benevolence."*

JAINISM: *"The days are of most profit to him who acts in love."*

Copyright permission courtesy of Marcus Bach

Chapter Sixteen

Healing and the Mind-Body Connection

"Disease is not an entity, but a fluctuating condition of the patient's body, a battle between the substance of disease and the natural self-healing tendency of the body." ...Aristotle

"We believe that every person directly participates, either consciously or subconsciously, in the creation of his or her own reality, including the reality of health." ...C. Norman Shealy and Caroline M. Myss

"The idea is to love because it feels good, not because it will help us live forever. Love is the end itself, not the means. Love makes life worth living, no matter how long it lasts. It also increases the likelihood of physical healing, but that is the bonus, the icing on the cake." ...Bernie Siegel

---

We are in the midst of an exciting new revolution. This revolution holds the promise of extending the health, longevity and happiness of every human being. This revolution is the open exploration of the mind-body connection by traditional scientists. You have seen the reports in newspapers, magazines and television.

What for centuries has been of interest only to religions, theologians and philosophers, is now being openly discussed by scientists. What is the nature of human consciousness? Are the brain and mind separate entities? How does the mind affect the body? What is the mind's possible effect on the rest of the physical universe? How can we help the ill use their minds to combat illness?

This revolution is not a new fad. It is the result of long-term scientific research, with many clinical studies now emerging that verify each other. A vast array of recent evidence indicates that what goes on in the mind has a direct effect upon the body. The mind has the power to produce and to maintain an illness as well as to heal an illness. Understanding the mind-body connection is crucial for the effective practice of healing prayer.

THE CASE FOR THE MIND-BODY CONNECTION

The medical term *"psychoimmunology,"* first used to describe the mind-body connection, was coined in 1966 by psychiatrist George Solomon of the University of Southern California. It was later expanded to the term used today, *"psychoneuroimmuniology,"* or PNI. Intriguing PNI evidence now exists showing that psychological factors directly affect recovery from cancer, heart disease, colds, asthma, ulcers, migraine headaches and broken bones.

In a recent Harvard Medical School medical study, a cold virus was sprayed into the mouths of one hundred volunteer college students. Only eleven students caught a cold. What prevented the other eighty-nine experimental subjects from contracting a cold from viral exposure?

A number of studies indicate that emotional stress places people at a greater illness risk. In one study, psychologists Janice Kiecolt-Glaser and Ronald Glaser at Ohio State University discovered that the spousal caregivers of Alzheimer's patients, over a period of time, experienced a decrease in cellular immunity and were more often ill from respiratory tract infections.

For years we have known that the stress of losing a spouse causes the surviving partner to have double the incidence of illness in the following year than others in his or her age group.

From many sources the evidence indicates that the ill who have the support of a group or a therapist either recover more quickly or prolong both the length and quality of their lives.

While studying wellness with Bernie Siegel, MD, in New Haven, Connecticut, I met dozens of previously terminally ill cancer patients who had participated in Siegel's Exceptional Cancer Patient (ECaP) support groups or applied the wellness wisdom of his books. These individuals now had been cancer-fee for five to ten years.

William G. Braud, PhD, of the Mind Science Foundation, San Antonio, Texas, has performed more than five hundred experiments designed to detect the influence of the consciousness -- pure thought -- on biological processes. Braud concludes that consciousness produces verifiable effects in distant human targets as well as in bacteria, neurons, cancer cells, enzymes, fungi, plants, larvae, insects, chicks, gerbils, cats and dogs. Therapeutic Prayer seeks to produce similar results.

The National Institute of Health has a new *Panel on Mind/Body Interventions.* It recently issued a report calling for a task force on the nature of consciousness, with representatives from many disciplines participating, including psychologists, neuropsychologists, artificial intelligence experts, physicists, physicians and philosophers. The panel will be exploring a new scientific model for health.

THE NEED FOR A NEW SCIENTIFIC MODEL

The science of life energies provides part of that needed new scientific model, as it deals with the existence of the human energy fields that interpenetrate the physical body.

Medical science is already aware that stress lowers the immune system's ability to fight illness by lowering defenses such as the production of white blood cells. What we think, feel, and say also influences the health of the human energy fields. Life energies scientists propose that negative thoughts and emotions distort the quality and power of the human energy fields, resulting in physical illness.

Illness does have organic and genetic causes, but the breakdown of energy fields usually occurs before the physical onset of an illness. Ramesh Chouhan's research demonstrates that the symptoms of cancer appear in the energy field three to six months before physical symptoms occur. During that period, something is causing the energy fields to be distorted, causing vulnerability to the cancer process. While environmental chemicals, viruses, bacteria and genetic predisposition are real causes of illness, the causes also involve mental and emotional states of consciousness. If the energy fields are strongly maintained, they apparently can prolong good health or prevent the onset of an illness.

During an illness, strengthened energy fields heal physical illness. Absent- and touch-prayer can heal the energy fields and produce health, but that does not mean a person is whole. A person's thoughts and emotions may remain unhealed, causing the mental and emotional energy fields to remain distorted. These distortions will continue to affect the physical energy field, causing the body to become ill once more.

This is not only an issue of healing prayer. Surgeons face similar problems. I remember one woman who complained that she had had twenty-five major surgeries in fifteen years. The surgeon would repair or remove a diseased organ, permitting the woman to heal herself. A few months later, the woman would again become ill and require another surgery. I asked the woman how she and her husband got along. She said, *"We get along fine as long as I am ill, but as I soon as I recover from a surgery, life becomes hell again. We fight constantly. The doctor said if I am to remain healthy I need to see a psychologist and a marriage counselor."*

THE THEORETICAL WORKING MODEL FOR HEALTH

Let us restate the whole case through this theoretical working model. Humans have at least seven energy fields which interpenetrate the physical body. Through prayer, God's healing love energy is transmitted to a living organism -- plant, animal or human. This energy enhances life because all living organisms have energy fields that receive the healing energy and utilize it effectively. These energy fields then interact with the human components of wholeness to produce healing effects. The existence of human energy fields scientifically explains how prayer affects human beings and makes them whole. When any of these components is impaired, it affects the other components.

Restoring wholeness is often accomplished through the combined efforts of several professional fields. Recovery from a heart attack is best made through the combined efforts of medicine, psychology, education, physical fitness, diet, a support community and healing prayer. If a person does not choose to remain physically, mentally and emotionally whole, illness can return within months or years. The logical extension of this line of reasoning is that one's thoughts and emotions play a major role in causing and maintaining physical illness.

If you wish to use healing prayer to restore health to yourself or a loved one, there is a need to let go of any anger, resentment, bitterness, fear, sadness or despair. Sometimes these emotions become so fixed that you feel enslaved by them. There are several explanations for this. They can become so deeply impressed on your brain memory tapes that you can't let go. A combination of counseling, hypnosis and healing prayer can heal these emotions. Sometimes these emotions develop a life of their own, taking on identity as energy fields or spirit entities. In this case, counseling, hypnosis, healing prayer and exorcism work. Or you can just shout in joy and defiance, *"I want to live and will let go of my past pain in order to do so."*

THE ROLE OF EMOTIONS IN PHYSICAL HEALTH

About twenty years ago, one study indicated that twelve to eighteen months prior to the onset of cancer, many persons had experienced a painful personal loss. It could be a divorce, the death of a loved one, the loss of a job, betrayal or personal rejection. This painful experience caused immense anger and resentment that they had not been able to resolve or heal over an eighteen- month period. If they had been able to let go of the anger and resentment within a year or so, cancer would not have developed. They could not, and they became the victims of cancer. Later studies confirmed these findings. So, one of the questions I ask the seriously ill is, *"In the past twelve to eighteen months, has something happened that created immense rage, resentment or hurt within you which you still carry around?"* Dozens of cancer-ravaged persons I have known fit this pattern.

It is normal for persons to react to crisis with any number of emotions. Most take months to work through emotional pain. This is normal. There is plenty of time. The human energy fields are extremely stable so it may take many months or years for physical illness to reflect the inner emotional and mental states. But ongoing unhappiness, stress and physical illness distort these energy fields. This affects the way we think, feel and interact. It is a downward spiral that can be altered only by some form of intervention. Physical illness, emotional illness, interpersonal estrangement and death are forms of intervention. *So is the intentional personal decision to become whole.*

Lola. Lola was diagnosed with cancer. She took the diagnosis so calmly that I was moved to ask the above question. Without hesitation she answered, *"For years I have been angry with my daughter for moving out-of-state and deserting me. Then, last year, my husband died. I am furious with him for also deserting me. Day and night I am consumed with anger at my husband for dying. I will never forgive him."* I shared with her the fact that her anger would hasten her death and that if she could manage to give up her anger she might survive. She responded, *"I don't want to live, but don't tell my sons about that."*

This situation involved two mind-body connections. First, her anger had enabled the outbreak of cancer. Second, Lola was choosing to die because life had become unbearable for her. Her cancer was a respectable way of committing suicide. During her dying, Lola was the happiest I had seen her in years. She was enjoying the sympathy of friends and the tender care of her family. She died graciously, just as the script she had written for her final months portrayed. Respecting her wishes, I prayed with her only for inner peace and protection from pain. Both requests were granted.

Norman Shealy, MD,[1] states, *"It is now widely reported that cancer often is diagnosed one to two years following a devastating illness. Indeed, 75% of the cancer patients I've treated have reported that they actually wanted to die for the six to twenty-four months previous to the diagnosis."*

Helen. Helen had been battling breast cancer for several years. By the time she came to me, cancer cells had entered the bone in several parts of her body, including the spine. The medical prognosis was that death was inevitable. She admitted that the only reason she had come to me, a healer, was that she had exhausted all other treatment options and was desperately seeking a way to recover.

When I insisted on accompanying the healing sessions with counseling, she reluctantly agreed. Like most of my clients, she saw no correlation between counseling and recovery. Helen viewed cancer only as a virus, like a cold virus. She wanted me to kill the cancer with touch-prayer in the same way that radiation or chemotherapy treatments destroy cancer cells. I told her that if she wanted to get well, the odds were eighty percent that our touch-healing sessions would make her symptom-free of cancer. I cautioned her that the cancer symptoms might return if she did not work on becoming mentally and emotionally whole.

We met for six two-hour sessions over a two-week period, spending most of our time in counseling. She held painful memories, leading to emotions of anger and bitterness. I told her during the sixth session that I sensed that she was free of cancer symptoms. Her distorted energy fields had been restored and strengthened, producing healing. I suggested that we needed to continue the counseling sessions. She refused.

Four months later she phoned and excitedly told me that recent diagnostic tests showed no trace of cancer. She thanked me. I urged her to undergo further counseling. She declined. Five months later symptoms of cancer returned. She refused further healing sessions. Several months later she died.

What happened? Helen needed to work through the inner anger, bitterness and pain. They were disrupting her emotional and mental energy fields, making them unable to maintain her newly acquired physical health and, thus, permitting the recurrence of cancer cells. To live free of cancer, she needed mental and emotional healing of her inner hurt. Helen stated that she wanted to become healthy. She wanted her body to be whole. She could not understand the need for her emotions and thoughts to become whole for her body to remain healthy. She chose to die because she was tired of living with the emotional and physical pain.

Some people cannot be healed through prayer because they are choosing at some level of the mind to remain ill. Their illness is beneficial to them in some way. Because of this free-will choice to remain ill, any healing energy is either rejected by their energy fields or not utilized properly for healing.

Other people become ill because they have been caught in a destructive emotional state that becomes the central cause of their illness. Unresolved destructive emotions can be the direct cause of illness. Unresolved destructive emotions can distort the human energy fields to the extent that they are incapable of fighting bacteria, virus and other causes of disease. In these circumstances, healing prayer may bring them temporary health or, with counseling, even bring them continuing health.

GAYLE. This recently became true for me as I worked with a professional colleague, Gayle, who had suddenly developed breast cancer. I practiced touch-healing prayer with her three times daily for four days with little reduction of the hard cancerous tumor. The fifth day was devoted to intensive counseling during which pain from deep hurts came forth accompanied by sobbing tears. By the following day the tumor had disappeared.

Gayle lived one of the healthiest and spiritual lifestyles I had ever observed. She was also an extremely competent wellness therapist. But, she was completely unaware of her deep emotional wounds. They were walled off in her subconscious mind and hidden from her conscious awareness. Her hurts had distorted her energy fields, causing the physical cancer in her breast. *Everyone with cancer or any life-threatening disease, no matter how mature and whole they feel, must undergo wellness counseling in order to fully utilize healing energy and become well.*

Sometimes loved ones cause illness. They do this through their lack of support, their put-downs and blaming, and the destructive energy they transmit. Their ill victims are usually sensitive, cooperative people who are incapable of defending themselves against such regular attacks. Because of this, their energy fields become poisoned and they become ill. These dynamics puzzle most psychotherapists. This has given rise to family therapists who specialize in these dynamics.

A *sensitive* in Poland, a medical doctor, is able to *see* the energy interactions between family members. In one case, a child was afflicted with one illness after another. Observing family energy interactions, the doctor noted that the mother was constantly stealing the child's life energy, producing energy depletions that made the child vulnerable to illnesses. Through counseling and energy field management, the doctor reported the child's health dramatically improved.

WELLNESS WISDOM

Bernie Siegel, MD, observed that some terminally ill cancer patients did not die. Exhausting all medical treatment, about ten percent got well. These survivors became Siegel's teachers and Exceptional Cancer Patients (ECaPs).

Siegel found specific survival tactics among ECaPs. ECaPs did not passively wait to die. They were determined to live. They took charge of their own lives by accepting responsibility for their own happiness and satisfaction. They focused upon living, not dying. This involved seeking to live every day to its fullest.

ECaPs examined themselves to see what was causing them emotional pain. They sought to satisfy their own personal needs before the needs of others. They asked themselves, *"What do I want out of life?"* They focused on two areas -- family life and vocation. They asked, *"Are these contributing to my happiness and satisfaction or are they sources of my pain?"* If the latter, they asked, *"What can I do about it?"*

Third, they developed a strategy for becoming well -- a special diet, exercise, meditation, a wellness support group. If they believed their strategy would make them well, it often would. This is the faith factor in wellness.

These approaches renew and strengthen the human energy fields. Finding unconditional love renews energy fields. Research indicates that using a wellness counselor or support group prolongs the quality and length of life. Loving and being loved makes one's burden bearable.

Letting go of negativity renews energy fields. Feelings of anger, resentment, fear and inadequacy distort and weaken energy fields, making one more vulnerable to disease. Most need help in letting go. Wellness counseling and support groups offer this help. Massage and other body-work can release feelings. Touch-healing also works.

Being ill is often a personal choice at some inner level. For some people, an illness fulfills personal needs. In other words, some people need their illness in order to cope or be happy. I have seen these dramas played out time and again by people I have served. Here is my own partial list of needs met by illness:

SOME REASONS FOR NEEDING AN ILLNESS

1. Unresolved guilt, grief or anger following a tragedy may give rise to illness as self-punishment.
2. Stress and bitterness due to the long-term care of a now-deceased loved one can cause life-threatening illnesses that offer an escape from despair.
3. Illness can provide escape from unhappiness in the family or in a vocation when one feels trapped in a hopeless situation.
4. A disregarded plea for help or reunion with a former spouse over an unwelcome divorce may lead to illness in the rejected partner.
5. The illness of one family member may serve a dysfunctional family's needs. Families may unknowingly seek to maintain the illness of a member because it balances and makes some family members happy.
6. Illness can be a means for manipulating loved ones, including permitting the ill person to be dependent and cared for, and keeping a family member from leaving home.
7. We can use an illness to punish those with whom we are angry, including ourselves.
8. Illness can represent an escape from boredom and the loss of meaning and self worth. This can happen when children leave home, in retirement, or as a result of poverty or unemployment.
9. A distorted or faulty life script may cause us to believe that illness and death will come at a certain age because it happened that way to other family members.

If you recognize yourself in these or similar situations, then you may be able to escape both illness and death by choosing life. Staying where we are is usually a matter of free choice. *We are responsible for our own health and life, and have the power to influence our circumstances.*

THE SHEALY-MYSS STRESS PATTERNS AND ILLNESS

C. Norman Shealy and Caroline M. Myss offer us immense insight on the causes and responses to disease in <u>The Creation of Health</u>.[2] They key in on a major understanding of alternative medicine, *"We believe that every person directly participates, either consciously or subconsciously, in the creation of his or her own reality, including the reality of health."*

They emphasize that being healthy involves using your own inner tools -- attitudes, emotions and belief patterns and the awareness of the spiritual self. Appreciating the power of the inner self permit two things to happen. First, the individual becomes receptive to learning *how* emotions, attitudes and belief patterns contribute in very specific ways to the creation of health or of disease. Secondly, the individual develops the capacity to keep healthy through being aware that *negative attitudes create negative responses within the physical body.* Negativity must not go unchallenged since the consequence is disease.

Eight Stress Factors. People who become ill identify with one or more of the following eight dysfunctional patterns.

1. The presence of *unresolved or deeply consuming* emotional, psychological or spiritual stress within a person's life.

2. The degree of control that negative belief patterns have upon a person's life.

3. The inability to give and/or receive love.

4. The lack of humor and the inability to distinguish between serious concerns from the lesser issues of life.

5. How effectively one exercises the power of choice in terms of holding dominion over the movement and activities of their own life.

6. How well a person has attended to the needs of the physical body.

7. The "existential vacuum" or the suffering that accompanies the absence or loss of meaning in one's life.

8. A tendency towards denial.

Getting well again is related to four factors: self-empowerment, taking responsibility for one's own life, having the wisdom to accept what we cannot change and having the courage to change when we need to change, and learning to thrive on love.

THE ROLE OF FORGIVENESS

The role of forgiveness is important. Every person should learn to forgive himself or herself as well as others. The concept of forgiveness includes being able to let go of a destructive feeling or attitude. We choose to forgive ourselves. We choose to forgive others. We choose to accept God's forgiveness.

Holding on to the pain fixates one's life. Letting go of pain through forgiveness allows us to move on and become whole. Learning to forgive can be developed through contact with a counselor, support group or pastor. Forgiving involves a conscious decision as well as understanding insight and love.

I have witnessed many persons who are stuck in their emotional states die of cancer and other diseases. Because I am a pastor, people feel safe in telling me things that they would tell no one else. They describe ongoing unhappiness, an inability to move on, an unwillingness to forgive or a wish to die. They are either defiantly holding on or imploring me to rescue them from these fixated states that hold them prisoner.

Sometimes I have served as an accomplice. In one instance, a wealthy seventy-three-year-old widow said to me, *"Walt, your healing prayers cured my cancer two years ago, but now, please permit me to die of this illness. I have been miserable since my husband died ten years ago. Death will bring me peace."* With tender understanding I honored that plea, believing in her free-will choice. I felt comfortable with respecting her decision because of my strong belief in the afterlife. For me, death is but a transition into a more beautiful state of existence.

Often, the ill admitted that they did not wish to get well and that the cancer was doing them a favor. For many, their decision or stance was fixed. Neither counseling nor prayer affected them. This is free will in action. When someone remains determined to die, no type of intervention works. However, when time permits, combining spiritual healing with counseling can lead to dramatic healing results.

Once the troubling issues are named and understood, prayer can heal that which has been brought out into the open. In the subconscious mind, emotional pain is used to program the energy fields in distorted ways. Counseling and group work can overcome negative emotions so that they can be released. Most persons with ongoing disease would be more capable of reclaiming health if they used these processes.

From both the religious and psychological perspectives, we must openly confront the deep wounds and scars caused by emotional trauma, negative feelings and confused thinking. The truth and strength of many religious traditions are rooted in the view that the unhappy person is filled with darkness and needs to be made aware of that darkness within, in order to make a conscious choice to be freed from the darkness, to deal with the issues of forgiveness, and to choose to live responsibly in God's light. Counseling and spiritual redemption are often key elements in moving toward wholeness.

The mind-body movement employs counseling, group work and spiritually redemptive approaches that are consistent with spiritual healing. These involve viewing a person as sacred, unique and precious before God -- a style that completely accepts, respects, and seeks the best for that person. It also shares the unconditional love that enables the transformation to take place. It is obvious that intellectual integrity requires a consistency between mind-body principles and spiritual healing principles.

ROLLING WITH THE PUNCHES

Some people roll with the punches better than others. They are obeying the folk wisdom that says when life hands you a lemon, you should learn how to make tasty lemonade. Others are more easily traumatized by the pains of life. These people are more rigid in defining what they want from life and do not easily make adjustments when troubles come. In other words, health and happiness may be directly related to mental and emotional flexibility.

PRAYERS FOR WORKING TOWARD INNER WHOLENESS

These prayers need to be used along with self-exploration. People often bury their pain so deeply that they are no longer aware of it. Explore the painful experiences of your life. Be open to the hurt involved. Repeatedly use the appropriate prayers. Further help will be provided in the other chapters of this Guide To Self-Healing.

1. *A THERAPEUTIC PRAYER FOR HEALING EMOTIONAL WOUNDS*

God, I continue to hurt. I have painful, unhealed wounds. *(Recall them here.)* **I realize I am only hurting myself as the hurt continues, but I have been unable to forget or to let the pain subside. I feel stuck where I am, filled with hurt. But I am willing to try.**

God, I forgive anyone who has caused me pain. *(Forgive them individually here.)* **I forgive myself for any role I played in the pain. I release the pain to you, God. I cut the ties that bind me to my pain. I give away my anger, my hurt, my bitterness, my fear. I no longer choose to live in the darkness as I accept your marvelous light and love into my life. I ask you to heal my pain and hurt. I ask you to fill me with your goodness, love, joy and peace.**

God, I thank you for the precious gift of life. Free me that I might be truly free of the past as I seek to move on into a happier future. I choose to take charge of my life, living it in your light. I choose a life of happiness and satisfaction. I thank you for the new life that courses through my veins. I rely upon your sustaining presence and guidance.

God, I ask you to make me whole by restoring my energy fields and making them healthy. Thank you. Amen.

2. *A THERAPEUTIC PRAYER FOR HEALING PAINFUL MEMORIES*

God, life was not supposed to be this difficult. I did not expect my life to be like a happy fairy tale of unending bliss. I knew life was a struggle at times. But I did not expect this much agony and pain. The pain continues to wash over me through unexpected flashbacks and nightmares. My happiness and inner security have been stolen from me. Painful memories overshadow my whole life, ruining each day and my relationship with others. I feel afraid. I am distrustful. Nameless fear haunts me daily. I am tired and often sad. I wish to end this seemingly endless agony.

God, I choose to take control of my life. I will no longer be a victim of my past. I let go of my painful memories. I ask you to heal the pain by erasing it from the memory tapes of my brain and my energy fields. God, heal my wounds.

I release my pain, my anger, my bitterness, my hurt, my fear. I forgive those who have caused me pain. I forgive myself for any role I have played in my pain. I release the pain to you. I cut the ties that bind me to my hurts. Heal my body, mind and spirit and set me free.

I breathe in your presence, your love, your joy, your peace. Recreate me and make me fresh and new. I accept your new life, your love and light. Thank you. Amen.

3. A THERAPEUTIC PRAYER FOR HEALING GUILT

God, guilt imprisons me and I seek release. I have made mistakes. I have hurt others. At times I have been out of control. I was doing the best I knew how to do at the time. My present sense of guilt tells me that I know how wrong I have been and that I have grown in my understanding.

God, I forgive myself for the pain I have inflicted upon others as well as myself. I seek to make amends by ending this cycle of guilt that only makes me miserable and unable to be a blessing to other. Free me, God, that I might be a better person. I accept myself for who I am. I am sacred, precious, unique and of infinite worth.

God, enable me to love myself. Bring healing to my mind and spirit. Fill me with your love and wisdom and peace. May only good flow to me and through me. Grant me the wisdom to care for myself and others in responsible ways that represent love and abundant living. Thank you. Amen.

4. A THERAPEUTIC PRAYER FOR COMFORT IN GRIEF

God, I am hurting from the loss of my loved one. I feel empty except for a constant sadness and ache. I am angry because this seems so unfair. I feel sorry for my loved one. I feel guilty because of my helplessness in preventing this death. I feel so alone and isolated. I have pain over unfinished business between us, of words unsaid and dreams never to be. I know the pain is good because it tells of the love and beauty we shared. I am thankful for the life we shared together and for good memories that will be with me forever. I am thankful for the life you gave my loved one and for all the good s/he shared with the world. Thank you, God, for the precious gift of life.

God, I thank you for the spiritual nature of life, that we are all eternal and can never really die. I thank you for my loved one's entrance into eternal life. I pray for your blessings in granting continuing opportunities for growth and becoming.

God, help me handle my enormous sense of loss and emptiness. Comfort me in my grief. I release my pain to you. Fill me with your comforting peace. Fill me with your love and light and provide for my needs. Thank you. Amen.

5. A THERAPEUTIC PRAYER FOR ENDING A RELATIONSHIP

God, it is so painful to end relationships. Each day holds an emptiness and a longing. This person meant so much to me. Our lives have been like one. I have so many beautiful and joyous memories. Now I feel only half here. It hurts terribly. It is almost unbearable. I am all emotions right now. I feel anger and hurt, loneliness and longing. I want to be through with this pain. I want to get on with my life.

God, to end the pain, I release the tie that binds. I sever the energy linking us together. I forgive all the past and release it to your care. I forgive myself. I let go of my anger, my hurt, my fear, my self- pity. I honor the love we shared and all the joy it brought. I am thankful for the life we shared. Let me hold to the good memories with no sense of pain. Heal me and make me new. Thank you. Amen.

6. A THERAPEUTIC PRAYER FOR DISCOURAGING TIMES

God, I sense life passing me by. I struggle and struggle to find happiness and fulfillment. I have worked hard at it. But so often everything turns to dust. Life seems so unfair. I have forgotten how to laugh, and resent the humor of others. Sometimes I just do not understand life. It is as if I am on a treadmill with no way off. Is there a way out for me? God, can you help me?

God, I am so confused. It is as if I am living in the dark. Is there a map that will lead me out so that I can see the light at the end of the tunnel? I try to please, but no one sees my efforts. I resent what is happening to me. I worry about my future. Sometimes I am angry at the way others steal my happiness and ignore my efforts. I am losing my trust in people. I fear getting too close to others because so many times I have been disappointed. Is there a way out? God, can you help me?

God, I feel so trapped -- trapped by my past, present and future. I keep trying and trying. I so want to make life work. In my darker moments I sense no purpose in my life. There is nothing to look forward to but more illness and struggle. Is there a way out? God, can you help me?

God, I hear that others have found a path, that there is a rainbow of hope. I need to tune into myself and discover my own needs. I need to nourish my yearnings, to encourage what brings me happiness and satisfaction. I need to do things that bring me a sense of fulfillment, joy and worth and make me feel good about myself. I need to take charge of my life and have the courage to follow my dreams. This is the path I must choose to find life. God, be with me on this new path.

God, I need to clean up my inner self. I need to come to terms with my negative feelings and with the inner pain. I need to give up my resentments and envies. I need to let go of fear. I need to release my sadness and anger. God, I am angry with you and with everyone around me and with myself. God, enable me to release my anger. I release my anger to your care. My feelings are important and I must express them responsibly if I am to be free. Bring healing to me. Fill me with your love, joy, peace and light. God, free me for my new path.

God, I need to learn of love. Enable me to love and appreciate myself. I have heard that I am sacred and precious, the only one like me. Aid me in believing that, in valuing your divine image in me. Help me to value my worth, my gifts, my abilities. Teach me to look into a mirror and tell myself, *"I love you. You are all right."* Fill me with your love and let love be my aim. Let me be love as I express caring in all its many facets. God, may love for myself and your whole creation be the focus of my life.

God, I need to learn spiritual wisdom. Teach me the lessons of my life -- that each experience I have ever had, whether painful or happy, has been an opportunity for understanding, learning and growth, molding me into the person I am today. Grant me insight and help me to grow like a newborn baby, beautiful for you. I forgive myself for all my failures and pains. I accept responsibility for my life. Help me to like the emerging me. God, enable me to grow and to become new and whole on this new path.

God, enable me to live fully. Teach me how to enter joyous, honest, loving relationships that help me to grow and become. Teach me how to be healthy and whole. I choose to be healthy. I choose to have inner peace. I choose to find wholeness and hope. I choose to claim them today. Heal me, God, my creator and sustainer, and make me whole in body, mind and spirit. Mold me into your spirit. Make me one with myself and with you. Make us one in unity and purpose. God, you are my strength and my salvation. Restore me and make me new. Thank you. Amen.

WELLNESS IS ALWAYS THE ILL PERSON'S RESPONSIBILITY

Wellness is always the ill person's responsibility.

These can come through as harsh, judgmental words. That is not their purpose. They are stating the truth. When you become ill, you must reach out to seek medical treatment. When decisions are required about your medical treatment, patients with sound minds are legally responsible for making their own decisions. When you are informed of factors affecting your health, you are responsible for maximizing the health factors in your life.

With the almost daily growth in medical knowledge and procedures, every consumer is responsible for keeping up with the new discoveries. When you become ill, you must research your illness using many sources.

PrayWell is seeking to educate you about the benefits of using the mind-body connection and spiritual healing for getting well again. No one can help you in these areas but yourself. Take control of your life. Reach out!

When I studied with Bernie Siegel in New Haven, I met dozens of people who had been terminally ill cancer patients. I met people who had suffered with multiple sclerosis and Lou Gehrig's Disease. These people were now well. Some had been well for five or ten years. They had taken responsibility for their own illness and won the battle.

Once you accept this truth, you can understand something even more difficult. Bernie Siegel states, *"There are no incurable diseases, only incurable people."* This is a message of insight and hope for everyone.

Chapter Seventeen

Therapeutic Prayers for Self-Healing

"We experience God most intensely when our despair is most intense." ...Anthony Bloom*

"Breathe deep into your strength to plan for tomorrow. Then, leave tomorrow to take care of itself and celebrate being alive today." ...I Can Cope, American Cancer Society

"Is any one among you suffering? Let him pray. Is any cheerful? Let him sing praise. Is any among you sick? Let him call for the elders of the church, and let them pray over him, anointing him with oil in the name of the Lord, and the prayer of faith will save the sick man...." ...James 5:13-16

There is more belief in the processes that heal the emotions than in prayers that physically heal the body. My experience is that the healing of the physical body through prayer is far easier than the healing of emotions. So, if these past two chapters have contributed to your wholeness, you can approach this chapter with utmost confidence. Physical healing is a relatively easy process.

You have chosen to use prayer for your own self-healing. Because of this choice, you are the only one who is responsible for your ongoing efforts. Do not expect others to have the same enthusiasm as you. You are in charge of your own healing efforts. Gain the cooperation of those you can but do not waste your energy trying to convince those who will not cooperate or support your efforts. This is your journey. Respect and enjoy it.

This chapter provides prayers and guidance for your own physical self-healing. It also tells how you can enlist others in contributing to your own prayer efforts. We begin with some basic teachings on the practice of healing prayer.

PRACTICING HEALING SKILLS

Practice in Transmitting Energy. With fingers straight, place the palms and fingers of both hands against each other. Then pull them apart about half an inch. Try to send energy through each hand to the other. Every person can be taught to transmit energy in this way. Sense the energy between your hands. Now, while continuing to sense this energy, slowly bring your hands apart, until you can no longer feel it. Then move your hands together until they touch.

An additional experiment is to cup your hands together as if you are holding an orange. Then move your hands rapidly in opposite circular motions. You will sense an energy build-up. When we care and we pray, this energy is transformed into God's healing love energy. By touching yourself during prayer, you transmit the healing energy to your own body.

Hand Polarity. In healing, your hands are like the poles on a battery. One is positively charged and the other is negatively charged. One hand sends and the other receives. The sending hand needs to be grounded elsewhere on the body by the receiving hand. The exception is when the hand transmitting healing can completely surround the injured area. In that case, only one hand is necessary.

Most spiritual healing experts insist that the right hand is always the sending hand. This is not true for me. My left hand is my natural sending hand. I also happen to be left-hand dominant. I am awkwardly able to change poles and transmit with my right hand. You can recognize your natural sending hand as the one with which you sense energy, heat, coolness or a tingling while transmitting healing energy. This is referred to as your favored hand.

Hand polarity is not always important. With a sprained ankle, I place my hands on either side of my ankle for five minutes and then switch hands to the opposite sides for another five minutes. I do this with any joint or muscle injury or a broken bone.

Your Own Healing Hands. Before each prayer, quiet yourself and attempt to be one with God. Use your hands for transmitting healing energy during each prayer. To heal a physical condition, if possible place your favored hand on the area needing healing, with the other hand on the opposite side or just touching your body anywhere. Or place your favored hand over your diaphragm and the other hand over your heart, then reverse hands. Life energy enters through the diaphragm and emerges through the heart in prayer. Leave your hands in place for fifteen minutes following a prayer so the energy can continue to flow. You can either remain in prayer or talk or even watch TV while doing so. Once the energy begins flowing, it just continues. When we stop working at it, our hands know what to do by themselves.

Halting the Flow. After any healing effort, stop the flow of the healing energy emitting from your hands by rubbing the palms briskly against each other or clapping your hands or rinsing them with water. If you forget this step, you may experience an energy drain.

SELF-HEALING FIRST AID

PrayWell's self-healing prayer can be used as first aid in daily living. This provides major opportunities for experimenting and practicing prayer touch-healing. It can also be done calmly, in contrast to the urgency of healing a major illness. Torn muscles, bruises, broken bones, damaged cartilage, cuts, burns and sunburn all respond to self-healing touch prayer. This is healing first-aid. The faster you begin healing treatment, the quicker the response. Do it within ten minutes of receiving the injury and you may be symptom-free within minutes or hours. Wait twenty-four hours and the results appear to be far more limited. You can practice healing while applying ice, lotion or aloe vera to the afflicted area.

Trauma Injury. An eighty-year-old physician, Dr. Hubert Hensel, survived a plane crash. But he required seven hours of reconstructive surgery on his face. He broke his right arm, sternum and eye socket and cracked seven ribs. Following the facial surgery, Dr. Hensel immediately began touch self-healing. Within a week his face had healed without a scar and his broken bones healed within four weeks.

A Cut. You can heal a cut on the finger by placing the fingers of either hand around the finger for fifteen minutes. If this is done within minutes of receiving the cut, it may be healed without a scar within forty-eight hours. There will be no pain or discomfort even if the cut was deep and needs a half-dozen sutures. Get the sutures and practice healing. Be one with God while focusing your intentions on transmitting healing energy.

For sunburn, touch each sunburned area for about one minute with your transmitting hand. Place your other hand over your heart area. To be effective, this procedure must be applied at the first symptoms of sunburn or even before. By the following day, the skin damage has been completed and your efforts will yield negligible results.

After any healing prayer, continue to concentrate on a oneness with God and the area being healed. Alternate this with the intention of transmitting healing energy, imagining the desired effects. Once you become experienced in performing these two procedures, you will learn to continue the healing flow while involved in other activities, like carrying on a conversation, reading or watching television. You will sense when you are able to do this.

Two People's Hands Are Better Than One

In practicing touch-healing prayer, invite one or two others to place their transmitting hands over yours. The healing flow, and results, will dramatically improve.

SELF-HEALING OF CHRONIC CONDITIONS

Several years ago, a sports medicine orthopedic physician x-rayed my swollen and painful left knee that had stopped me from participation in recreational sports. He reported that my bone loss was worse than that of seventy percent of men my age. He recommended that I quit racquetball, volleyball and golf and stop all recreational walking. If I did not, he said, an artificial knee replacement would be needed and he added, *"You are much too young for that."*

Even as a healer, I had not thought of using self-healing before seeking medical care. Now I had no choice. By practicing touch self-healing prayer, I had my knee symptom-free within three days. In the six years since, my knee has functioned normally in all situations.

Arthritis is a good model for healing a chronic condition. Initially, work on only the worst arthritic joint, such as a knee. Place your hands for ten minutes on one side and then reverse hand positions for another ten minutes. Do this once daily for five consecutive days. You will then notice the beneficial effects and can begin working on other arthritic joints.

Note once again, this is a process that works somewhat like an antibiotic, as the effects build up over a period of time. Apply the same procedure for hearing and sight losses, skin diseases, heart damage, cancers and other diseases.

ALL THE PRAYERS YOU NEED DURING A HEALTH CRISIS

This first prayer covers everything involved in a health emergency. Before beginning, place your hands on the affected area. If you do not know what needs to be healed, place your transmitting hand on your diaphragm and the other on your heart.

1. A THERAPEUTIC PRAYER DURING A HEALTH CRISIS

Divine Creator, out of love you created the physical universe and it was good. You created human beings in your own image; we are spiritual beings with life-giving energy fields which when healthy contain all the information needed to provide us abundant living.

God, you granted me the precious gift of life and then invited me to travel with you through the years of my life's journey. All too often I have ignored your invitation. When I have welcomed your Spirit, you have been with me in my pain and struggles, my disappointments and failures, my happiness and fulfillment, my love and joy, guiding and sustaining me. You have been my teacher, molding me into the person that I am today.

Divine Creator, too often I have ignored your presence, your guidance and your offer of New Life. But I know that you are always present with me when I open myself to you. You want me to be well and whole. I invite you into my life to restore my energy fields with your creative powers. Make me whole in body, mind and spirit.

Divine Creator, I am intensely aware of my ailing body. I am out of balance. I release my worries and cares to you, accepting your calming presence. I ask you to protect me from physical pain and discomfort. Preserve my life and renew me. I place this body of mine into your care, knowing that you wish to restore its perfect blueprint for the healthy me. Transform me and make me whole once more. I choose to be well and welcome your aid. Provide for my needs and protect me from all harm.

Divine Creator, cleanse my inner being and fill me with life anew. Let your creative, renewing power flow through my hands, renewing all my energy fields, that they might reflect the perfect form you intended. Heal me in body, mind and soul and grant me your peace. Thank you for the renewal that is beginning to flow through me.

God, as I pray, may my hands flow with your healing presence. I thank you for those who are caring for me. I trust their loving intentions and accept their care. Provide me with the resources for continuing on the path back to wholeness. Renew my faith in your goodness and will towards wholeness. I ask you to continue the process of making me a renewed person, vibrant with divine life, filled with your love and confident of all that is to come. Amen.

Now imagine God's presence as a pure white healing light flowing from your favored hand. Say the following prayer as you seek to merge and become one with God:

God, I ask you come into my life and merge with me. Enable me to be one with you as we unite in Spirit. Let your healing white light flow from my hand throughout my whole body. I sense your presence and light pervading my whole being. I accept this healing. I accept your peace. I ask that wherever your light and love touch, I become whole. Let my healing begin now. Thanks. Amen.

2. YOUR THERAPEUTIC PRAYER DURING A HOSPITAL STAY

God, I am thankful to be in this hospital where I am receiving the special care I need. I am thankful for the doctors, nurses and others who are here to help me. Guide and sustain them as they care for me and for others who need their care. I accept their care in love and appreciation. Yet, enable me to remain in control of the decisions about my care. Grant me the wisdom to make the right decisions. Keep me safe and enable me to return home soon in the process of becoming whole.

Creator and Sustainer, I ask you to fill me with your love. I release my frustrations, fears and anger. I let go of all my earthly concerns and responsibilities that I might fully concentrate on becoming well. I forgive every person who has ever hurt me. I release all anger about events in the past. I ask your forgiveness for the pain I have caused others. I will seek to make amends to all persons and institutions that I have hurt. Forgive me, God, for the pain I have caused any other person. Make me aware of any responsibility I bear for my present medical condition that I may make any needed changes in becoming and remaining well. I ask your guidance on the path back to health.

God, take away my darkness and fill me with your marvelous light. Satisfy me with your love, joy and peace, that your calming presence may sustain me. Grant me inner peace in the midst of uncertainty. I place my life in your hands. I want to be restored and become well. I have the assurance that nothing can ever separate me from your love and care.

In God's name, I pray that any spirits of illness depart from me at this time. I deny their power over me. God, I ask that you heal me in body, mind and spirit. Begin the healing that I need and let it continue until I am well. Thank you for the healing that is taking place throughout my whole being. I accept it with deep appreciation. Amen.

Now place one or both hands on either side of the area needing to be healed. Or place one hand on your heart and the other on your forehead. Do this for ten minutes at a time, morning, afternoon and evening. Pray:

God, use my hands as channels for your healing love, so that wherever I place my hands, your healing flow enters and heals me. May this healing begin now and continue until I am well. Amen.

3. YOUR THERAPEUTIC PRAYER BEFORE SURGERY

Before praying, place your hands close to the surgical area. If this is not possible, imagine you have done so. Now offer the following prayer:

God, I thank you for the upcoming surgery that will permit my body to heal itself. I thank you for the skills of each member of the surgical team. I trust them and place my life in their hands. Guide them in the use of their skills. Thank you.

God, I care about myself. I wish to be well again. I pray that you will use me as a channel of my own healing. Let your healing energy flow into the surgical area and into my lungs and heart. Fill these areas with your life energy and increase the oxygen levels in my tissues. Enable all the cells of my body to fight for health as they communicate with each other. Protect me from pain and bleeding during surgery and afterwards. Enable the surgical wound to heal quickly. Fill me with the calm and power of your presence. I open myself to a oneness with you. I rest in your care and wisdom. Thank you. Amen.

You may repeat this prayer after surgery several times daily using the last paragraph of the prayer.

4. YOUR DAILY PRAYER DURING A HOSPITAL STAY

Place your hands on your heart and diaphragm before you begin.

God, as I pray, use my hands, enabling them to flow with your healing power. I thank you, God, for this stay in the hospital and the professional care of the entire staff. Provide me with the resources I need to be content and get well. Renew my faith and hope in your goodness and your intentions to help me be restored and recover.

God, I am thankful for everyone who has supported me during this ordeal. I pray for my loved ones who have worried about me and been under great stress. Grant them your calm, strength and assurance. Provide for our daily needs and unite us in love. May this be a time of personal renewal.

God, create a grateful spirit within me. Permit me to be content this day and to greet the future with optimism. I am thankful for this pause in my life, enabling me to gain new perspective and wisdom. As I have been forced to stop and smell the roses, enable me to taste, savor and enjoy life. May I be nourished in the beauty that is mine for the seeing.

God, fill me with your presence and enable me to live life to its fullest. Grant me the ability to give and receive love fully, to appreciate the joys of each moment and the fulfillment of each day. Let me not forget this experience as I have been forced to live faithfully and courageously. I am happy to be alive.

Heal me in body, mind and spirit that I might be well once again. Thank you. Amen.

5. A THERAPEUTIC PRAYER BY LOVED ONES

When ill, ask visiting family and friends to pray with you. They may appear to be reluctant. This has nothing to do with not wanting to pray with you. It is just that most persons have never prayed aloud with someone. They feel awkward in doing something new. In the same way, most people lack the skills of prayer as well as the knowledge to offer it in the special form of healing prayer.

You might approach loved ones in this way: *"I have decided that I want to be soaked with prayer as I cope with this illness. Prayer provides an energy for healing that I need. This book (PrayWell) has a prayer which I would like you to offer for me. Would you pray with me? While doing so, can we join hands?"* Then provide them with the following healing prayer. Note that they may know how to pray without this prayer, but ask them to use this therapeutic prayer because its focus is upon healing.

A THERAPEUTIC PRAYER FOR HEALING BY LOVED ONES

Join hands. Take a deep breath. Then say, "Let us pray:"

God, the giver and sustainer of all life, we thank you for your gift of life to _____. We ask you to strengthen _____ and each of us in this special time of need. Provide for our needs, fill us with your love and bind us to one another in mutual caring. Bring healing to _____ in body, mind and spirit.

Protect _____ from pain and fear. Bring us calmness that we may face this crisis with confidence. Surround him/her with the love of all who care. We know that your will is that s/he become well. Grant _____ your wholeness and let it begin now. Thank you. Amen.

6. YOUR PRAYER WELCOMING THE PRAYERS OF OTHERS

Human energy fields may be closed, guarding us from others. This prayer intends to open your energy fields. It also gives permission for the energy to be used for healing.

God, I joyfully open myself to the love and healing energy that is being sent me through prayer. I accept the healing that is flowing into me. I pray that it will be effectively used in healing my body, calming my feelings and filling me with your peace and love. I am thankful for all the people who are spiritually caring for me. Thank you. Amen.

REQUESTING ABSENT PRAYER

If at all possible, at the onset of illness, request prayer from family, friends, strangers, churches, prayer groups and prayer chains. You or your family can write a prayer or use prayer seven which follows this introduction. Distribute the printed prayers to every individual. The promise, *"I will pray for you,"* should seldom be taken literally. Translated, it has come to mean, *"I will be thinking caringly about you."* Clearly state, *"I am counting on you to pray for me every day. I need the energy of your prayers to help me get well."*

In requesting prayers from groups, have someone phone every known prayer group and prayer chain in the area. Keep the groups informed of your progress, motivating their concern and continuing prayers. Intentionally open yourself to receiving the prayer message. We have voluntary control of our energy fields' reception of healing energy. To open yourself, use prayer six, above.

This first step of having people pray with you will bathe you with healing energy. This will place all the organs in your body in optimal condition. It is likely to increase the oxygen in your blood by about ten percent, and your body's normal healing ability will be enhanced by two to seven times. It will reduce any pain or discomfort. It will calm you and place you in a state of emotional well-being. You will probably not need tranquilizing medication. These intercessory prayers may result in complete healing. Remember that, if unexpected wellness occurs.

ABSENT THERAPEUTIC PRAYER FOR HEALING

Directions: This person has requested your prayers. Your prayer will provide an energy for healing that scientific data shows enhances the health of each organ in the body, increases the blood oxygen level and provides emotional calming. Your efforts are crucial because the power of prayer is the square of the number of persons praying. God is willing to use you as a channel for healing because you care enough to offer a prayer. Your specific prayer is needed. Simply feeling concerned does not work. God does nothing except through prayer. Prayer is the medium for God's miracles of healing.

A. If possible, provide others with copies of this prayer, telling them of your concern.
B. If possible, ask others to join you in praying, gathering in a circle. If you have only one copy, do *"pray-along"* -- saying a phrase and having the others repeat it after you.
C. Before praying, recall the situation of the prayee. Compassion enables the power of prayer.
D. Then, recall the person. Just the first name is all that is necessary.
E. Then, in your mind, imagine you, God, and the prayer recipient being united and blended into oneness. In this state of union, picture the intended results, a picture of the person transformed back to wholeness. If possible, offer this prayer aloud in your normal speaking voice.

7. AN ABSENT THERAPEUTIC PRAYER FOR HEALING

God, I thank you for _____. I thank you for her/his birth, life, hopes and dreams. I am concerned for her/him. S/he wishes to get well. You are the Creator and Sustainer of all life. Sustain her/him in this time of need. Recreate a right spirit within her/him. Heal _____ in body, mind and spirit and grant her/him your peace. Unite me with God and _____, making us one in Spirit. Make us one with you and each other. I send this prayer to _____ through you. Thank you. Amen.

Now, sense God and visualize the person or the name and then, in your mind, unite God, the person, and yourself into one -- a merging of the three of you into one -- the Healing Trinity. Pray again, saying:

God, make me one with _____ and you. Thank you.

Hold that sense of merged oneness in your mind for five minutes. Now, deeply feel your deep concern for _____. Gather up all the love you can. Visualize that love being transmitted to _____ form your heart as a white laser beam of light. This is God's healing energy in prayer. As you do so, pray aloud:

God, let this healing love energy fill and aid _____. Thank you.

Concluding prayer:

God, fill _____ with your presence. Let this healing begin now and continue throughout the coming hours and days. Thank you for the healing that is now taking place. Amen.

DIRECTIONS FOR TOUCH-HEALING PRAYER BY LOVED ONES

Invite people to practice touch-healing prayer with you. The following instructions provide all the information they need.

A. Before praying, all pray-ers should rinse their hands in water to neutralize their existing energy. This enables the healing energy to be purer and more effective.

B. You need to practice. With fingers straight, place the palms and fingers of both hands against each other. Then pull them apart about half an inch. Try to send energy through each hand to the other. Every person can be taught to transmit life force in this way. Sense the energy between your hands. Now, while continuing to sense this energy, slowly move your hands apart, all the while sensing the energy, until you can no longer feel it. Then, bring your hands together until they touch.

When we care and we pray, this energy is transformed and becomes God's healing energy. Through touching a person during prayer, the healing energy is transmitted to the body. The fingers and the palms of the hands transmit the energy. You may sense nothing. Some persons sense heat, some cold, some an energy flow. With experience, your sensings are likely to become more consistent. Such sensings provide reassurance that you are passing the healing energy, and bolster confidence. Trying hard can stem the healing flow. Just relax and allow it to happen.

C. The recipient may have similar sensings where you are touching. Sometimes the body area needing healing grows warm. Sometimes there is tingling throughout the body. Reports of this tingling usually are followed by a complete alleviation of all symptoms. Do not be disappointed if you feel nothing at first. You will sense something within a week of daily praying.

D. The imparted healing energy enhances the vitality of all organs, increases the oxygen in the blood, decreases pain, initiates healing in circumstances resistant to medical treatment, enhances the healing rate by two to seven times and creates a sense of inner calm. Healing energy is capable of producing genetic engineering and of regenerating tissue. It causes all tissue to function at optimum potential. The healing energy knows what to do to restore wellness.

E. This is a process taking place over time. The healing energy is only being imparted while prayer is being offered. It must reach a specific threshold or level of power to initiate and maintain the healing process.

The healing energy is empowered by love, compassion, intimacy, faith and hope. The power is also increased by the number of persons praying, the power being the square of that number.

F. Healing energy works like an antibiotic. It must be constantly replenished because it is used up by the process of healing. Replenishing must take place every day. If a person is acutely ill, several daily applications are encouraged. Once the healing process is initiated or begins, the healing energy must be regularly applied until complete healing occurs. Like an antibiotic, the healing energy masks the symptoms of an illness, so keep praying for several days after all symptoms disappear. If complete healing has not occurred, the illness returns.

G. The hands are the most efficient means for transmitting the healing energy. If one person is praying, there are several ways of placing the hands. For a specific area needing healed, place your hands on either side of the area. If the illness is generalized, either hold both the person's hands or place one hand on the forehead and the other on the nape of the neck. Be sure your arms are in a comfortable position so that they do not tire over a period of time. The comfort of your body during healing prayer is important. A second person can hold an ankle in either hand. A third person can place hands on the forehead and nape of neck. Other persons may stand or sit in a circle around the recipient, praying.

H. After the prayer, your hands will continue to transmit healing energy, so leave them there until you no longer sense an energy transmission. Twelve minutes is minimal. During this time, seek to sense a oneness between you, God and the person, or seek to transmit the healing energy. Either approach works. With experience, you will be able to carry on a conversation with the recipient while transmitting the energy. This also helps to attune and empower the energy. Afterwards, stop the healing energy emitting from your hands by rubbing the palms briskly against each other, or clapping your hands or rinsing them with water. If you do not, you may experience an energy drain.

I. During the healing encounter, the recipient silently states, *"I choose to be well. I open myself to the healing flow and will utilize it for my own healing."* The recipient should open him/herself to a sense of God's presence within, in love and peace, and imagine what it would like to be completely well.

J. Who leads the prayer? It could be the person who is emotionally closest to the recipient. It could be the person who is the most outgoing and friendly. It could be the person who feels the most comfortable in offering the prayer. Begin by saying, *"Let us pray."* Pause for a moment to center upon God, touch the person with your hands, then begin the prayer.

8A. A BEGINNER'S TOUCH-HEALING THERAPEUTIC PRAYER

God, the Creator and Sustainer of all life, I thank you for bringing us together in prayer. I thank you for your sacred gift of life to _____. I know that you want her/him to be well. S/he chooses to accept your gift of wholeness and open herself/himself to your care. Provide for her/his needs and protect her/him from all harm. Create in _____ a vision of a new day, a day when her/his life has been transformed and made whole.

I ask to be used as a channel for your healing power. Enable me to enter into her/his pain and hurt, her/his hopes and dreams, that I might have compassion and oneness with this person whom I love. My intention is that your healing energy flow through me and be effectively utilized to make _____ well.

God, heal _____ in body, mind and spirit and make her/him well. Let this healing begin now and continue until wellness is achieved. Deepen our faith, our hope, our expectations, that your healing energy may be empowered. Attune me to _____'s needs and to her/his essence as a person. Grant her/him your love, joy and peace. We thank you for the healing that is taking place. We trust you. Amen.

As you silently continue, alternate between these three styles:
  A. Sense the energy flowing through your hands.
  B. Sense your oneness with God and the recipient.
  C. Visualize the intended results within your mind.

8B. A BRIEFER TOUCH-HEALING PRAYER

Begin by saying, *"Let us pray."* Pause for a moment to center upon God, touch the person with your hands, then begin the prayer.

God, I ask you to use me as a channel for healing. Use my hands for your healing flow. _____, be healed in body, mind and spirit. May God bless you with love, joy and peace. Thank you for the healing that is taking place. Amen.

As you silently continue, alternate between these three styles:
  A. Sense the energy flowing through your hands.
  B. Sense your oneness with God and the recipient.
  C. Visualize the intended results within your mind.

9. A TOUCH-HEALING PRAYER FOR YOUR OWN HEALING

Touch yourself in the needed areas or place your favored hand on your diaphragm, the other on the heart, then after five minutes reverse hands..

God, I thank you for the gift of life and for this marvelously engineered physical body of mine. I come to you, God, seeking healing. I offer my hands as channels for my own healing. Let your healing flow be imparted to my body that I might become well. Heal me in body, mind and spirit and make me whole.

I visualize this area as healed. Remove any pain and restore all tissue to normal. I quietly await your healing. May it begin now and continue until I am well. Enable me to be one with you and the healing flow. Thank you, God, for the healing that is taking place. Amen.

10. THE SELF-HEALING OF INFECTIONS

First, express your will. State,

I do not want this infection. I do not need this infection. I choose to be well. Virus (bacteria), go away.

Then center yourself, sensing a peace and harmony within you. Place your hands on either side of your head and command:

Virus, in God's name, depart from me. God, make this virus disappear. Protect me from this illness. I ask you to heal me in body, mind and spirit. Let all symptoms of this illness disappear now. Amen.

11. HEALING CHARGED MATERIALS

Water, cotton and wool cloth and surgical gauze can all be charged with healing energy. These have many practical applications. I once incurred deep bruises to my back and torn ligaments along my spine as the result of falling down steps. I charged a cotton dish towel by holding it in my hands for fifteen minutes after praying for healing. I then placed the towel on my back under my shirt. I experienced a constant flow of heat and energy into my back, which diminished pain and enhanced the rate of healing.

Healing-charged towels can be placed for long periods of time on areas needing healing. Surgical gauze used for medical dressings can also be charged with healing energy. A glass or plastic container of water can be charged with healing energy and be ingested two ounces at a time at meals and bedtime. The healing water then flows into every cell of the body, making it excellent for use in many diseases or for the healing of negative emotions. The healing charge lasts up to two years, but dissipates in sunlight, extreme heat or handling by others. You can charge up your own medium or ask someone who seems proficient to do it. I hold cotton dish towels or gauze for fifteen minutes and water for thirty minutes.

RESOURCES BEYOND YOUR HOME

There are at least five sources of spiritual healing beyond your home. Traveling to these resources will supplement the daily healing efforts taking place in your home. Each resource adds it unique energy for healing. Combining any of these resources strengthens your possibilities for finding the healing you need.

12. A Support Group. One source is a support group, some of which use the Twelve Step program. Some are led by professionals, like Bernie Siegel's Exceptional Cancer Patient (ECaP) groups, and are for persons with any illness. Most are self-help groups designed for persons with a particular illness. They can be found in hospitals, churches and other places offering meeting space. The energy for healing in support groups derives from the caring that occurs. Anytime people selflessly care, it releases an energy for healing which pervades a group. Adding healing prayer would be the next logical step. Attend regularly. This is a process, not a one-step cure.

13. A Prayer Group. Prayer groups are my preferred setting for spiritual healing. Everyone is caring and praying, which therapeutically enables an ill person to offer his love to others. There is the healing energy. And there is a personal identity for everyone present which helps to attune the energy for healing.

14. A Healing Service. Healing services can be found in churches throughout most communities. The charismatic renewal movement has led to healing services in some Roman Catholic, Episcopal and Lutheran churches. Healing services can sometimes be found in the mainline United Church of Christ, Presbyterian and United Methodist churches. All Church of the Brethren congregations, which are in the holiness tradition, offer healing. All Pentecostal churches offer healing services including the Church of God, Four Square Gospel and Assemblies of God. Among evangelical churches, the Church of the Nazarene often offers healing services, as do a few Baptist churches. Spiritualist churches always offer healing services. Some New Age churches offer healing services. Feel free to phone a number of churches, and find the one that feels right for you.

You need not be a member to attend a healing service. The variety of styles and messages is immense. Unfamiliarity may make you feel awkward at first in most settings. Some churches seek converts through healing services. Be aware that not only does the sacred group energy field encompassing most healing services hold healing energy; the information within it is also quietly converting you to the religious beliefs of those sponsoring the service.

The healing service's intention to offer healing creates a powerful group healing energy field that is attuned to healing and is thus ideal. In such a service, open yourself to the energy present. Silently say to yourself, *"I open myself to this energy and pray that it heals me in body, mind, and spirit."* Fill yourself with hope, with expectancy, with miracle-readiness. Sit quietly and visualize the healing energy pervading every part of your body. Imagine it touching your illness and transforming it. See yourself as well. If the opportunity is there, accept any touch-prayer that is offered. When you stand, sit or kneel to be touched, open yourself to the healing power that is offered.

Again, healing is a process taking place over a period of time. Keep returning to the healing service. Do this long after you think you have been healed. Your body or emotions may have been healed, but your energy fields may still need further help for a total restoration.

15. A Religious Service. When the people of a particular religion gather together in ritual, they create a group energy field that can be used for healing. The information in a group energy field includes the love, goodness and spirituality of each individual gathered, the power of the beliefs of the ritual and the people, and the powerful energy of the rituals themselves. The sacred group energy field revitalizes the human energy fields, enhancing the power of your own self-healing meditative prayer. If you do not sense anything you need in one religious gathering, explore others until you find what you need.

16. A Healer. The previous sources of healing energy were groups. But individual healers can be found in every community. Certified healers can be found in Christian Science and Spiritualist churches. Anyone offering healing during healing services is capable of providing individual sessions. Some of the most proficient healers can be found in England, Brazil, the Philippines and among native North and South Americans.

Healers can also be found outside of organized religion. Most of these healers use techniques they have learned at workshops. Touch for Health has five thousand instructors in thirty-seven nations, including many health care professionals. Reiki, an oriental technique, has many able healers. Therapeutic Touch has been taught to thousands of nurses in many nursing schools. The cleansing and balancing of chakras and energy fields is practiced by many healers and some health care professionals. Acupuncture, acupressure and reflexology are forms of energy healing. Many chiropractors, some osteopaths and a few medical doctors practice various forms of healing, often cloaked in terms of medical technology like *energy medicine.* Homeopathic and naturopathic physicians offer forms of spiritual healing. Some massotherapists and physical therapists offer healing. The staff at health food stores can often refer you to a local healer.

While you can count on groups to produce large quantities of energy for healing, this is not the strength of individual healers. Working with a competent healer offers better odds for healing than does a group because of the healer's attuning skills and the extra time permitted in individual care. Before making an appointment, ask the healer for the name of one person he or she has healed who had a disease similar to yours. Do not accept the excuse that such information is confidential. If you cannot find confirmed healings by a healer, you might consider looking elsewhere. If you are suspicious of a healer who takes money and you have the resources, make a double or nothing bargain. In this agreement you pay nothing if not healed but double the charge if the agreed-upon levels of healing occur.

Outside of religious groups, healers usually charge, though a few ask only for a donation. Be happy and willing to compensate a healer fairly for his or her professional time and efforts as you would a doctor, lawyer or therapist. If you are reluctant to pay, it is probably because either you object to a healer charging or you do not trust that healing will result. If you remain unwilling to pay or are resentful about paying, then cancel your appointment. You would be unable to accept and utilize the healing energy well. Payment is a statement of trust and faith. Note the chapter six observations on how long it takes for a healer to heal a particular illness. Agree beforehand upon what results are acceptable and upon the maximum number of sessions necessary. Let no one shame you into not seeing a healer or into quitting in the midst of the process. But, if in your own judgment, the healer is not helping, quit.

THE ONGOING ADVENTURE

By your own experience of self-healing, you will have been convinced of the healing reality. What is your next step? Do not expect everyone to believe you. Do have the courage to tell your story. A simple telling of your experience is far more convincing than giving your audience all the knowledge you have acquired about healing prayer. Opportunities will arise for you to help others to be healed. Offer them a copy of PrayWell. Offer to do touch-healing with them. Continue the ongoing adventure.

HEALTH & HEALING in the *World's Great Religions*

CHRISTIANITY: *"The prayer of faith shall heal the sick, and the Lord shall raise him up."*

HINDUISM: *"Enricher, Healer of disease, be a good friend to us."*

ISLAM: *"The Lord of the worlds created me... and when I am sick, He heals me."*

BUDDHISM: *"To keep the body in good health is a duty...otherwise we shall not be able to keep our mind strong and clear."*

BAHA'I: *"All healing comes from God"*

JUDAISM: *"O Lord, my God, I cried to you for help and you have healed me."*

SIKHISM: *"God is Creator of all, the remover of sickness, the giver of health."*

JAINISM: *"All living beings owe their present state of health to their own Karma."*

ZOROASTRIANISM: *"Love endows the sick body of man with firmness and health."*

TOAISM: *"Pursue a middle course. Thus will you keep a healthy body and a healthy mind."*

Copyright permission courtesy of Marcus Bach

Chapter Eighteen

Healing Through a Shift in Consciousness

*"Synchronistic fate: The coming together, as if by design, of evidently unrelated phenomena in order to form a clear pattern." ...*Tristan Jones

*"It is generally as painful to us to discard old beliefs as for the scientists to discard the old laws of physics and accept new theory." ...*Lin Yutang

"Birth is not one act; it is a process. The aim of life is to be fully born, though its tragedy is that most of us die before we are thus born. To live is to be born every minute." ... Erich Fromm

The past seventeen chapters have explored Therapeutic Prayer. The life energy released by prayer causes healing by restoring the human energy fields, making them healthy. The healthy energy fields then restore physical, emotional and mental health.

Prayer can also cause healing by altering brain-wave patterns. This produces a shift in consciousness that dramatically restores both the human energy fields and physical, emotional and mental health. This process may be an essential element of many life energy healings.

Religious rituals use the same mechanisms for restoring health. For Christians, these rituals include healing services, worship services, the eucharist, baptism and confirmation.

The signatures of all illnesses appear to become engraved in the brain and mind. This could explain why quick treatment of a physical injury is more effective than a delayed response. If we can get to the injury before its signature is engraved into the brain and mind, healing is rapid. If we delay, then the brain and mind become programmed to maintain the condition. The same process seems evident in viral infections.

If I had an acute, chronic or life-threatening condition, I would use Therapeutic Prayer, prayer groups, healing services and a shift to a peak state of consciousness. They complement one another.

Neurologist Dr. Robert Nash, MD, thinks that the greatest breakthrough in the neurosciences will be the understanding of how we can self-tune the transceiver we call the brain. In *Pathways* (Fall, 1989), he is quoted as stating, *"Through a variety of mechanisms which are yet to be elucidated scientifically, we will most likely be able to bring electromagnetic homeostasis to our brain, which will bring us health. There is some evidence for this already, where studies have shown that those who do Transcendental Meditation have a far lower incidence of disease, bordering on eighty percent, in cardiovascular disease and diseases of the nervous system, compared with those who do not practice this technique....The brain, as we begin to understand how the electromagnetic aspects of it function, is like a finely tuned heterodyne receiver for radio communications. We may be able to transgress our space-time continuum and attain knowledge and capacities now relegated only to science fiction."*

ALTERED STATES LEAD HUMANS TO A HIGHER WISDOM

Various altered states of consciousness do far more than enable healing to occur. Altered states produce peak states of consciousness, including the peak experience of God (PEG). Altered states can put us into contact with God. They make us aware of our flowing oneness with the universe. Here is where religious miracles occur.

From peak states of consciousness, great creativity flows and outstanding human performance happens. In that state of flowing awareness of unity with the universe, Tchaikovsky, Beethoven and Handel must have composed great music, Edison and Einstein made their discoveries, athletes win championships, lovers rejoice and a hundred pound woman lifts the fifteen hundred pound rear end of an automobile to free an injured child.

We have thought of miracles, including healing, as happening only when we are experiencing the presence of God or the spiritual state of being. The evidence indicates otherwise. Healing takes place in many ways never before considered. If you know that healing is possible through a peak state of consciousness, then entering one offers the possibility of healing your illness.

There are dozens of ways of shifting one's consciousness in order to re-program the brain and thereby alleviate all symptoms of illness. It does not follow that doing so once, using one approach, produces instant healing. One must explore various altered states over a period of weeks or months.

Shifting consciousness for healing is a process just like Therapeutic Prayer. With prayer, you can reprogram your brain and mind without reaching a peak state of consciousness. The energy released by prayer bathes you with a constant frequency that produces healing.

Complete healing can occur through reaching just one peak state of consciousness. In this peak state, reprogramming can be perfect. But, just as in Therapeutic Prayer, I would continue seeking to achieve peak states to improve and strengthen the new brain programming.

Look for mental, emotional and energy improvements that might precede physical change. The initial improvements would involve a growing sense of inner calm and mental clarity, stronger emotions, an increasing sense of humor, and more physical vitality as indicated by less time needed for sleep, less effort needed to concentrate on reading or television and less fatigue from visitors. Combine these with mind-body work and prayer.

Keep a daily record in a journal. Note your initial physical, mental, emotional and spiritual states of being. We usually forget how bad we originally felt. Rate each state by number, with ten being the highest level and one the lowest level. You might find yourself initially to be emotionally at a four, physically at a two, mentally at a six and spiritually at a two. From this baseline, you can measure future daily or weekly progress.

CLINICAL EVIDENCE

Neurologist Robert Nash's vision of a breakthrough *"to self-tune the transceiver we call the brain"* has recently occurred. Chapter ten briefly reported this.

During the past three years, accumulated scientific evidence indicates that any time a person is able to achieve a peak state of consciousness, personal transformation and empowerment can occur. Using biofeedback, you can learn to enter the low theta brain-wave state of four to eight frequencies per second. At that point, you get into a state of consciousness where you can move up and go into a state of revelry. This state is called the autogenic shift. You are operating at the back of the head in the left cortex or the left occipital lobe of the brain.

Elmer Green, PhD, who set up the Psychophysiology Lab at the Menninger Clinic in Topeka, Kansas in 1964, reports that through biofeedback a Westerner can attain the mystic state of the Tibetan or Hindu yogi in two to three days. The body, emotions and thoughts are quieted as you enter the unconscious upper four levels of consciousness. This is known as self-mastery.[1]

At this consciousness level, you can focus your intentions downward for the transformation of the body, emotions and thoughts. When alcoholics get into this theta state, they can turn their attention downwards to the hypothalamus and are able to rewire that gland so that they no longer want to drink. This has been successfully done with six thousand alcoholic subjects to date.

Scientific evidence indicates that any time a person is able to achieve a peak state of consciousness, personal transformation and empowerment can occur. The limbic area of the brain is the emotional brain. The limbic area of the brain must have activity in it for us to feel emotions in our physical bodies. The emotions are connected to our unconscious, so we enter the unconscious through the limbic area.

Dr. Green states, *"Sensory information from the outer world enters through the limbic brain which is the master of the mechanical brain which is the master of the body. If you take the information from the body and put it back into the outside world -- that is biofeedback -- and you look at it and you imagine what you would like to happen -- the limbic brain is not smart enough to know that what you are imagining is not the real thing. It responds to it as if it was information of your sensory perceptions of outside the skin events, acting as if it was the real thing.*

"The body responds to our visualizations as if they were the real thing -- the real world. That is the power of visualization. The reason visualization works is because the limbic system implements it -- controlling the hypothalamus, the pituitary and the physiological responses. All you have to do is get some feedback and you can learn to control it.

"There is a spectrum of consciousness from sleep, delta (1-4 bps [brainwaves per second]), to theta (4-8 bps), to alpha (8-13 bps), to beta or wide awake (13-26 bps). If you get into a state of consciousness where you can move UP and go into revelry, you can go into this state called the autogenic shift. You are in theta (4-8 bps) and at the back of the head in the left cortex or the left occipital lobe -- a visual lobe. It is also concerned with analy-

sis or reasoning. You have to be awake, in beta, to analyze. You cannot analyze very well in alpha and not at all in theta. If you can get the left cortex, the visual part, to go into theta, then you free the rest of the brain to do some very interesting things.

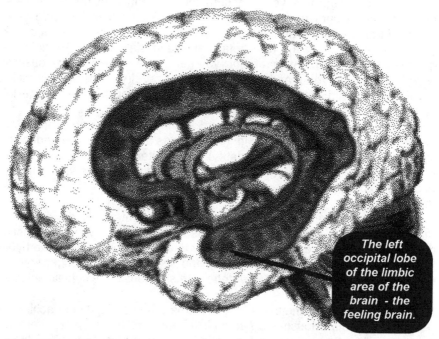

The left occipital lobe of the limbic area of the brain - the feeling brain.

Figure 10. The left occipital lobe of the limbic area of the brain can be programmed for physical, emotional and compulsive-addictive healing.

"I am talking about yoga -- deep Tibetan yoga, deep Hindu yoga -- that is what it is all about. A yogi is sitting there getting his body quiet, getting his emotions quiet, getting his thoughts quiet. When that happens, people go into theta.

"In theta brain-wave training, people are able develop this profound trance-like state in Westerners in two to three days. The reason it works so quickly is that, by meditation alone, you do not know exactly when you are in the theta state. In biofeedback, when the tone beeps, you know you are in theta. If, when the tone beeps, you say, 'Oh, I am in theta,' then you are no longer in theta. You cannot have theta when you mentally know it is there. [When you use the mental rational state of conscious, theta disappears and you return to beta.] In order to be at theta and notice it is there, you have to become a witness -- a witness above yourself to transcend your normal self -- above your body, emotions and thoughts."[2]

Consciousness is in the lower three levels. All the levels above these lower three levels constitute the unconscious. The first level, E4, is the subconscious, the intuitive. The top three levels are the superconscious. This is the level where you become conscious of during Theta Training.

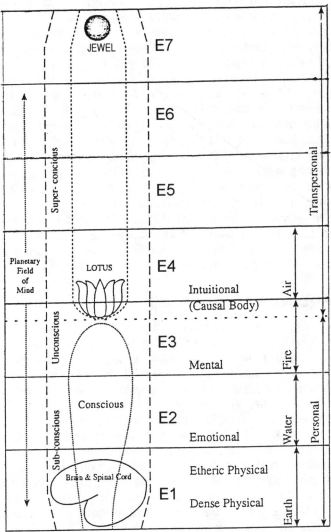

Figure 11. Levels of Human Consciousness. This is a *symbolic* representation of the levels of human consciousness. The vertical dotted line from top to bottom on either side of the figure represents the human mind. The horizontal dotted line below the lotus represents the normal states of human consciousness: the conscious, subconscious and unconscious minds (E1, E2, E3) We have full access to only part of the conscious mind, and little access to the subconscious and unconscious. The Planetary Field of Mind on the left represents the different frequencies of matter, with each E representing a different one. These seven levels also represent the boundaries between different kinds of possible perceptions and actions.

When we enter the lotus level (the white light) of the mystic consciousness that begins with E4, the transpersonal, we are in a peak state of consciousness or the peak experience of God. At this higher state of consciousness, personal transformation becomes relatively easy. Here we can reprogram ourselves for physical, emotional, mental and spiritual health. This is the end goal of the personal growth or spiritual journey.

When you get the body, emotions and thoughts quiet, you find that you are still here. You are at this entrance to the mystic state -- the white light -- and at that point, you can focus the intentions downward, and you can start to get the body, emotions and thoughts under control.

Many of the biofeedback subjects, without knowing anything about it, have the tunnel experience. They can have OBEs. One subject said, *"I felt like I had electricity shooting out of the top of my head. I saw this bright light on the other side. I realized I had to go there. I started running down the tunnel and I saw the light coming from a figure of me. It was upside down and on top of another figure of me."* That is the temple with the angels and the demons. *"The light was so intense it was too painful to continue."* Those who have this experience have difficulty putting it into words. This is the ineffable zone. But you know it without words.[3]

Those who work with LSD have been able to get up there and go through, but they could not stay up there because it was a chemically-induce shot, and inevitably they came back to earth.

Biofeedback research provides the scientific data and rationale needed for us to trust altered states of consciousness as a reliable means for achieving health and wholeness. Similar claims for hypnosis, autogenic training, visualization and meditation are also validated by biofeedback research.

1. BIOFEEDBACK THETA TRAINING

You may want to use biofeedback on your own path back to health. The first step is finding someone certified in biofeedback theta training. Many college psychology departments have a certified biofeedback professor. Some hospitals use biofeedback. You might find biofeedback theta training among psychologists, psychiatrists or physicians. If not, these sources may refer you to someone. Try the Yellow Pages of your phone book.

Not all certified biofeedback technicians may be familiar with the Menninger Clinic work. Ask if they offer theta training and can help you achieve a peak state of consciousness or the mystical state.

You will not achieve your goal while learning on a biofeedback machine. Elmer Green states that once you have been trained to enter the theta state, you must get off the biofeedback machine. The real work begins after your biofeedback theta training. While in theta, gently reprogram yourself to be healthy. Use your own imagination.

2. HYPNOSIS

Hypnosis was the first technique used to reprogram the brain. During the 1950s, German psychiatrist Johannes Schultz became convinced that hypnosis could be used to control the cortical and subcortical brain processes. He helped patients visualize their way to health. With hypnosis, Schultz produced many of the results clinically verified in biofeedback training.

This approach was hampered by the human problem. People did not want to be hypnotized. So Schultz developed a self-help technique, Autogenic Training, that people could induce for themselves. This produced results similar to those of hypnosis. Autogenic Training will be covered in the following pages.

While one is in a hypnotic state, suggestion can program the brain. Thirty years ago, my colleague Hubert Hensel used hypnotism to eliminate pain during the surgery of Cesarean sections, holding conversations with the mother as he delivered the baby.

Hypnosis can be used in dentistry for pain-free dental work. Kay Thompson, a Philadelphia dentist, reported that people with hemophilia could prevent themselves from bleeding during surgery and extractions, using self-hypnosis.[4]

Wadden and Anderson found in their review of clinical uses of hypnosis that suggestion does affect the stomach functions, brain blood flow, bronchial airway activity and wart remission.[5]

I have used hypnosis to remove the addictive-compulsive cravings of smoking, to lower stress levels, to heal sexual dysfunction, to release traumatic memories, to internalize counseling insight, to promote physical healing following strokes, heart attacks and cancer, and to make people more receptive to touch-healing prayer.

A professional hypnotist can program you to regularly enter a hypnotic state through post-hypnotic suggestion involving a triggering word. This enables you to do your own suggesting and visualization. Elmer Green suggests that you can make all kinds of things happen in the body through hypnosis. All you need is an *"Organ Specific Formula"* -- directions fitting your specific condition.

3. RUSSIAN HYPNOTIST PRODUCES A FOUNTAIN OF YOUTH

Dr. Anatoly Gerasimov, MD, of Moscow, Russia deserves special mention because of his hypnosis research with senior citizens. Gerasimov cuts an impressive figure with his booming voice, large physical stature and black beard. He is a physician, healer and internationally renowned hypnosis researcher.

Gerasimov's staff at a Moscow hospital clinically determined the chronological ages of seventy-five senior citizens in their seventies and eighties. He then hypnotized them as a group and suggested that they had the bodies of fifty-year-olds. A month later, clinical exams showed an average physiological age reduction of fifteen years for the group. The clinical results indicated improved muscle tone, lowered pulse and blood pressure, improved agility, more endurance and energy, and more youthful skin with a dramatic decrease in wrinkles and crow's feet.

As with touch-healing, few people believe his reported results. I have offered this process to dozens of senior citizens during the past year with only about ten percent accepting the offer. My results are identical to those Gerasimov reported to me. It is not known at this time whether all hypnotists can achieve these results. Might healers possess special qualities that would account for such dramatic responses? Further investigation will help to answer this question.

4. AUTOGENIC TRAINING

In 1975, I used autogenic training as the basis for healing my damaged heart muscle, as described in the last chapter. Once in this self-induced state, you must employ a conscious technique. I used meditation, visualization and prayer for more than an hour daily for six weeks. Within two weeks, I was completely relaxed, with my stress and fear replaced by inner calmness. In the sixth week, I had a peak experience of God (PEG) that included perceiving a brilliant white light in my mind during which my heart muscle was healed. This also involved touch-healing, as my own hands on my chest produced an incredible amount of healing energy.

Dr. Johannes Schultz, the creator of autogenic training, called it a psychophysiological skill. Through autogenic training, many patients could produce within themselves the same phenomena found in subjects of hypnosis research. At the time, Schultz's clinical findings were dismissed by most physicians and psychologists as placebo effects.[6] Biofeedback researchers have now provided the physiological answers for why autogenic training works. Autogenic training can be trusted to reprogram the brain and mind, just as do biofeedback and hypnosis.

The drawback to both hypnosis and autogenic training, according to Elmer Green, is that you do not know when you have reached the theta state of brain-wave activity as you do in biofeedback when there is a "beep" telling you so. However, Green is mistaken. When you see a bright white light in your brain, or a tunnel, you know you are in theta and can quickly reprogram the brain for health and wholeness. When you have a peak experience of God (PEG) in which you are filled with the Holy Spirit, the bright white light and the tunnel are usually missing, but you are still in the effective theta state of brain-wave activity needed for healing transformation and empowerment. My experience confirms that during any noticeable religious experience, even if only if you are just short of theta, you are still quietly and slowly reprogramming the brain and mind over a period of time.

4A. MEDITATION

Here we need to introduce the role of meditation. To most people, meditation is a bore. But, when combined with autogenic training, meditation flows far more easily. That is why I have introduced the subject of meditation at this point. Daily meditation produces the theta state on its own.

Until recently, meditation, the traditional tool of Hindu yogis, Tibetan monks, and Christian mystics has been thought of as only a religious endeavor. Using mental techniques, one concentrated upon the revealed image of God. The purpose was to draw closer to God and thus become more like the revealed image of God upon which one focused.

Now meditation is also seen as having the potential to bring about a shift of consciousness and lead one to wholeness and health. In this context, meditation involves focusing in such a way as to transform one's awareness or consciousness. It requires turning inward in concentration on those images and symbols that arise from our unconscious depths, as we pause for a time of silence or inner focus.

Meditation can help sharpen thinking processes and memory, diminish fatigue and stress, put one in touch with one's feelings and heal them, restore the brain function of recovering chemical addicts, increase the body's defense system, produce physical healings, provide personal direction, increase the intuitive-creative process and create meaning and joy. More rapid progress can be made in group meditation sessions.

All meditation techniques produce the same results. The least expensive leadership can be found within organized religion. Other leadership is not usually excessively costly. Meditations, as simple as breath-counting or repeating a word or phrase for twenty minutes, can produce all the results you are seeking. Lawrence LeShan's small book, How To Meditate (Bantam), is one of the best guides available.

4B. VISUALIZATIONS AND AFFIRMATIONS

Visualization and affirmations can also reprogram the brain and mind, but for that to occur, they must be done while one is in the alpha and theta states. That is why I include them under autogenic training.

4C. BEGINNING AUTOGENIC TRAINING

The following autogenic training process, which I call meditative prayer, can be used for the self-healing of an acute, chronic, life-limiting or life-threatening illness. It can also restore mental, emotional and spiritual health. This ultimate healing process includes meditation, visualization, affirmation and prayer. Motivation and commitment are important because this process requires a daily commitment of thirty to sixty minutes.

If you are in the midst of a medical crisis, you have both the necessary commitment and plenty of time. Be expectant but do not be impatient. Your energy fields are extremely stable. This is not a quick fix like taking an aspirin or an antibiotic. It takes time for their transformation to occur. It took an hour or two each day for six weeks before a peak healing experience completed the healing of my heart muscle. The meditative prayer process would be my first choice for the healing of any major illness or condition. It can work when all other approaches have failed.

Throughout this process, follow your doctor's instructions. Do not assume that you have been completely healed because all the symptoms have disappeared. Continue contributing to the balance and strength of your energy fields and brain/mind for at least three weeks after you are symptom-free. Return to your doctor to confirm results.

If diagnostic tests indicate that you still have the illness in your system even though you feel great, this indicates that you have increased the strength and balance of your energy fields, but still need to continue practicing meditative self-healing prayer. In rare cases, your healing attempts may mask the outward symptoms of the disease while your body is still being damaged by the disease. With other conditions, your healing efforts may not result in a cure but will still permit you to function as though in normal health. This is like the action of insulin, which does not cure diabetes but helps to maintain normal living. In one case of Crohn's Disease, no cure resulted but the patient remained symptom-free while continuing healing treatments.

Do not accept any doctor's or loved one's ridicule of your reclaimed state of health. Rejection could completely undo the results. Your beliefs are a powerful force for reclaiming health. They can also make you ill again, often immediately following ridicule and the insistence that you are still ill because you have an incurable disease. If you are living among scoffers, the best approach is to tell no one what you have been doing to reclaim your health. If you sense that your illness has been completely healed but your doctor refuses to accept your testimony, find a new doctor who knows none of your medical history. Request a physical exam that includes tests for the illness you had.

4D. BENEFITS OF AUTOGENIC TRAINING AND MEDITATIVE PRAYER

If you master the procedures and stay with them for several weeks, meditative prayer will become a joy for you. You are motivated by your focus on becoming well. You will also become the beneficiary of a number of pleasing side-effects. Meditative prayer slowly produces changes in you. Meditation is a secular mental exercise that sharpens your brain functioning and guides you towards emotional wholeness. When a religious or spiritual context is added to meditation, it deepens your contact with God. Meditative prayer produces optimal functioning of the mental, emotional and spiritual energy fields, which then affect the physical energy field, producing physical healing.

Daily meditation quiets random thoughts and emotions. The chatter in your brain-functioning grows silent. If you choose to think nothing, there is silence. You mentally gain control of your thinking and emotions. Your ability to concentrate, remember and create sharply increases. Barriers to action are removed. Procrastination ends. You set a goal and find yourself easily acting to accomplish it. You sleep more soundly, feeling refreshed in the morning.

Meditative prayer provides more energy. An inner sense of calm begins pervading you. You become more able to choose how you would like to feel. Your emotional responses become more spontaneous and vital. Painful buried memories and emotions surface, not to hurt, but to be healed. You develop the ability to study a situation or problem from an emotional distance. You lower stress levels. In doing so, you may lower your pulse and blood pressure, as well. Adding spiritual content and prayer to meditation brings one into more direct contact with God. It can strengthen the reality of your religious beliefs. It can transform you into your image of God and empower this divine image in you. It can heal both life's hurts and those of the physical body.

You will find some exercises easier for you than others. Just because an exercise is difficult does not mean you cannot and should not master it. Mastering the difficult exercise may fulfill your greatest need. Try every exercise at least twice before choosing those parts that are most helpful for you. Before beginning, warm up with this imaging skill exercise.

Visualizing. Forming a picture in the mind and holding it is hindered by strong effort. It happens best through passive action. To practice mental imaging, place a simple object before you. Look at it. Close your eyes and form a mental picture. Hold that image as long as possible; only a few seconds is likely at the beginning. Then repeat this process time after time.

Suggested images: *Simple:* An orange, an apple, a ball, a color, like green, red, blue, yellow. *More complex:* a chair, a table, a kitchen appliance, a tree, a flower, an animal. *Advanced:* an entire room, a familiar human face.

| 4E. | AUTOGENIC TRAINING: BEING HEALED BY GOD |

This exercise is intended to heal you physically and emotionally.

Find a quiet place with a calming light. You may need to maintain one position for up to an hour, so find a comfortable place to sit or to lie down with your back straight. This is a place set apart from the responsibilities and business of the world. Arrange not to be disturbed. Quiet the phone. Focus solely upon what you are about to do. Have a timer present so you will not have to keep track of time yourself. Hold these instructions on your lap or in a hand so you can follow them conveniently. Are you comfortable? Move around until you are confident of your comfort. Breathe deeply and relax. With repetition this process will move smoothly. You might ask someone to lead you through the instructions the first time.

A. Autogenic Training: The purpose of this exercise is to place you in a relaxed state similar to hypnosis. In order to do this, you will be moving and flexing various muscle groups. This makes you aware of that area. Then you will be telling each body part that it will relax as you count from ten down to one. This worked for me the first time but other professionals caution that it may take a dozen trials before it works.

Right Leg: Flex once the muscle groups of your right leg -- your toes, foot, ankle, calf, thigh, and buttocks. Then silently speak to your right leg:

As I count from 10 down to 1, my right leg is going to relax, beginning with the tip of the toes and flowing right up through the foot, the ankle, the calf, the knee, the thigh, the buttocks. This relaxation will feel like a heaviness or tingling.

Then while breathing slowly and deeply on each inhale and exhale, count silently, *10, 9, 8, 7, 6, 5, 4, 3, 2, 1.* Then silently say, *My right leg is now relaxing and will continue to relax as I proceed.* Then proceed to the left leg.

Left Leg: Repeat instructions given for the right leg.

Torso: Now you are going to relax your torso. Flex the muscles of the lower back, middle back, upper back, shoulders, rib cage, diaphragm and tummy. Then silently speak to your torso:

As I count from 10 to 1, my torso is going to relax, beginning with my lower back up my back to my shoulders and then down the front through my rib cage, diaphragm and tummy. All my internal organs are being relaxed - my heart, lungs, liver, stomach, intestines, bladder and kidneys.

Then while breathing slowly and deeply on each inhale and exhale, count silently, *10, 9, 8, 7, 6, 5, 4, 3, 2, 1.* Then say, *My torso is now relaxing and will continue to relax as I proceed.*

Right Arm: Flex once the muscle groups of your right arm -- your fingers, hand, wrist, forearm, elbow and biceps. Then silently speak to your right arm: *As I count from 10 to 1, my right arm is going to relax, be-*

ginning with the tips of my fingers and flowing up my arm to my shoulder. This relaxation will feel like a heaviness or a tingling.

Then while breathing slowly and deeply on each inhale and exhale, count silently, *10, 9, 8, 7, 6, 5, 4, 3, 2, 1.* Then silently say, *My right arm is now relaxing and will continue to relax as I proceed.*

Left Arm: Repeat the same procedure as on the right arm.

Neck and Head: Now you need to relax your neck and head muscles. Flex the muscles in your neck, throat, jaw, cheeks, forehead, temples, scalp. Then say, *As I count from 10 to 1, my neck and throat, jaws and cheeks, forehead and temples, and scalp are going to relax.* Then while breathing slowly and deeply on each inhale and exhale, count silently, *10, 9, 8, 7, 6, 5, 4, 3, 2, 1.*

Final Countdown: Do not flex any muscles here. As you count from ten to one, go through all the muscle groups, beginning with the right leg. Sense, and then quietly tell each muscle group to relax. Say: *As I count from 10 to 1, each muscle group I tell to relax will relax even further, doubling my state of relaxation.* Then count *10, 9, 8, 7, 6, 5, 4, 3, 2,1.*

B. Entering the Mystical Room. You are now unclothed and have an imaginary body. Let your imaginary body stand up. Before you is a doorway. As you look through the doorway, you see steps leading downward. The steps are well lit and covered with purple carpet. You are going to walk down these steps and as you do so, you will find yourself going deeper into your mind. There are twenty steps. As you walk down the steps, you will count each of the twenty steps. 1, 2, 3.... You are now at the bottom of the steps. Before you is a room, a mystical room. It has white walls, white ceiling and white carpet. In the center of the room is a white chair. Walk to the chair and be seated. In this chair, you have complete access to God.

C. Being with God. Seek out God. Sense his immensity. Be filled with the sweetest, purest love you have ever known -- God. Sit quietly and enjoy God's presence. Then wait silently, listening for God's voice to speak to you.

D. God's Cleansing. When you are ready, you feel a mist of warm rain falling upon you. The rain is God cleansing you. The rain enters the top of your head and flows through all parts of your body. Every organ and cell the rain touches represents God cleansing and purifying you. Let the rain cleanse your mind and all your thoughts and feelings. Let it flow into the chest cavity and cleanse your heart and lungs, your liver and stomach, and each organ of your body. Let it flow through your arms and out your fingers, through your legs and out through your toes. You are being cleansed and made pure as God touches every part of you.

E. God's Healing Light. The rain has stopped. You have been purified. You are now ready to be healed by God's healing white light. As you sit in your white chair, you sense a warmth like that of the sun bathing you. But it is not the sun but a shaft of God's healing light. The white healing light enters your body through the top of your head. You welcome the warmth and love as God's healing light slowly begins flowing throughout your mind, healing it. God is recreating you and making every part of you new and healthy. You let the healing light slowly flow throughout your body, healing every organ and cell. Eventually, the healing light flows down your arms and out through your fingers, then down through your torso, down your legs, and out through your toes. Every cell in your body has been renewed. You sense your energy fields, filled with healing energy, radiating in a strong and balanced fashion.

F. God Empowers your Hands. God calls your name: *"_____, your hands are now filled with the power of my healing flow. Your hands now radiate the power of my love. Lift your hands and move them over your body, pausing at places that need special healing. This is a double blessing of healing. You feel the healing flow radiating from your hands and entering every cell, regenerating and making all things new. You sense the healing taking place. You rejoice in the healing. You now feel so light, you feel that you could float. You are being restored...."* Then pray:

G. A Prayer for Healing. *God, out of love you created the universe and made it good. You created human beings in your own image, meaning that we are spiritual beings like yourself. You granted me the gift of life. You have traveled with me throughout my life's journey. Thank you.*

God, I wish to reclaim your perfect image. Help me to touch your presence within me. I release my pains and my hurts, my worries and my fears to your care. I release to you all my negative thoughts, attitudes, feelings. I relax and place myself in your hands. You are the potter and I am the clay. God, cleanse my inner being and mold me into your love.

God, I know your will is for me to be well. Renew all my energy fields so that they reflect your divine plan for perfection. Heal me in body, mind and spirit, making me whole. I choose to be well, vibrant and fully alive. I accept the healing that is coursing through me. I sense your wholeness filling me. Thank you.

God, bless me that I might become a blessing to others. Provide me with a vision of what the future needs to be for me. Teach me that I might know. Thank you for the health that is slowly transforming me. Amen.

H. Closing. You are now ready to leave the mystical room. Arise and walk to the stairway. Climb the steps, counting each of twenty steps as you do so. Return to your body. When you return to the normal state of being, you will feel refreshed and renewed. You will be aware that God's healing love energy is coursing throughout your body as the healing process continues. Now count to three and you are back. Thus ends this meditative self-healing process.

4F.   A SECOND MEDITATIVE PRAYER: INTENTIONALLY HEALING

This exercise is intended to heal you physically and emotionally.

Find a quiet place with a calming light. You may need to maintain one position for up to an hour so find a comfortable place to sit or to lie down with your back straight. This is a place set apart from the responsibilities and business of the world. Arrange not to be disturbed. Quiet the phone. Focus solely upon what you are about to do. Have a timer present so you will not have to keep track of time yourself. Hold these instructions on your lap or in a hand so you can conveniently follow them.

Breathe deeply through your nostrils and relax. With repetition this whole process will move smoothly. You might ask someone to lead you through the instructions the first time.

A. Centering: If possible, begin by standing and gently stretching and flexing every muscle in your body while inhaling and exhaling deeply through the nostrils down into your diaphragm. Do this three times. Let's begin. Inhale - stretch and flex - exhale. Inhale - stretch and flex - exhale. Inhale - stretch and flex - exhale.

B. Praying Mantis Exercise: While inhaling, place the palms of your hands facing each other at about one-half inch apart. Beginning at the groin, move them straight up the front of your body until your arms are outstretched straight over your head. Then, while exhaling, keep arms straight, and bring them down in an arc along your sides until your hands are at your groin again. Do five repetitions. Praise God mentally while doing this. Now sit straight or lie down.

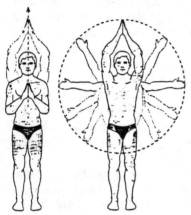

Figure 12. The Praying Mantis Exercise.

C. A Focusing Meditation: All meditation exercises have the same effects as the ones already listed. They go by many names. In this focusing, sit with your eyes closed and repeat a word or phrase aloud for ten minutes. Let the pauses between speaking take about the same time as the speaking. Make no attempt to think about the meaning of what you are saying, saying, just say it. You will have distractions. These commonly include an itching nose or cheek, the hardness pressing into your buttocks or back, your mind wandering to something you have to do, or thinking through something. These are your mind's attempts to interrupt your focus. Ignore them and gently bring your focus back to speaking your word or phrase over and over. It is the attempt which counts, not your perfection in doing it. Your instructions are these:

* Choose a word or short phrase to say. Suggestions: *Love, Peace, God, One, All is One, God is Love, Grant me your peace, Be still and know that I am God.*
* Set your timer for ten minutes.
* Begin.

D. Imaging Relaxation. When the mind relaxes, one's body also relaxes. Imagine you are relaxing alone in a secluded outdoor place like a warm sunny beach. Remain there for at least four minutes. *You are alone on a warm sunny beach in your bathing suit. You lie down and feel the sun gently warming your skin. Close your eyes. You have taken a vacation from worries and responsibilities. You are at peace with yourself and the world. You can hear birds singing and the water is lapping at the shore. Just relax and be. The present moment is filled with love and peace.*

    E. The Meditation of Breath Counting. Close your eyes and, while breathing normally, count your exhales in your mind in groups of four. Inhale-exhale-1, inhale-exhale-2, inhale-exhale-3, inhale-exhale-4 then repeat inhale-exhale-1. Begin with five minutes and work up to fifteen minutes. Use a timer. While doing this, seek to keep your mind free of all sensing, thoughts, and feelings.

    F. Waterfall Cleansing. Imagine a waterfall of sparkling water at a comfortable temperature. Enter the waterfall and imagine the water entering your body through the top of your head. Let it flow through your head, down your arms and out your fingers, through your torso, down your legs and out your toes. Imagine the water cleansing every organ it touches. Take your time.

    G. God's Healing Light. Think of the most loving person you know. Imagine this person placing his/her hand on the top of your head. S/he says: *"In the name of God, be healed!"*

    You sense the love of God surrounding and entering you. You feel the healing white light of God pervading your body from his hand. Let it bathe your whole being. Sense it surrounding and entering every organ of your body. Let it surround every area where there is illness. Wherever God's healing light touches, say: "I *am being healed.*" God's healing white light is regenerating your body, mind and spirit.

    H. Your Own Healing Hands. Place your hands on areas needing to be healed. Pray: *"God, use my hands as channels for your healing love. Wherever I touch, the healing energy is regenerating and renewing me. I am being healed. Thank you. Amen."*

    I. Imaging Wholeness. You are as you believe. Imagine you have been healed and you are now taking part in joyous physical situations. See yourself dancing, biking, running, playing, creating, being vigorously alive, healthy and happy.

    J. Centering On God. Now quiet your mind. Sense your inner calm. Be open to any message which may come to you.

    K. Closing Prayer: *God, Creator, Sustainer, Healer, thank you for the hope that wells up within me. Thank you for the healing that has begun and continues to restore my body, mind and soul. I accept this healing because I want to be well. Continue to fill me with your presence, with your love, joy and peace, that I might continue to have faith and trust in your care. Amen.*

5. BRENNAN'S HARA DIMENSION, TAN TIEN AND THE CORE STAR

In her new book, Light Emerging - the Journey of Personal Healing (Bantam, 1993), Barbara Ann Brennan breaks amazing new ground for our understanding of the healing and empowerment of the human energy fields. Never have I been so astounded by creative theological insight. While I think of PrayWell as applied theology, Brennan's work may make her the most significant theologian and religious teacher of the twentieth century.

At the end of Light Emerging she focuses upon intentionality. She states that highest spiritual intentions (and life purpose) are present in the hara dimension. This is a straight energy line originating about three and a half feet above the human head and moving down and attached to the energetic core of Earth. The "hara line" has energy centers in the human body at the "tan tien," about one and a half inches below the navel and at the "soul seat," in the upper chest around the sternum. The hara exists on a dimension deeper than the auric field. It is the source of your physical body's energy and of your manifestation as physical. The tan tien is the source of power in the martial arts, like tai chi. It is also the source of power of all personal intention and life purpose. When the tan tien is healed, a person becomes energized and directed for creative, fulfilling living.

Beneath the haric dimension lies the dimension of your deeper core. This is the eternal self, the true self. This is where the divine spark of God dwells in every person. This is the "core star," located about one and a half inches above the navel on the hara line. It is the eternal source of your essence. Where the core light emerges, it brings health. Where it is blocked, disease occurs.

As I read of the tan tien and core star, I knew this was a deeper understanding of healing than I had ever known. It made more sense of the Word of God that I have quietly equated with the divine intention of our lives. Intention through the Rational Word, intention expressed in vocal prayer, intention during the healing encounter -- all these are the basis or at the heart of effective healing. When that intention takes on a life of its own within the healer, as divine intention is empowered by the Holy Spirit, all healings become possible. Brennan is describing a means for both wholeness and religious salvation.

In a similar way, when I become aware of the essence of the healee during the healing encounter, either from the tan tien or core star or both, then complete healing is probable.

As I read Barbara Ann Brennan's words, I understood the troubling personal energies within myself in what I learned were my own tan tien and core star. I understood why my core star vibrated with more energy and joy when I am with certain colleagues. The exercises she describes worked well for me. Buy her book, Light Emerging, to see for yourself.

I must note that the tan tien and core star can be restored through other methods including wellness counseling combined with simple touch-healing and some of the other methods described in this book. Since Brennan has described their existence and function, this awareness begins living and renewing within spiritual persons.

6. NEAR-DEATH EXPERIENCE (NDE)

In a 1982 Gallup poll, about eight million Americans reported having near-death experiences. The near-death experience is considered by researchers to be only a peak experience of God (PEG) that proves the existence of an afterlife. As a healing researcher, I have reached a different conclusion. A key element completely ignored by other researchers is that traditional NDEs have resulted in the restoration of a clinically dead physical body. Thus, I am led to conclude that the real significance of an NDE is that it is a healing experience.

The report of traditional NDEs is of the consciousness leaving the physical body while one is clinically dead. The consciousness travels through a tunnel of light at the end of which one is greeted by a religious figure or by loved ones who encourages one to return through the tunnel and choose life over death. A minor variation is to go through a dark tunnel and at the other end have a negative experience. Some persons report reviewing the key elements of their life history. Some report viewing their body lying dead while medical personnel work to revive it. For most, it is a deeply religious experience.

The presence of a white light and/or tunnel indicate that this is a peak state of consciousness. Participants are now in the theta state in which they can reprogram the brain/mind and be healed.

Those undergoing a positive near-death experience are usually permanently transformed, psychologically and spiritually. They have no further fear of death. They are filled with an inner serenity, a love of everyone and a sense of spiritual purpose. This makes the NDE a peak experience God (a PEG) that produces spiritual transformation and salvation.

The Philadelphia-based International Association of Near Death Studies adds a new perspective on NDEs. Their survey indicates that only twenty-three percent of reported NDE experiences occurred during clinical death. The rest occurred during illness or trauma or out of nowhere during normal living. The personal transformation remains the same. These other seventy-seven percent are not NDEs. They are theta state peak experiences of God (PEG) or peak states of consciousness.

I must admit that I am a minority advocate of the NDE as a healing experience. Those members of the International Association of Near Death Studies with whom I have spoken angrily deny such a conclusion. They point out that those who have survived clinical death have reported normal recovery time and are often left with limited health. They do not consider their miraculous recovery from clinical death to be a result of an enhanced healing mode triggered by the experience.

This reaction, of course, is to be expected, considering the prevailing attitudes in our culture toward spiritual healing. Here is another instance where we encounter automatic resistance and rejection. Yet, NDEs possess many similarities with healing encounters. With both phenomena, participants report the overwhelming awareness of immense inner love and white light. With both, individuals report being emotionally and spiritually changed. After both experiences, a few report discovering the ability to heal. In both instances, those involved report loved ones being troubled by their stories and by the new person who emerges.

Just consider the NDE to be a healing experience. Might it be possible for more people to survive clinical death if they knew that their death experience might be a means for enhancing vital signs and returning to life? If you, the reader, should have an NDE, will the knowledge that it may be a healing experience alter the script and, thus, the outcome of the experience?

In the midst of an NDE, might it be possible intentionally to exert more control over the healing process, enabling a larger percentage of persons to survive clinical death and report NDEs? A new script could involve asking God to heal the physical and emotional wounds that have occurred, and visualizing your body becoming whole. Your consciousness might be able to intentionally touch your own physical body to induce wholeness.

When I heard Elmer Green lecture about biofeedback in May, 1993, he too identified the NDE as the theta state of peak consciousness. My heart warmed as he said, *"People who have out-of-body experiences and near-death experiences -- their brains are not working, but their minds and emotions are working."*

Those who have experienced NDEs likely possess latent healing abilities. The NDE began their healing process. Now they can continue that healing process to fully restored health by using the resources in PrayWell.

7. OUT-OF-BODY EXPERIENCES

One of my parishioners, Gib, struggled with multiple sclerosis for seven years. The disease had progressed to the point where he was bedridden, with his only locomotion, as he said, "*being to squirm across the floor like a snake.*" One day, Gib experienced an instant miracle of healing and was cured of his MS. Here is the story in Gib's own words:

"It was December. As Christmas music filled our home, my wife and her girlfriend were baking Christmas cookies. I was lying in bed as usual with my MS, savoring the smell of baking cookies as it wafted in from the kitchen. Suddenly, I found myself up at the ceiling looking down at my physical body on the bed. I was completely at peace. Then the strangeness of the situation sank in. I became fearful and found myself back in my body. I was so excited by what had happened that I wanted to tell my wife. Without thinking, I got out of bed and walked into the kitchen. Boy, was she shocked to see me! I hadn't walked in a year. Being curious, I had two different medical doctors examine me. Both could find no trace of the disease and called it a misdiagnosis."

Gib had a spontaneous out-of-body experience (OBE) in which one senses the mind or consciousness leaving one's physical body, often hovering at ceiling level, but capable of traveling quickly to almost any place. History is replete with stories of spontaneous OBEs. Many report having OBEs, also known as astral travel or second-body travel, during sleep. Often, it is a once-in-a-lifetime experience arising from moments of great emotional stress or physical illness. This is definitely a peak state of consciousness that holds the potential for restoring the energy fields and the physical body through a shift in awareness. It is, therefore, another medium for healing miracles.

Modern Explorations. The modern intentional experimental exploration of out-of-body experiences began in 1958 with businessman Robert A. Monroe of Virginia. He reported his OBEs in his books <u>Journeys Out Of the Body</u> and <u>Far Journeys</u> and established the Monroe Institute of Applied Sciences, P.O.Box 57, Afton, VA 22920, to involve others in OBEs.

The Monroe Institute has never considered OBEs to be a healing experience and maintains no records of any possible reported healings. This was to be expected, because paranormal researchers wear the same blinders as the rest of society in dismissing the subject of healing, in spite of the fact that healing is classified as a paranormal experience by both religion and parapsychology.

Monroe refers to OBEs as a universal human experience, generally of a once-in-a-lifetime variety, a most profound experience, extremely joyful, and sometimes an extremely accurate means for distant information-gathering. He wrote his books to provide others with a how-to-do-it procedure and to provide insights into expanded human knowledge of the paranormal reality.

Here are some suggestions for using an OBE for your own healing:

A. Find a means for inducing an OBE. Books are available in your public library.
B. While hovering over your body, *think* the physical body well. Imagine it to be whole and healed.
C. State your name, saying, "_____, *in God's name, be healed in body, mind, and spirit.*"
D. From the ceiling area, extend your hands to your physical body, enter, and move your hands to produce the desired changes.
E. Replace any sexual desire with compassionate love for yourself. Project that love desire to your body without returning.
F. Experiment on your own. Take many journeys and explore what works.

8. LAUGHTER

One of the most celebrated cases of health produced by a shift in consciousness was reported by Norman Cousins. In his book, <u>Anatomy of an Illness</u>, Cousins describes how laughter, intention and courage cured him of a serious collagen illness, a disease of the connective tissue.

Cousins watched comedy films by the hour believing that the laughter that affected his state of mind also could cure his body. He stated that the changed emotional state created by laughter affected the chemical imbalance that produced his body's disease. What happened to Cousins extends far deeper than Cousins' explanation. Laughter triggers an altered state of consciousness. His shift in consciousness brought healing to his mind and energy fields and they affected the chemical imbalance, bringing about a miraculous cure.

Intentionally focusing upon humor and laughter has been a part of my own wellness therapy through the years. Being able to joke good-naturedly about your own misery produces relaxation and a change of mental and emotional perspective. Reproducing Cousins' design within your own personal context may offer improvement of your health.

9. SENSING THE PRESENCE OF GOD

Spiritually sensing the sacred and the holy and being touched by God are transformative experiences. Any experience that produces an inner sense of awe, wonder, faith, hope and love can produce inner wholeness. Make these available to yourself on a daily basis by drawing upon your own religious beliefs and practices.

10. USING ABUNDANT LIFE ENERGY

During the past year, I have used Gerasimov's hypnotic technique in an attempt to reduce my own physiological age. I have also used an abundance of life energy. In the past year, I have encountered four unusual healers -- two from Russia, one from Brazil and a fourth here in the United States. All four transmitted an unusually high amount of energy that stayed with me for days and improved my brain-functioning. None of the four actually healed me. Their energy was different from that of the hundreds of other healers I have known.

Of this group, the late Mauricio Panisset of Brasilia, Brazil was the most remarkable. His energy stayed with me for more than six weeks. During that time, all I had to do was to lie down, take two deep breaths and I was in a deep altered state of consciousness. I then mentally did what I might do under hypnosis, making suggestions to myself about health and personal growth. Without reciting the details, I assure you that it works.

I mention this because I believe the same process can be used in the midst of any healing service where immense energy is bathing you. Let this energy flow through you and use it for your own transformation and healing.

11. DREAMS AND VISIONS

Throughout the centuries, literature has been filled with references to the dreams and visions of religious, political, military, scientific, artistic and literary figures. During eight hours of sleep, the average person has five to eight dreams. With practice, one can learn to recall most dreams.

All dreams are meaningful and have a purpose. Dreams are a window through which one can focus upon the subconscious mind and upon all the unresolved issues with which a person has not consciously dealt. Dreams offer hope as they bid us to live life more fully than it is consciously lived in the daily awake state. It is estimated that more than ninety percent of dream content is attempting to cope with unresolved personal issues. Thus, one path to wholeness lies in dream therapy or dream work. If one is struggling to survive, exploring one's dreams may lead one onto the path back to wholeness. This is especially helpful for persons seeking to recover from chemical addictions, neurotic behavior, depression, traumatic memories and acute or chronic illnesses.

Procedure. Dream work is surprisingly simple, though it does require nightly preparations. If others sleep in your bedroom, plans must be made for not disturbing their sleep. Because dream content is quickly forgotten, it must be immediately recorded upon awakening. Keep a cassette recorder or paper and pencil, plus a light, next to your bed. Before going to sleep, program yourself to remember dreams by saying something like: *"I will begin remembering dreams tonight and will briefly awaken after each dream in order to record it. Then I will quickly fall back to sleep for further dreaming. I will awaken rested in the morning."*

My personal experience is to awaken rested in the morning after having recorded four or five dreams. The first few nights you may recall few or no dreams. Be persistent. You will succeed. A fifteen-minute daily session of meditation facilitates dream recall.

Being part of a weekly dream group can be helpful. During sessions dream content is shared. One New York City dream group reported members receiving dream information that resolved the issues of other members' lives.

Dreams come to us in symbolic pictures, sounds and voices. Afterwards, one must interpret what these symbols mean. Trust your own personal understanding. Dreams may have a beginning, a middle conflict and an end resolution. Many dreams are ordinary, dealing with daily inner and outer life issues. These dreams can provide helpful insight into the issues troubling us.

Anxiety dreams or nightmares cover areas of life in which we have not faced our fears. As a parish pastor, my recurring Saturday night dream was that of standing before my congregation to lead them in Sunday worship without my pants. I interpreted the dream as meaning I had the fear of revealing myself in my sermons in a way that might be embarrassing.

Affirming dreams mirror new steps we are taking in our lives, or they support our present spiritual journey. Several times, an authoritative voice identifying itself as the Heavenly Father affirmed my spiritual journey with one or two sentences. Sometimes, that voice has given me orders on how to fulfill my hopes and dreams. My first book was written following such an order. I view that voice as either my own higher consciousness speaking to me in terms my human mind can understand or as an actual message from God.

Intuitive-creative dreams can resolve real life issues. Psychic dreams can forecast one's own or another's future -- like moving, getting a new job, becoming ill, becoming well. They may also become self-fulfilling prophecy when we choose to let them influence our future.

Another type of dream is a lucid dream. A lucid dream is so vividly real that we think it represents reality. Some persons have become capable of intervening in their own lucid dreams, controlling the ending, whether these endings involve anxiety, unresolved personal issues or creativity. Others report being able to program themselves on the content of their dreams. Before going to sleep, they say, *"I need help with this issue in my life, so I ask that my dreams tonight deal with this issue. How can I get myself together?"* Persistent dream work over a six-week period of time can be a very rewarding path toward wholeness.

12. GENEROUS LOVE

The receiving and the sharing of generous love leads to wholeness. In religion, this is known as divine love or *agape*. In secular terms, it is called altruistic love. Nothing leads to a change of consciousness and eventual wholeness more effectively than receiving and sharing a quality of love that liberates, empowers and restores.

Loving and serving others is great wellness therapy. This should be done with no expectation of wages or of being paid back. Acting as a volunteer caregiver in a meaningful way serves this function. This could involve volunteer work with a daycare center, senior center, medical center, with shut-ins, the grieving, a religious group, family and neighbors.

13. FALLING IN LOVE

Romantically falling in love causes a shift in awareness. This experience is described as *"being on cloud nine,"* or as *"floating ten feet off the ground."* Falling in love is not reserved for singles. Marriages of all durations can experience this. Genuine affection between persons releases an energy for healing. Expressions of sexual passion also energize and balance the human energy field while leading to a momentary shift in consciousness.

14. INTENSE SUFFERING

Recently a male friend in his mid-forties experienced a medical crisis. Within hours he could no longer breathe on his own. Quick action placed him in a hospital intensive care unit. For ten days he lay in a semi-comatose state, kept alive by a breathing machine. No viral or bacterial agent was diagnosed. He suffered from *"shock lung"* and none of the medical staff expected him to recover.

We bathed him in healing prayer and he survived. During this period of suffering, he had three near-death experiences and several out-of-body experiences. He was also bathed in the presence of God. Emerging from this immense suffering, he spiritually glowed. He dramatically changed his lifestyle into a healthier one and deepened his vocational purpose, changing to a job that brought him satisfaction.

Intense suffering can shift one's consciousness into a higher wholeness. It can result unexpectedly in many of the psychic and religious experiences already noted. Yearning to be rescued, one can intentionally call upon God's help with words like, *"Lord God, please come to my aid. I want to be well; please heal me."* Following the sending of such a request, the answer can later come through experiences of divine healing while one is either asleep or awake.

Chapter Nineteen

The Final Healing

"In death and in grief we do not as much need protection from painful experiences as we need the boldness to face them. We do not need as much tranquilization from pain as we need the strength to conquer it. If we choose to love, we must also have the courage to grieve." ...Elizabeth Kubler-Ross

"Prayer is a sense of the Presence of God." ...Brother Lawrence*

"And whenever you stand praying, forgive, if you have anything against any one; so that your Father also who is in heaven may forgive you your trespasses." ...Mark 11:25

Even with the best of understanding, intentions and effort, your illness may result in death, the Final Healing. Our knowledge of healing prayer is still in its infancy. What we do know is that when we immerse ourselves in prayer, God enables us to face death with inner peace and outer serenity.

Skeptics of healing prayer ask the taunting question, *"You do not expect to keep people alive forever with prayer, do you? We all die someday."* My response is that no matter what the final outcome, the quality of life improves immensely through the use of healing prayer.

A Presbyterian minister told me how his wife faced spreading breast cancer. The medical prognosis was eighteen months. With healing prayer, a loving family and the support of her religious community, she lived twelve years. These were not closed-in years of waiting to die, filled with unhappiness, fear and depression. They were joyous, satisfying years. She had worked through any feelings of fear, anger and self-pity. She had faith and hope that God was with her in life, in death and in life beyond death. She daily experienced God's presence, peace and joy. She continued living a full life of caring love and warm supportive relationships. Healing prayer prolonged her life and provided abundant living for both herself and her husband.

We are eternal and never die. Death is but a transition. In death, we sleep and awaken as though into the next morning. We find that the ravages of illness and aging have been erased. We are vital and whole once more, living in a spiritual body that is just as real as the physical body we left behind. There is joy and security in that knowledge. Healing prayer produces a sense of God's power and presence within people. This is the most convincing personal evidence as the Unseen and the Eternal transform us into New Persons, able to live victoriously even to the moment of physical death.

PREPARING FOR THE DYING PROCESS

Chapters fifteen and sixteen provide resources and prayers for facing death. If you have not done so, explore those chapters. The emotional issues we face during illness, covered in chapter fifteen, are the same as the five stages of dying.

Dying can become a lonely, isolated journey, or it can be a joyous and fulfilling journey shared with loved ones. Just as you have taken charge of your own emotional and physical healing, there is merit, should the need arise, in taking charge of your own dying process.

I observe that loved ones have a harder time dealing with dying than does the dying person. Because most people do not cope with dying often, they have little understanding of the process, and few coping skills. Loved ones tend to avoid talking about death unless the dying person brings up the subject. There is often a conspiracy of silence about discussing the subject of death with the dying loved one. Commonly there is complete avoidance, using the mechanism of false assurances, such as, *"You are not dying. You are going to be all right. You will feel much better tomorrow. You are getting well."* This can be maddening to the dying person who has sensed the truth.

During prolonged periods of dying, loved ones can work through their grief prematurely before the impending death occurs. In doing so, they emotionally separate themselves from the dying. To the dying, this comes through as, *"My family no longer cares about me. They have already buried me and I no longer matter. I am all alone during the Final Healing."*

Taking charge of your own dying process means that you do not play a passive role. You assert what you want from your loved ones. You bridge the gap of silence. You talk to loved ones about your own dying and death. You tend to their anguish and pain as well as your own. Talking to loved ones about your impending death provides courage, meaning and support for everyone. Here are some suggestions.

1. Repeatedly state to loved ones, *"All the evidence points to fact that I am closing in on death. It would be helpful to me if we talked about the issues involved. Are you willing to cooperate with me on this?"* If a talk with your physician refutes your evidence, reconsider and back off. If you receive false assurances that you are not dying, then.

2. State, *"That is not helpful to me. Are you so afraid of my death that you cannot face it?"* Even this assertive question will not persuade some to talk about it. Subjects to discuss include:

3. Closure. Initiate conversations with individuals about your life together. These include:

    A. Forgiving and letting go of any past pain and differences.

    B. Affectionate reminiscing about past shared events.

    C. Talking about the loved one's future beyond your physical death.

4. Your Needs. What do you want from loved ones? Let this not be a brave, *"I will take care of my own needs alone."* Make honest requests that meet your needs and enable them to express their love in practical ways.

Consider making out a Living Will that limits extraordinary medical steps to maintain your life when there is no longer any hope for living.

5. How do you feel about the dying process? Honestly share your fears, doubts and concerns. Tell about your growth in facing death. Talk about the positive elements of your dying and death.

6. Death and After. Express your own understanding of what occurs at death and after death. Ask others to share their beliefs.

7. Your Funeral. Talk about what you want for your funeral.

8. Affirmations. Express your love to everyone. Say your good-byes.

9. Prayers. By this time, you know what you want to say and have your own unique way of praying. Take charge of your prayer life and flow in faith with God. Prayers are appropriate as a part of any and all of the above suggested steps. Here is a Therapeutic Prayer for the dying process:

A THERAPEUTIC PRAYER IN THE MIDST OF DYING

God, I thank you for the gift of life. I thank you for your presence during my journey. Enable me to look back upon my life with a sense of satisfaction. It is strange how my priorities have changed -- how the things that seemed so unimportant now have deep meaning.

Help me to complete any unfinished business. I choose to die in peace. I release my angers, my resentments, my hurts, my disappointments and my fears to your care. I forgive anyone who has ever hurt me. I forgive myself for any misgivings I have. Fill me with your presence, love and joy and grant me your peace.

I place my life in your hands. I know that you are with me in life, in death and in life beyond death. I trust you. Tend to my needs. I rest in your care. Thank you. Amen.

IMMORTALITY in the World's Great Religions

CHRISTIANITY: *"So is it with the resurrection of the dead. It is sown a physical body, it is raised a spiritual body. If there is a physical body, there is also a spiritual body. Just as we have born the image of the man of dust, we shall also bear the image of the man of heaven."*

JUDAISM: *"The dust returns to the earth as it was, and the Spirit returns to God who gave it."*

ISLAM: *"Those who have believed and done the things which are right, these shall be inmates of Paradise."*

HINDUISM: *"He becomes immortal who seeks the general good of man."*

BUDDHISM: *"Earnestness is the path to immortality."*

JAINISM: *"I know there will be life hereafter."*

SHINTO: *"Regard Heaven as your father, Earth as your mother, all things as your brothers and sisters, and you will enjoy the divine country which excels all others."*

CONFUCIANISM: *"All the living must die and, dying, return to the ground, but the Spirit issues forth and is displayed in light."*

SIKHISM: *"Why weep when a man dies, since he is only going home?"*

TAOISM: *"Life is going forth. Death is returning home."*

BAHA'I: *"Make mention of Me on earth that in My Heaven I may remember you."*

ZOROASTRIANISM: *"The soul of the righteous shall be joyful in immortality."*

Chapter Twenty

Therapeutic Prayers During Crisis

"The most beautiful people....are those who have known defeat, known suffering, known struggle, known loss, and have found their way out of the depths. These persons have an appreciation, a sensitivity and an understanding of life that fills them with compassion, gentleness, and a deep loving concern. Beautiful people do not just happen." ...Elizabeth Kubler-Ross

"Prayer is God's breathing in us, by which we become part of the intimacy of God's inner life, and by which are born anew." ...Henri J. Nouwen*

"Let love be genuine; hate what is evil, hold fast to what is good; love one another with brotherly affection; outdo one another in showing honor. Never flag in zeal, be aglow with the Spirit, serve the Lord. Rejoice in your hope, be patient in tribulation, be constant in prayer. Contribute to the needs of the saints, practice hospitality." ...Romans 12:9-13

To be human is to know hurt. To be human is to wonder fearfully how we are ever going to get through this particular hurt. To be human is to moan, scream and cry as the hurt goes on and on. To be human is to die a little with each dose of hurt. To be human can mean to become numbed -- unfeeling of the awful hurt. Then come hurt's destructive cousins -- anger, bitterness and depression. Wounds and scars are impressed upon the hearts of many people.

Is there another way? To be human is also to reach out to God for help. To be human is to pray for help, for relief, for some light of hope at the end of the seemingly endless tunnel of darkness and despair. Can we overcome our hurt? Can we heal our wounds? Can we become free to be happy and satisfied? Millions have done so.

I remember the prayers I offered for those who were hurting. Most of all, I recall the hundreds of hurting people who afterwards asked me to write a prayer for them -- like the one we had just shared -- for their daily use. Then came the wonderful reports. People were finding wholeness and renewal through simple prayer. Those memories motivate this chapter.

Elizabeth Kubler-Ross stated it best when she wrote, *"The most beautiful people...are those who have known defeat, known suffering, known struggle, known loss, and have found their way out of the depths. These persons have an appreciation, a sensitivity and an understanding of life that fills them with compassion, gentleness, and a deep loving concern. Beautiful people do not just happen."*

Prayer cannot prevent a hurt. It does not always rescue one from a painful situation. Prayer *can* make an otherwise unbearable hurt bearable.

Prayer can seek to heal the hurt. Prayer can help you out of the depths. Prayer can convince you that with God, all things are possible. Yes, prayer can provide hope and power for your life.

FINDING YOUR PRAYERS

These Therapeutic Prayers are in alphabetical order. Therapeutic Prayers for healing and personal renewal can be found in other chapters. See the Index at the back of the book for more help.

You can use these prayers with others in several ways. You can use them as they are, saying them in unison with others. You can use *"Pray-Along,"* with one person saying the prayer in phrases and everyone repeating the phrase.

THERAPEUTIC PRAYERS THAT ADDRESS YOUR HURT

---

1. ACCIDENT, AUTO. God, I am having flashbacks about the accident. My calm has been shattered. It was so sudden and unexpected. Heal this painful memory and grant me your peace. I am happy to be alive. Thank you. Amen.

2. ADDICTIVE-COMPULSIVE BEHAVIORS. God, I am imprisoned by a satisfying behavior. I like doing it. It makes me feel good. But, there is a downside. It gets me in trouble with my loved ones. It gets me in trouble with my personal life. It gets me in trouble with society. Others tell me it is wrong and is hurting me. I don't like myself because of it. But I can't stop and I am not sure I want to stop. It is so satisfying. I am constantly deceiving others, even myself, about my addictive-compulsive behavior.

God, I turn to you because I am helpless before this behavior. I need the help of a power greater than myself in order to stop. It seems like this behavior is the best friend I have ever had. God, I renounce the spirit of my addictive-compulsive behavior. I feel sadness and loss about its leaving. Remove this spirit from my soul. Fill me with your Spirit -- the Spirit of Freedom and Truth. Help me to take control of my life. Guide me to any help I need. Remove any withdrawal symptoms. Fill me with your love and peace.

God, I am in this battle for the long haul. Strengthen me daily. Remind me of where I have been. Provide me a clear picture of where I am going. Keep me free and whole. Thank you. Amen.

3. ANGER. God, I am angry. I am being treated unfairly. I am not understood. I am not respected. I do not feel as if I belong here. I want to lash out in anger and hurt others. I have been nasty in many ways. I know that I am hurting others. I feel trapped. I do not know what else to do. Anger is consuming me.

God, I know that family members are not the cause of all my anger. It is as though I have a volcano within me that keeps erupting with hot, angry lava. Help me to understand the sources of my anger. I know I blame others for my own frustrations. I know that I am unhappy.

God, I release my anger into your care. I let go of it. Fill me with your love and light. Enable me to take responsibility for my own feelings, words and actions. Help me to find happiness and satisfaction. Help me to responsibly take charge of my life.

God, transform me into a new person. Help me to understand and care for family members. I love them and want life to be good for all of us. Abide with me throughout this journey. Amen.

4. <u>BETRAYAL, MARITAL.</u> God, I feel so betrayed. I had invested all the love and trust I have into my marriage. Now I feel so foolish and stupid. The lies, the cover-ups, the words of love and reassurance are so painful to me. All I have treasured between us is now gone. How can I ever handle this? All the tender experiences of passion, companionship and commitment have turned to dust; they are nothing now. I am raging with anger, hurt and embarrassed. I am frightened. I am depressed. I feel worthless, like a nothing. My confidence has been shattered. God, help me in this time of trouble. What shall I do?

God, I place myself in your care. Be my strength and my salvation. I thought I had been a good spouse. For my own peace of mind, I re-fuse to put myself down. I know I am still sacred and precious. I am a competent, caring, attractive person. I let go of my anger, my hurt, my self-pity. I let the pain be washed away in your love and peace.

God, I do not know the future of my marriage. It may be over, or we may have to struggle to a new understanding and relationship. If my spouse is truly sorry for the betrayal, I will seek to forgive him/her. If not, I will choose to let go and get on with my life. Provide me with the strength I need. Bring people into my life to comfort me. Enable me to take control of my own life. Surround me with your love and guide me through this painful and uncertain time of my life. Empower me to be the person I need to be. Thank you. Amen.

5. <u>CONFLICT.</u> God, I am upset with _____. I do not yet know the final results. I open myself to your presence in this conflict. I forgive everyone who has hurt me and will make amends to all I have hurt. Fill me with your peace and understanding. I also ask you to surround _____ in your love and light. *(Visualize this.)* May only fairness, harmony and wisdom flow from what has happened. Bless us in this time of pain and hurt. Make us one with you and each other. Thank you. Amen.

6. <u>CRIME VICTIM.</u> God, I feel violated, raped. My calm and security have been destroyed. I am angry, enraged. My privacy has been invaded. Parts of me, my possessions, have been stolen. I am also frightened. This is so much more painful than hearing about other victims. This is personal. This happened to me.

God, my life feels out of control. I could not prevent this crime from happening. I am anxious. I still hurt. I feel weak and helpless. God, I place my hurt in your hands. Heal me and make me whole in body, mind and spirit. Bathe me with your love that I might be whole once more. Grant me your peace and protect me from harm. Thank you. Amen.

7. <u>CRIMINAL BEHAVIOR</u>. God, I have grown into my criminal behavior from earliest childhood. I know most of the tricks of my trade. I have distanced myself from my victims and see them as the source of my livelihood. I am proud of my accomplishments. Many of my friends are criminals. They are like family, sharing my values and skills.

I know that if I continue in this vocation, I will spend most of my life behind bars. This is a given of my trade. I have dreamed of going straight, of avoiding time in prison. I have thought of settling down and getting a regular job. I doubt if I can.

Is there another way, God? Can I do it? Can I change my life and go straight? God, I renounce the spirit of criminality. Remove this spirit from my life. Fill me with your Spirit, the Spirit of truth and responsibility. May your Spirit protect and guide me throughout life.

God, help me to feel the pain of those I have hurt. Help me to make amends for what I have done. Free me of guilt and fill me with compassion. Grant me a clear mind filled with the Word and the Spirit. Lead me to people who can help me. Open up a new future for me. Thank you. Amen.

8. <u>CRISIS, INTERPERSONAL</u>. Lord God, I am upset, frustrated and confused. I feel a gulf between _____ and myself. I have mixed feelings: wanting to maintain distance and yet wanting to have harmony between us again. Open us to our own higher wisdom. Enable us to draw back and look from a distance, that we might discern the truth and fairness of what is happening. Fill us with your love, compassion and peace. Protect us from all harm. Thank you. Amen.

9. <u>DANGER, IMMEDIATE</u>. God, come to my aid and save me!

10. <u>DANGER, ONGOING</u>. God, I am concerned about the dangers in my neighborhood. Violence, shootings and death have become all too common. I am afraid night and day. God, fill me with your love that it might cast out my fear. I pray for the residents of my neighborhood. Keep them safe from all harm. I ask that you fill our neighborhood with your love and peace. Stop the violent people. Fill them with your love and peace. Let them feel the pain of their victims and of their victims' loved ones. Place a protective bubble around my home and the homes of all my neighbors so that no harm can come to us. I trust in your care. Thank you. Amen. *(Then visualize yourself and others enclosed in a protective bubble.)*

11. <u>DECEASED LOVED ONE</u>. God, I pray for a loved one in the afterlife. I am struggling with my own terrible sense of loss, but I want to be sure that _____ is safe on the other side. I thank you for her/his life, for all the good s/he did and for the satisfaction of our relationship. Guide _____ into your light. Heal her/his hurts and grant her/him wholeness. Let her/him know how much I love her/him. Thank you. Amen.

12. <u>DEPRESSION</u>. God, life seems so bleak and useless right now. I don't have any energy. I have no ambition to do much of anything. I am really feeling down. I feel "down on" myself and "down on" everyone around me. Even as I pray, I don't sense your presence. I am going through the motions, knowing that you are still with me.

I know that I am sacred and precious but they are just words right now. I know that my life has been worthwhile, full of many wonderful people and experiences, much happiness and joy. I feel little of this right now. God, all I can do is affirm the goodness of life and try to hold on until the darkness is replaced by your light and love.

Help me to spot the lies that my depressed emotions are telling me. Life is good. I am good. You are good. Grant me hope. My loved ones love me. Life will be beautiful again. Soon, I will see the beauty around me again. Soon, I will again know vitality and purpose, happiness and love. Until then, give me the strength and hope to survive this day.

Help me to smile and laugh, even if just for a moment. Be my strength and salvation. I ask you to restore me and make me whole. Fill me with the Word and the Spirit that I might be recreated anew. I praise and thank you. Amen.

13. <u>DIVORCE, IN THE MIDST OF</u>. God, I have been linked to my spouse in so many ways. There is a tie that still binds us. I release the tie that binds. I ask you to sever the spiritual link between us. I ask you to sever the emotional links that bind us. Remove the pain of the conflict with my spouse from my life.

God, I let go of the pain involved in our marriage. I forgive my spouse for the pain that was caused. I ask your forgiveness for the pain I inflicted. Free me, that I may move on with my life. Fill me with your love, joy and peace. Guide me into my new future. Provide for my needs. Protect me from all harm. Bring new people into my life who will meet my various needs. I trust in your love and care. Thank you. Amen.

14. <u>DIVORCE, AFTER</u>. God, it is over. I am a single person. I thought it would be easier than this. I have so many beautiful and joyous memories. My spouse meant much to me. Our lives have been intertwined, even in our pain and struggles. I feel only half here. Sometimes it hurts terribly. It is almost unbearable. I am all emotions right now. Anger and hurt. Loneliness and longing. I want to be through with this pain. I want to get on with my life.

It is so painful to end relationships. God, to end the pain, I cut the tie that binds. I sever the energy linking us together. I forgive all the past and release it to your care. I forgive myself. I let go of my anger, my hurt, my fear, my self-pity, my bitterness. I honor the love we shared and all the joy it brought. Let me hold to the good memories with no sense of pain.

Enable me to move on now, to find renewed happiness and satisfaction. Heal my hurts. Guide me into my new future. Provide for my needs. Protect me from all harm. Bring new people into my life who will meet my many needs. I trust in your love and care. Create in me a clean heart. Enable my energy fields to be whole as you renew me in body, mind and spirit. Thank you. Amen.

15. <u>FEAR AND ANXIETY</u>. God, my life has changed abruptly. Nothing will ever be the same again. I am tense. I know that much of that tension is due to fear. I fear the present. I fear the past. I fear the future. I fear the limitations that have been placed upon my life. I fear for my loved ones. I fear about money matters. I fear death. I fear fear. I am not sure I have the strength needed to handle my life as it is.

God, I know that fear is draining me of energy. Rather than seeking to defeat the fear through my own strength, I let go of my fear. I place my fear in your hands. I release my fear to you. God, I place myself in your hands. I accept your peace. Fill me with your love, your strength, your assurance, your peace. Make me aware of my own sacred and eternal nature. Your power and presence course throughout me and dwell within me.

God, grant me confidence. I know I am competent in many areas. I know I can handle my life. It would be easier with your help. Enable me to rely upon you. I ask for your guidance and care. Enable me to live this day peacefully and calmly. Thank you, God. I rest in your care. Amen.

(Then sit or lie down while using this calming exercise. Breathe deeply for ten minutes, as follows: While inhaling, silently say "Peace." Each time you exhale, let peace flow throughout your body. The peace is God's peace entering you.)

16. FIRE, HOUSE. God, I did not think this could be so painful. It is a living nightmare. I lost treasures in the fire. All those possessions represented me and my history. It is like losing part of my identity, part of me. I feel numb, as if I had just lost a loved one. I grieve for my loss. God, begin healing the pain and the loss.

Be with my loved ones who are feeling much as I am. Take away their pain as you surround them in your love and light. Grant them your peace.

Provide for our needs as we prepare for a new home. Guide and sustain us in all the financial issues. Enable us to rebuild our lives as we love and support each other. Thank you. Amen.

17. GRIEF, GENERAL. God, the creator and sustainer of all life, I thank you for your gift of life to _____ and for the fullness of the years we shared. I am thankful for the life you gave my loved one and for the good life s/he shared with the world. Thank you, God, for the precious gift of life. I entrust her/him to your loving care and thank you for her/his transition into your heavenly kingdom where s/he is being restored and made whole.

God, I am still hurting terribly. The pain of my loss is almost too intense. There is a huge emptiness within me. It doesn't seem fair. I miss her/him immensely. Many emotions threaten to overwhelm me. I feel angry that this has happened. I feel uneasy about unfinished business. I feel so alone and vulnerable. My life is now completely different. Adjusting and coping is so difficult.

God, I need your support and presence as never before. I ask you to dwell with me and fill the huge emptiness within. Please comfort and strengthen me and grant me your peace. Remove my weariness and make me whole.

God, guide me this day. Help me to handle each day. Guide and sustain me, and protect me from all harm. Enable me to reach the place where I can recall the love and life we shared together without breaking into tears. Heal my wounds this day and enable me to have faith and hope in your goodness. Provide for my needs until life returns in all its fullness and joy. Thank you. Amen.

*(Now sit or lie down. Close your eyes. Take three deep breaths. Then, slowly repeat over and over again, **"You are my strength and my salvation,"** for 15 minutes.)*

18. <u>GRIEF, CHILD</u>. God, it is so tragic to lose a child. I loved her/him more than I loved myself. I poured out my life for her/his life and future.

Thank you for her/his life. I will always remember the different stages of her/his life, the times we spent together, the dreams s/he sought to fulfill.

I commend her/him to your care. May s/he be guided into your light and love. Enable her/him to continue to grow and to become in your heavenly kingdom.

This is one of the most painful things a parent can bear. I know life goes on, but I feel such deep sorrow. Comfort me in my grief and restore me to fullness of life. Thank you.

19. <u>GRIEF, PARENT</u>. God, I have lost my mother/father. It hurts far more than I thought it would. I will miss her/him.

I thank you for the love we shared through the years. S/he did the best s/he knew how to do as a parent. I will always appreciate the lessons s/he taught me, the affection we shared, and just being with her/him. Help me to express my grief with tears of love. Comfort me in my pain. Thank you.

God, I pray for her/his entrance into the afterlife. Restore her/him with a new spiritual body that is healthy and vigorous. May s/he dwell with you forever. Amen.

20. <u>GRIEF, SIBLING</u>. God, I will miss my sister/brother. We shared many moments together and loved each other deeply. I am thankful for the years s/he spent with us here on Earth.

I have a rough time dealing with death. It hurts so much to lose a loved one. I am hurting. Help me to express the pain of my grief. May the sadness be a tribute to our love. Comfort me with your Spirit. Heal me that I may once again rejoice in the happiness we shared.

God, I pray that _____ is now with you in your heavenly kingdom. May her/his spiritual body continue to live, grow and become as s/he enjoys the Company of Heaven. Thank you. Amen.

21. <u>GRIEF, SPOUSE</u>. God, it is such a shock, such a hurt, such a pain to lose _____. I know that you do not willingly cause suffering, illness and death. Your will is to bring us goodness and health. God, thank you for your gift of life to my husband/wife. I am thankful for our many years of marriage, for the struggles we faced together, for the love and affection we shared. I will always miss him/her.

The hurt keeps rolling over me. I have this tremendous ache -- this inner emptiness. My life is a shambles. Nothing will ever be the same again. God, give me the strength to handle all that is before me. Provide me with the support I need. Guide me in the decisions I need to make. Protect me from all harm. Comfort me with your presence and grant me your peace. Hold me in your love and renew me. Thank you.

God, I commend _____ to your care, knowing that s/he is now safe in your heavenly kingdom. Restore him/her to wholeness in his/her new spiritual body. Surround him/her with the love of family and friends on the other side. Help him/her to find new life on the other side. I trust that we will one day be united. Thank you.

Our Father, who art in heaven, hallowed be thy name; thy kingdom come, thy will be done, on earth as it is in heaven. Give us this day our daily bread. And forgive us our trespasses as we forgive those who trespass against us. And lead us not into temptation, but deliver us from evil, for thine is the kingdom, and the power, and the glory forever. Amen.

21a. GRIEF, SPOUSE: HEALING THE ANGER. God, I am feeling angry since my spouse's death. I am angry that _____ died. It was not fair that s/he left me alone. Everything in my home reminds me of her/ him. I feel only half-alive.

God, I want to work through my anger. I release my anger to your care. Replace it with your peace. Comfort me in my loss. Fill me with life anew. Thank you. Amen.

21b. GRIEF, SPOUSE: HEALING OF FEAR. *"Yea, though I walk through the valley of the shadow of death, I will fear no evil, for thou art with me, thy rod and thy staff they comfort me."*

God, at times I feel fearful. Making all my decisions alone is scary. At time, being alone at night makes me feel uneasy. Knowing that I must depend upon myself, with no one to support me day-to-day, sometimes makes me fearful. I feel vulnerable and alone.

God, I know I am competent to handle life. It is just that living alone is so new to me. Strengthen me and build my confidence. Help me to build life anew. Take my fear and replace it with your love and peace. Enable my life to be full of people, of caring, of sharing. I trust in your power and guidance in my life. Amen.

21c. GRIEF, SPOUSE: HEALING THE GUILT. God, I feel guilty since my spouse's death. I feel guilty because I could have been more supportive than I was. I feel guilty about things left unsaid. I could have been a better partner to _____. Now, I will never have another chance. I feel guilty about wanting to move on with my life without him/her. I feel guilty about doing new things without him/her. I feel guilty when I laugh and have a good time in the midst of my grief. I feel guilty when I think of enjoying the company of the opposite sex, as if I were being unfaithful.

God, I know my guilt is unnecessary. Our marriage was good. Our love was strong. I did the best I knew how to do and know I did well. Relieve me of my guilt. I place my guilt in your hands, God. Heal me and grant me life anew. Thank you. Amen.

21d. GRIEF, SPOUSE: HEALING THE PAIN. God, I have lost my spouse who is so dear to me. I am filled with terrible pain to the point of numbness. I feel so alone, isolated. Even you seem so distant and uncaring. My life has fallen apart. My peace and security are gone. I feel angry and hurt, guilty and helpless. God, free me of the pain. Comfort me with your Holy

Presence. Surround me with your love. Heal and strengthen my inner being. Grant me the courage to go on.

I am thankful for the life I shared with _____. I celebrate the love and the struggles we shared, the goodness of our life together, and his/her entrance into Everlasting Life. Grant me, God, the assurance and strength of your love as I seek to cope. Comfort me. Amen.

21e. GRIEF, SPOUSE: FOR PEACE. God, I can no't sleep tonight. Partly I am restless. I feel a bit lonely. I feel a bit lost. Breathe on me, breath of God. Fill me with life anew. Guide me into a new and fulfilling life. Grant me your peace. Thank you. Amen.

22. GRIEF, SUDDEN DEATH. God, I am numb. It seems like an endless nightmare, like a dream from which I cannot awaken. I have never been so shaken. The pain continues to roll over and through me. I am hurting badly. I do not know if I can handle this. Strengthen me in this terrible time of crisis and grant me your peace.

God, bless _____*(naming the deceased)* and grant her/him calmness in the midst of her/his shock. S/he is alive and aware on the other side. Enable her/him to be aware that s/he has made the transition into the next life. Heal the shock of death. Grant her/him help in finding the Light that leads to your Kingdom. Thank you.

God, provide for my needs during this tragedy. Guide and sustain me. Increase my faith in your love. Enable me to cope with all that is before me. Help me to survive. I rest in your calming peace and presence. Thank you for comforting me in my loss. Amen.

23. GUILT. God, guilt imprisons me and I seek release. I have made mistakes. I have hurt others. At times I have been out of control. At times, I was doing the best I knew how to do. My present sense of guilt tells me how wrong I have been. I want this cycle of guilt to end, for it makes me miserable and helps no one.

God, I forgive myself for the pain I have inflicted upon others as well as myself. I seek to make amends to everyone I have hurt. I seek to end this cycle of guilt that only makes me miserable and a blessing to very few. Free me, God, that I might be a better person. I accept myself for who I am. I am sacred, precious, unique and of infinite worth. God, enable me to love myself. Bring healing to my mind and spirit. Fill me with your love and wisdom and peace. May only good flow to me and through me. Grant me the ability to care for myself and others in responsible ways that represent love and abundant living. Thank you. Amen.

24. HANDICAPPED. God, it hurts to realize that I am handicapped. I feel cheated. I can't do things most people do. My life is limited. It is not fair, but I am trapped in this body and must make the best of it.

God, sometimes I hurt over the insensitivity of others. Sometimes I am angered and saddened by my situation. Sometimes I sink into a sense of fear and helplessness. That is not all of me. I am a multidimensional person. I know happiness and satisfaction. I know the fullness of life. I possess strengths many people do not. I have learned to be self-reliant in many ways. I dream and I fulfill my dreams. Thank you for the gift of life.

God, I place my life in your hands. Fill me with your love and light. Bring me wholeness in body, mind and spirit. Provide for my needs and protect me from all harm. You are my strength. Amen.

25. HONESTY. God, I want to become more honest. I don't know what happens to me. I keep deceiving people, even when it is unnecessary. It has become a way of life. I am even proud of my deceptions, how I got away with it. Help me to become uncomfortable with lies. Help me to see how they drain my strength and hurt my relationships.

God, I know there are reasons for my dishonesty. Sometimes I do no't want to have an argument with my loved ones. Sometimes, it is to please people and make them feel good about me. Sometimes, it is for self-preservation at work and with my friends.

God, I renounce the spirit of deception. Remove this spirit from me. Fill me with the Spirit of Truth. Help me think clearly. Help me have convictions. Help me speak the truth in love. Transform and make me into a new person -- a person of integrity and truth. Thank you. Amen.

26. LONELINESS. God, I feel so empty. I feel so isolated. It is as though I am not connected to anyone. At times, my loneliness is almost unbearable. Enable me to make contact with you. Fill me with your love and presence. Restore my wholeness.

God, provide for my needs. I open myself to your care. Bring the people I need into my life. Open me to the sharing of love and friendship. Connect my energy fields to loving energy fields that can restore me. Guide and sustain me this day. Fill me with life anew. Amen.

27. MEMORIES, PAINFUL. God, life was not supposed to be this difficult. I did not expect my life to be like a happy fairy tale of unending bliss. I knew life was a struggle at times. But I did not expect this much agony and pain. The pain continues to wash over me through unexpected flashbacks and nightmares. My happiness and inner security have been stolen from me. Painful memories overshadow my whole life, ruining each day and relationships with others. I feel afraid. I am distrustful. Nameless fear haunts me daily. I am tired and often sad. I wish to end this seemingly endless agony.

God, I choose to take control of my life. I will no longer be a victim of my past. I let go of my painful memories. I ask you to heal the pain by erasing it from the memory tapes of my brain. God, heal my wounds. I release my pain, my anger, my bitterness, my hurt, my fear.

I forgive those who have caused me pain. I forgive myself for any role I have played in my pain. I release the pain to you. I cut the ties that bind me to my hurts. Heal my body, mind and spirit and set me free. I breathe in your presence, your love, your joy, your peace. Recreate me and make me fresh and new. I accept your new life, your love and light. Thank you. Amen.

28. MENTAL ILLNESS. God, I am emotionally troubled. I am trapped and can't let go of it. I ask you to release me from this condition. I forgive all persons who have ever hurt me. I forgive myself. I let go of my anger, hurt, fear and anxiety. Take from my soul the strain and stress and let my ordered life proclaim the beauty of your peace. I entrust myself to your care. Provide for my needs and protect me from all harm. Fill me with your love, joy and peace. I accept your power to transform and empower me. Thank you for the calmness that is coming over me. Amen.

29. <u>NATURAL DISASTER</u>. God, I place my life in your hands. Protect me from all harm as this situation develops. Place a protective bubble around me so that only good can come to me and flow through me. Protect the lives and belongings of my loved ones and everyone in our community.

Divine Creator, the source of all the energy in the universe, in your love, stop this crisis from happening. Let peace dwell within in both the heavens and the earth. Thank you. Amen.

30. <u>OVERWHELMED, FATHER</u>. God, I was so proud to become a parent. I thought this was the best thing that had ever happened to me. But I have become unhappy. Life seems to be work, work, work, with no fun at all. My time is not my own. I feel as if I am losing out on life. I am unhappy. I am tense, filled with anger and becoming bitter.

God, I find myself avoiding my family. I love my wife but she is always busy, tired and irritated. I no longer find the responsibilities of home to be satisfying. What am I to do? Leave? Remain unhappy? Or find some answers?

God, help me to be a responsible husband and father. I know my wife is hurting and my child(ren) need me. Enable me to hear my wife's anguish and frustrations. Enable us to find some answers. I release my anger and my frustrations to your care. Provide me with new understanding that I might learn how to handle this situation. Fill me with your strength and guidance, with love and concern. Thank you. Amen.

31. <u>OVERWHELMED, MOTHER</u>. God, I am burned out, exhausted and overwhelmed as a mother. I love my child(ren) but at this moment I wonder if I am capable of being a caring parent. I feel angry and trapped with no way out. I feel sorry for myself. It is as if life is passing me by. I feel I have to give up my own needs in order to be a good parent. I need help but don't know from where it might come.

God, I forgive everyone with whom I am angry. I release my anger and frustrations to you. In my present mood, I have been unable to think clearly. Fill me with your power and refresh me. Clear my mind and enable me to take control of my own life. Enable me to reach out and find solutions that will produce the happiness and satisfaction I need. I rest in your care. Restore me and provide me with the resources I need. Fill me with your love. Enable me to love myself and my child(ren). Thank you. Amen.

32. <u>PANIC</u>. God, at times I am filled with terror. I can hardly breathe; my lungs stop working; I gasp for air. My heart beats rapidly in my chest. My hands sweat. I am having a panic attack. I have no control over it. When it happens, I want to run and scream. At that time, I need a safe, familiar, peaceful haven. Afterward, I feel embarrassment and shame.

God, this is destroying me. Please remove this burden. Provide the resources I need to overcome my panic attacks. Heal the past that burdens my present. Provide me with insight about my panic. Heal me in body, mind and spirit and restore me to normal living. I accept your love and light into my life. Grant me your peace. Amen.

33. PET, LOSS OF. God, I thank you for _____. S/he has been a good friend. I will miss her/him. I know that pets survive physical death just as people do. Bless ____ in the afterlife.

God, I am hurting. Comfort me in my grief. Remove the pain of my loss. Help me to gently remember the good times we had together. Thank you. Amen.

34. POSSESSIVENESS. God, my possessions and loved ones are important to me. I want them all for myself. This sometimes gets me into trouble.

I do not like to share my possessions with others. I want to keep them for my use only. I have often been shamed for fighting to keep my possessions for myself. I would like to change. Release me from my possessive nature. Help me to be generous in sharing my possessions with others. Possessions can be replaced, but friends can't. Free me, God, from my possessive nature.

I do not like to share my family and friends with others. I become upset when people I love are enjoying other people. This annoys others. I lose friends over this. I know this behavior seems childish, but I cannot help myself. God, free me of my angry reactions of jealousy. Remove this spirit from me. Help me to be generous in sharing my loved ones with others. Grant me calmness and confidence in my relationships. Thank you. Amen.

35. POVERTY. God, I feel so helpless and out of control. I feel trapped with no way out of my situation. It is as if no one cares. I am angry at a society that will not help me. I feel so helpless and weak. I try not to be bitter and passive. God, empower me for a new day.

God, I pray for a way out. I accept responsibility for what is possible in my life. Please provide for my needs. Bring opportunities into my life. Bring people into my life who may help. May I recognize the path I need to take. I live each day, trusting in your care. Thank you. Amen.

36. RAPE VICTIM. God, I hurt. The pain keeps rolling through me. This is an unending nightmare. I have been violated, raped by an evil man. I did nothing to deserve this, yet I feel shame and humiliation. I have been terrorized. I am an innocent victim, in the wrong place at the wrong time.

God, I am still shaking in terror. I didn't think anything could hurt as much as this. I feel dirty. The sacredness of my body and soul have been violated. I also feel anger, a rage at this man who has violated me. How dare he do this to me for his own sick and perverted purposes. I pray that he be arrested, convicted and punished. I pray that no one else will be hurt by him.

God, I have flashbacks and nightmares. I would like to put this behind me as though this had never happened. I want to get on with my life. I know that it is going to take time for me to heal. I have been unable to forget or to let the pain subside. I feel stuck where I am, filled with hurt. But I am willing to try.

God, I refuse to take my anger and pain out on my loved ones. I accept their concern, their loving care. I refuse to become bitter and sad. Life remains good. Life can still be fulfilling. Enable me to feel pure, whole and strong once more. Cleanse my soul. Help me to be unafraid of my passion; to distinguish between the violent attack of a sick man and the love and tenderness of a lover.

God, I release my pain and hurt to your loving care. I cut the ties that bind me to my pain. I give away my anger, my hurt, my bitterness, my fear. I no longer choose to live in the darkness as I accept your marvelous light and love into my life. I ask you to heal my pain and hurt. I ask you to fill me with your goodness, love, joy and peace.

God, I thank you for the precious gift of life. Free me that I might be truly free of the past as I seek to move on into a happier future. I choose to take charge of my life, living it in your light. I choose a life of happiness and satisfaction. I thank you for the new life that courses through my veins. I rely upon your sustaining presence and guidance. Thank you. Amen.

37. <u>RESPONSIBILITY</u>. God, I want to take responsibility for my life. Life seems to be passing me by. Help me take control of my life. Help me seek happiness and satisfaction. Help me see clearly my responsibilities to myself and others.

God, quiet my inner being and grant me peace. Show me my priorities. Empower me to follow through on my commitments. I renounce the spirit of irresponsibility. Remove this spirit from me. Fill me with your creative Spirit and make me a responsible person. Thank you. Amen.

38. <u>SEPARATION, MARITAL</u>. God, my life is so uncertain right now. I do not know what the future holds for me. I have a sense of loss, of grief; a sense that the past is over forever and whatever is before me will be new and different, whether there is reconciliation or divorce. Yet, I have so many memories of shared love, of passion, of companionship, that I am haunted by flashbacks to better days. I don't know whether to try to make my marriage work, or plan to move on with my life. I am frightened. I know that there will be financial problems. I know that I have been dependent upon my spouse for so many things. Fill me with the strength and wisdom I need to survive. Comfort me with your love and peace. Thank you. Amen.

39. <u>SEXUAL ABUSE, ADULT</u>. God, I hurt! My body has been used against my will. I am in pain. I feel angry and degraded and worthless. My sense of personal power has been stolen from me. I have been violated! I am filled with fear. How will I ever trust again?

God, these feelings are more than I can bear. I know I must release them to you. Heal my hurt so that I may live in happiness again. I release my pain to you. I release my anger toward the person who did this. I release my anger toward myself. Give me back my self-esteem. Fill me with your peace and love.

God, I don't want this to ever happen again. My body is my own. My love and passion are mine to share only as I choose. Guide me in what I do now. Provide me with the strength and wisdom I need so that I can change the present and future. Thank you. Amen.

40. SEXUAL ABUSE, CHILD. God, I hurt. What is happening is completely wrong. I do not deserve this and have not caused this. At a time when I should be an innocent child enjoying life, this terrible nightmare continues. I feel dirty and used. Heal me in body, mind and spirit. Enable me to feel clean and innocent once more

God, I care about my abuser but I also hate him/her. I feel shame. I feel trapped. I do not want to hurt my abuser, but the abuse must stop so I can end this nightmare.

God, come to my aid. Protect me from any further attacks. Place a bubble around me to protect me from further harm. Break the need my abuser has to touch me. Awaken his/her compassion and make him/her aware of the pain s/he is inflicting upon me and the whole family.

God, help me to be wise. Bring people into my life who can help me. My abuser has threatened me with the harm s/he would do if I told anyone. But, this is a crime and laws protect me from having to endure this. Give me the courage and means to report this sexual abuse to a teacher or the police.

God, release me from further pain. Fill me with your love and peace. Guide me into a good future and provide for my needs. Thank you. Amen.

41. SEXUAL ABUSE, YOUTH. God, I have been sexually abused. I feel dirty about this -- violated. I am frightened because I do not know how to stop any possible future sexual abuse. Help me reach out for help. Nothing ever justifies what has happened to me. It is illegal. No matter how it hurts my abuser, I must report this to a teacher, a doctor or the police. Give me the courage to do this.

God, protect me from further abuse. Come to my aid. Heal my hurt and restore my sense of self-worth. Fill me with your love and peace. Restore my innocence and integrity. Thank you. Amen.

42. SUBSTANCE ABUSE. God, there is someone in my family who gets high on chemicals. Then all hell breaks loose. Life is so unpredictable in our family. Sometimes there is love. Other times our home is filled with shouting, arguing, anger and violence. Promises are made but seldom kept. We never know when our loved one is going to even be around, especially during holidays and birthdays.

God, I hurt. I know other families don't live like we do. I am always covering up, keeping appearances. I am often embarrassed and ashamed. Sometimes, I am angry and want to hurt others. Sometimes, I want to run away. Sometimes, I am terrified.

God, help me find answers for my life. I have done nothing to deserve this. Fill our family with your love and peace. Provide for our needs. Bring people into our lives who can help. Heal my pain. Enable me to think straight. Guide and sustain me day after day. Be my strength.

God, heal my loved one who is so sick. Release her/him from bondage. Free her/him from the spirit that has imprisoned her/him. In God's name, I command this spirit to release her/him. Heal her/him in body, mind and spirit. Thank you. Amen.

43. TRAPPED. God, I feel trapped. I do not know how to get out of this situation. Help me to understand what is going on. Help me to examine myself to see my responsibilities. Help me to be free.

God, I hurt. I release my anger and resentment towards the person(s) and situation. Help me to take charge of my life. Provide the courage I need to take whatever actions will free me of this sense of being trapped. Thank you. Amen.

44. VIOLENCE, FAMILY. God, I hurt physically. I feel fear and terror. My soul is wounded. I am confused. I did nothing to deserve this. There is no excuse for this to happen to any human being. It is barbaric. I have deeply loved and cared for this man/woman. I have shared my friendship and passion with him/her. I do not deserve this. Yet, I feel shame and embarrassment. This is not the way a family is supposed to live.

God, I am also feeling furious anger. Concern and anger battle within me. Which will win? Is there a way out? Dare I defend myself? Dare I seek help? Dare I leave? Dare I desire a different way of life?

God, I am sacred and precious in your sight. I am competent and worthwhile in so many ways. Yet, I feel trapped. God, protect me from further harm. Place a protective bubble about me so that only good can flow to and through me. Help me to use all the resources at my command. Provide for my needs and free me from the ups and downs of this relationship. Free me. Enable me to move beyond where I am to build a new life. Heal all that hurts within me. Bathe me in your love and light. Sustain and guide me. Thank you. Amen.

45. UNEMPLOYMENT, JOB LOSS. God, I have just lost my job and I am afraid. I don't know what will happen to me. I am angry and hurt. I invested everything I could into my job. I was competent. In the end, no one cared. God, heal my hurt, remove my fear and grant me courage to face the future. Provide for my present financial needs. Guide me to a new job, a job even more rewarding than the one I lost. Teach me to accept help and charity from others until I can care for my own needs.

God, I know that I am a competent, creative and responsible worker. I know I have value beyond my vocation. Enable me to face my loved ones honestly and openly. Let me care for them as they, too, make adjustments. Mold us in love and protect us from hurting each other. Thank you. Amen.

46. UNEMPLOYMENT, SEEKING A JOB. God, I need employment. Please provide me with a job to meet my needs. Guide me to places and to persons who can help me. I need this employment by _____. Enable this to be.

God, I am hurting. My life has been turned upside down. I am afraid to face today and terrified of tomorrow. What if I never work again? God, fill me with your presence and peace. Take away my worry. I know that I am competent and worthy. Let me always remember that. Thank you. Amen.

47. <u>VIOLENT PERSON</u>. God, fill me with a heart of compassion. I have hurt many people. I have hurt those who love me and care about me the most. Let me feel their hurt. Open me to their pain. Enable me to be concerned about their welfare.

God, I am filled with anger. I have lashed out with my anger. I am selfish. I have not cared about others. Often, after my violence has hurt others, I have felt remorse. I was sorry I did it. Later, I do the same violence over again. I justify it. It is way of exerting control. It is my response to exploding.

God, this is hurting me. It is hurting my loved ones. It is as though I am possessed. I have no control over this. I want to change. I turn to you, a power greater than myself. Fill me with your love and peace. Heal my anger and fear. I place them in your hands. Enable me to establish control over my angry feelings and actions. I renounce the spirit of violence. Remove the spirit of violence from my soul. I accept your Spirit into my life. The Spirit is the source of your peace, your light, your love, your goodness, your healing. Bathe me in the Spirit and free me from all violence.

God, free me and I will truly be free. I place myself in your hands. I will seek to make amends for the violence of my past. Fill me with your love, joy and peace. Guide me to the help I need. Enable me to be a new person, filled with fairness and love. Thank you. Amen.

48. <u>VIOLENCE VICTIM</u>. God, I am shaken. My nerves are raw. I live in fear. I do not sleep well. I do not like being a victim. I am furiously angry. I did not deserve what happened to me. I was innocent. I have been violated. I am thankful to be alive, yet the nightmare continues.

God, I pray for justice. May those who hurt me be found and punished for their crime. I release my pain, my fears to you. Heal my body and restore it to its previous health. Heal my soul and remove the pain of the memories. God, I let go of my pain. Heal my inner hurt and fear. Grant me a sense of security through your peace. Renew me in body, mind and spirit.

God, enable me to share my hurt with loved ones. I know I must talk and get it out of my system. I accept their care. I accept their concern. I accept their sympathy. I need their love. Thank you. Amen.

49. <u>WAR, CITIZEN PRAYER</u>. God, we are at war. I have mixed feelings. I want my country to do what it needs to do for justice. I am also concerned about innocent people dying. I pray for you to protect our military troops from all harm. Be with the families of our fighters, strengthening them and providing for their needs.

God, as in all wars, I know my nation will pump up the propaganda releases to make all the people on the other side appear to be evil. But, people are human throughout the world, just like me, sacred and precious.

I pray for the innocent victims of war wherever they are. Protect them from all harm and provide for their needs.

God, I pray for the political leaders on both sides. Give them a heart of wisdom and compassion. May your Spirit and the Word make all wars unnecessary in the future. Amen.

50. <u>WAR, COMBATANT</u>. God, I am in a war. I have mixed feelings. I want to serve bravely but I am also frightened and want to be at home. I know that innocent people are going to be wounded or die. I know that the fighters on the other side are people like myself with loved ones awaiting them at home. Yet, I have a mission to accomplish. Help me to serve my unit well.

God, protect me from all harm. Place a protective shield around my unit and myself so that no harm will befall us. Give me the strength and wisdom to survive the rigors of combat. Let this war to be short and merciful that I may soon return to a world of peace. Fill the political and military leaders with your Spirit and Word so they will have hearts of compassion and wisdom.

God, be with my loved ones in my absence. Provide for their needs. Fill them with calmness and hope. If anything should happen to me, comfort and guide them. I pray that when I return home I can resume life and pursue my dreams. Thank you. Amen.

51. <u>WAR VICTIM</u>. God, will anything ever be the same again? The fighting is destroying everything. People I love are being killed. Food, water and fuel are scarce. I am angry. I want revenge. I also want peace. I am frightened. I am losing everything that has ever meant anything to me. Life is not worth living, yet I struggle to survive another day.

God, stop the fighting. Enable the killers to know the pain of the people they wound and murder. God, I pray for peace with justice. Find a way to stop the killing.

God, heal my pain, my loss. Comfort me. Provide for my daily needs. Protect my loved ones from all harm. Protect me. Place a bubble of protection around us that no harm may befall us. I spread your love and light daily to all my countrymen. Help me bring your power into the life of the world. Help me to be an instrument of your peace. Use me. Guide me. Sustain me. Thank you. Amen.

52. <u>WORKING MOTHER</u>. God, I find it almost impossible to find a balance between working and mothering. Often I am exhausted. Sometimes I feel guilty. Sometimes I am overwhelmed when there is a crisis at home or at work, or both places.

God, give me the strength and the wisdom to be a working mother. Help me be the best mother possible. Provide for my children's needs and protect them from all harm. Guide and sustain me that I might do my best. Enable me always to remain healthy in body, mind and spirit. Grant me your peace. Thank you. Amen.

PRAYWELL

THE PRACTICE OF
HEALING PRAYER

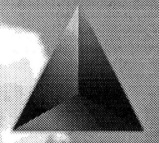

PART THREE

BASIC BELIEFS ABOUT HEALING PRAYER

God is the Source of all healing.

God desires health and renewal for all persons. Spiritual healing is a free gift of God to all persons regardless of their goodness, worthiness, status. or holiness.

God works almost invariably through human channels to produce healing. All persons can be channels for God's healing. Through Therapeutic Prayer, people become priests, bringing the power of God into the life of the world. Anyone can act as a priest. The only qualification is loving enough to express caring through prayer.

A person who compassionately cares automatically accumulates, attunes and transmits a healing energy that produces the optimum conditions for all life. This occurs naturally in any caring human interaction. Intentional efforts to produce healing increase the effectiveness of the energy.

A person who is a cynic or scoffer hampers all healing efforts by neutralizing the energy of prayer. Such persons must be screened out of all healing efforts. They also distort the life energy frequency of the ill.

Healing energy works as a process somewhat like that of an antibiotic, needing to accumulate a therapeutic threshold level that must be maintained until all symptoms of the condition have been relieved.

A therapeutic threshold level of healing energy can be accumulated and maintained by the regular Therapeutic Prayers of an individual, by the increased power of two or more persons in prayer (the square of the number involved), and by soaking prayer that constantly bathes a person in healing energy. Healing best takes place in a compassionate community that bathes participants in love and prayer.

Therapeutic Prayer expresses a universal form of caring that can be used by persons of all religious beliefs.

Therapeutic Prayer bathes people in an energy that produces quality individuals and relationships by reprogramming chaos and evil with God's Word and Spirit. Using this knowledge provides the greatest present hope for the renewal of individuals, marriages, families, classrooms, groups, communities, nations and all life on Earth. Therapeutic Prayer invariably fills people with God's peace and presence.

Negative feelings and thoughts contribute to and help to maintain illness; thus, ongoing health requires inner transformation.

God uses many agencies for healing, including medicine, psychology, and prayer.

If one can overcome the fear of dying, one need never fear living. God is with us in life, in death, and in life beyond death.

Chapter Twenty-One

Competency in Spoken Prayer

"Healing is only answered prayer and anyone can learn to pray."
...Agnes Sanford*

"In the experience of prayer we sense our oneness with others; we are filled with compassion; we know the love that henceforth will animate our activities outside of the time of prayer." ...M. Basil Pennington*

"And whatever you ask in prayer, you will receive if you have faith." ...Matthew 21:22

Few world-class healers employ spoken prayer in their healing efforts. Nor have most healers used it in laboratory experiments. With the record of their positive results, spoken prayer appears unnecessary for healers. Yet, most healers within organized religion employ spoken prayer. Since I grew up in the Christian faith tradition and have served as a clergyperson for more than thirty years, silent and spoken prayer are second nature to me. Because of this, spoken prayer is always my choice during the practice of healing.

Is spoken prayer for you? At the present time, surveys indicate that silent prayers of petition are used by ninety-nine percent of all Americans. In encouraging you to proceed, it can be stated that when you are praying for healing with family, friends and other hurting persons, the use of spoken prayer enhances the healing results. Spoken prayer is the best means for achieving oneness with the person and for attuning the healing energy. If you have not read chapter twelve, now is the time to do so. Note there the eighteen reasons for using spoken prayer.

Spoken prayer is essential for family devotions and group prayer, which surround us in God's love, peace and power. The easy, step-by-step learning skills taught in this chapter will enable you to utilize fully the chapters in Part Four. In terms of satisfaction and joy, spoken healing prayer with others is one of the most bliss-producing activities known to humanity. This experience of inner bliss is missing from silent group prayer. Bliss involves the sensing of joy, elation, ecstasy and rapture. In spoken prayer, there is also oneness, love and peace. Once you have experienced this spiritual bliss, your appreciation and respect for spoken prayer will lead you to seek its use throughout a full range of settings.

Francis MacNutt has polled hundreds of thousands of his prayer workshop participants about their spoken prayer usage. The results revealed that only about one percent had ever prayed aloud with a spouse to address a need, four percent of fathers had prayed aloud for their child's needs and twenty percent of mothers had prayed aloud with their children. These figures indicate that mothers are twenty times more likely to pray aloud with their children than with their spouses. So, you are not alone if you do not feel you have the ability to pray aloud.

Therefore, it comes as no surprise that for most persons, learning to pray aloud seems like a formidable task. Three primary reasons come to mind. First, it triggers a fear similar to that of public speaking. Second, never having done it, you may feel awkward about beginning. Third, you may believe you do not know the appropriate form and wording for spoken prayer and, therefore, may look bad.

PrayWell addresses each of these obstacles to spoken prayer. You will learn to pray aloud competently within a few weeks. Before we get to that, I would like to share the story of my own personal embarrassment as I began to practice spoken prayer. Thanks to PrayWell you will not have to experience the torture I did.

MY JOURNEY INTO PRAYER: AN AWKWARD, SCARY EXPERIENCE

I stumbled badly when I was suddenly forced to learn how to pray. Most people think the clergy are born competent. That was surely not true of me. As a twenty-two-year-old seminarian, I became the student pastor of a three hundred member church. I knew no more about praying aloud than most young adults. Not only was I ignorant about praying out loud; I was extremely shy, socially and verbally awkward and sometimes stuttered in stressful situations.

As a parish pastor, I quickly discovered that clergy, no matter how inept, need to offer prayer with people in crisis. Every week parishioners were sick, dying, grieving and struggling in various ways. They expected and needed their pastor to pray with them. I had a problem. I had never prayed with anyone. I did not know how to pray aloud.

What would you do? My solution was to buy books of prayers, type the prayers on small index cards and read them while praying in various crisis situations. I also had to take the heat. Not everyone closes their eyes when praying. The word got around quickly in that small rural community. *"We have a pastor who does not know how to pray."* During those three years of apprenticeship, I became verbally skillful in prayer. In the process, I was able to discard my learning tools.

PRAYER: A SPECIAL FORM OF COMMUNICATION

From that painful experience, I learned that prayer is a specialized form of communication not used anywhere else in society. It involves a unique prayer language and phrase compositions that are not used in everyday conversation. To pray also requires knowing who and what God is and how God works through prayer. You also need to have a certain wisdom about life. Many books explain what prayer is and how to pray, but none teaches us how to pray aloud with others. Teaching means coaching persons in the practice of prayer.

Prayer has become privatized, an activity performed alone by one person with God. This is partially because spoken prayer has become a social taboo; it labels one as deeply religious, a label most persons prefer to avoid. This taboo originated, in part, to justify many people's inability to pray aloud.

Learning to pray is like learning to play a sport. One may watch others play a sport a thousand times. This provides no practical skills preparing you for participation in the sport. Learning to play baseball involves practicing basic skills, building upon those skills and practicing at a specific skill level. It helps to have a coach teaching you. It is essential to have people with whom to play. This is also true of prayer.

If one has not mastered the skills of a sport by adulthood, most people give up on that particular sport. That is why I gave up on both baseball and basketball. I played poorly. If you reached adulthood without learning the art of spoken prayer, you may not want to begin at this stage of your life.

You may harbor certain reservations. There is a resistance among many to praying aloud with others for religious reasons. Most Christians cite the biblical admonition of Jesus to go and pray in secret where your Father, who hears in secret, will answer. That verse is taken out of the context of what Jesus was teaching. He was attempting to deal with the public show of piety when it was nothing more than human pride showing off. Seek to discern between this excuse and the possibility that you may be suffering from stage fright.

The primary motivation for offering a spoken prayer for healing is because your concern has prompted you to offer an act of love to a hurting person. If the purpose of your prayer is to show off, to express an ego need, to manipulate or to please someone else, then don't pray. Every pray-er feels inadequate for the task. Before praying with others, I usually request God's guidance. The following prayer of preparation includes many of my concerns:

A Prayer of Preparation

God, my concern has led me into becoming a channel for your healing power. Please use me as a channel for your healing flow. I feel inadequate in this role. I am not sure how well I will do. I might stumble. I place myself in your hands. Guide me in my efforts. Enable me to be a clear channel for your healing power. Let your healing energy flow through me that I might become a blessing to others. Amen.

LEARNING TO PRAY ALOUD WITH OTHERS

For fifteen years, I have been teaching what I call "A Course in Prayer." In five sessions, people meet in small groups to become competent and confident in spoken prayer. Seventy-five percent of those participants reported physical healings during their brief time together. If you have the opportunity to learn spoken prayer in a small group setting, skip this chapter. Chapter twenty-six details a group prayer learning process. The following is a tutored course in prayer for individuals. It enables you to begin your journey of praying aloud with others.

STEP ONE: BECOMING COMFORTABLE WITH PRAYING ALOUD

Find three persons with whom to pray. Approach each individually with a memorized prayer. Say, *"I am taking a course in prayer through PrayWell. I need someone with whom to practice prayer. Would you let me pray with you? I need to hold your hand and ask that you be quiet, while I do the praying."* Use a familiar prayer from your own religious tradition or the religiously neutral Christian's The Lord's Prayer that is printed below.

The Lord's Prayer

Our Father, who art in heaven, hallowed be thy name. Thy kingdom come, thy will be done, on earth as it is in heaven. Give us this day our daily bread. And forgive us our trespasses as we forgive those who trespass against us. Lead us not into temptation but deliver us from evil. For thine is the kingdom, and the power and the glory, forever. Amen.

This assignment can be scary. Most persons will cooperate if you do this in an appropriate setting of privacy without time pressures. It is normal to forget parts of a familiar or memorized prayer when doing it orally. Be willing to chuckle at yourself.

STEP TWO: PRACTICE BY WRITING TWO PRAYERS

Write prayers for two persons of your choice. Writing out prayers is the most important step in learning to pray. This teaches you to organize your thoughts and practice in privacy. How do you win cooperation? The most direct approach is this:

"I am taking a course in prayer through PrayWell. I need your help in learning to pray. Will you let me write a prayer for you? This will help me learn to pray. This involves interviewing you about your needs, preparing the prayer, and then returning to pray aloud with you."

A personal prayer differs from other forms of prayer. It focuses upon a person. It is difficult to offer prayer unless you know something about a person and his or her needs. Interview each person so that you know what to pray about. A few suggested questions:

SUGGESTED INTERVIEW QUESTIONS

A. Tell me about yourself.
B. What brings you happiness and satisfaction?
C. What are your hopes and dreams?
D. Where are you struggling with your life? Do you have an illness or medical condition which hampers you? If so, what?
F. Do you have any physical aches or pains? If so, where?

Write down the answers. Then in private, list the positive traits of the person, his/her pains and hurts, and the positive results you seek to address in your prayer. Then write a prayer for each person.

COMPONENTS OF PERSONAL PRAYER

G. Address God and praise him as the source of all wholeness.

H. Acknowledge the person's sacredness and preciousness before God.

I. Acknowledge his/her hopes and dreams.

J. State your intentions, the Word of God for this situation, by clearly expressing the needed positive results.

K. Offer a healing blessing.

L. Offer a spiritual blessing.

M. Thank God for the wholeness that is taking place.

The following prayer example is lengthy. It explores the whole range of possibilities in healing prayer. It provides you with maximum complexity as a learning tool. It places you in prayer long enough to yield healing results. This example is an expression of my personality, training and experience. You are free to alter this style to express your unique self.

A PERSONAL PRAYER MODEL

N. Address and Praise God:

God, we praise you for your creative and sustaining presence in the universe. We thank you for your love that is the basis of all life. We know that you are far more willing to give than we are to receive. Enable us to accept humbly and joyously all of your gifts. Be with us as we pray.

O. Affirm the Person's Relationship with God:

We thank you for your gift of life to John, for your presence along his life's journey, for the struggles and the celebrations that have molded him into the person he is today, and for sustaining him along the way.

P. Affirm the Person's Sacred Uniqueness as a Person:

We thank you for John's love that he shares with his wife and children, for his hard working and responsible style, for his appreciation of nature, for his craftsmanship with wood, for his sense of humor, for his helpfulness with family and friends.

Q. Acknowledge the Hurt:

God, John has hurts that need to be healed. He still grieves over his father's death. He is filled with anger. He is frustrated with money problems. He has pain in his lower back. His dreams are not being fulfilled.

R. Clearly State your Intentions:

God, we ask that John be made whole. He wishes to live life to its fullest -- to be able to enjoy family life, to work and play, to express joy and happiness, to offer love and caring to others.

S. Offer a Healing Blessing:

God, express your great love for John by healing his inner hurt. Comfort him in his grief. Enable him to understand the source of his anger; enable him to release it and grant him peace. Provide for his financial needs. Relieve the pain in his back and heal him in body, mind and spirit. As he pursues his dreams, enable them to coincide with your will for him. Guide and sustain John as he seeks to express his true self.

T. Offer a Spiritual Blessing:

God, fill John with your love and light that he might rejoice in the journey. Bless him that he might become a blessing to others.

U. Thank God for the Wholeness that Is Taking Place:

Thank you, God, for your love that is restoring John and making him whole. May your presence abide with John now and forever. Amen.

Write your prayer and then go back and rewrite it with more clarity and forcefulness. Read over the prayer four times to yourself so that it becomes natural to you.

STEP THREE: PRACTICE PRAYING ALOUD

Return to each person, saying something like, *"I have written this prayer for you. Because I am new at this, I may need to read it. May I hold your hand while praying with you?"*

Have your written prayer before you. By this time, you will be familiar with what you have written and probably will not need to look at your written prayer. You may be tense. That is normal in any new venture. Remember, pausing in the midst of prayer is normal. It comes through as the thoughtfulness it is. Say, *"Let us pray."* Pause for several moments of inner quiet and centering on God. Ask God guidance for your prayer. Then offer the prayer. Afterwards, thank him or her for letting you pray.

There is rarely a negative reaction to a personal prayer. If you sense one, explore it. Say, *"I sense that I've touched a tender spot during the prayer that upset you. Will you help me to understand what happened?"* This will be a learning experience. Two sources of negative reactions come to mind. The person may believe you have used the prayer to manipulate or control him, or the person may not be ready to recognize his hurt and the need to be healed.

STEP FOUR: GAIN EXPERIENCE IN PRAYING WITH PEOPLE

Make appointments with three persons. Choose these people because of their need. These persons could be in the hospital, ill at home, elderly, alone, grieving or going through a divorce. Just tell them you would like to visit them.

Once there, be your normal friendly self. Listen to their hurts. Care in natural ways. Avoid giving advice. It does not work. It is perceived as a lack of trust and comes through as judgment. It places people in a bind by imposing the decisions that are rightfully theirs to make. It is not helpful.

Before leaving tell them this. *"I am just learning to pray. I would like to have a prayer with you if you do not mind my stumbling a bit."* Naturally take his hand. Say, *"Let us pray."* Pause for a moment of inner quiet and centering on God. Offer the prayer.

STEP FIVE: EXPERIENCE CLOSENESS IN PRAYER

Ask God to make you a channel for his love and healing. Again, find three persons who are hurting. Go through the same procedure as in Step Four, with this addition. After saying, *"Let us pray,"* pause before beginning. Seek to become one with God and with the person with whom you are praying. Then offer the prayer in the midst of that oneness.

THE CONTINUING PRAYER JOURNEY

At this point you should be feeling more competent with prayer. It is among family and friends that your praying skills are most likely to be used. You are now prepared for the next chapter.

PEACE in the World's Great Religions

CHRISTIANITY: *"Blessed are the peacemakers, for they shall be called the children of God."*

ISLAM: *"God will guide men to peace. If they will heed him, He will lead them from the darkness of war to the light of peace."*

HINDUISM: *"Without meditation, where is peace? Without peace, where is happiness?"*

JUDAISM: *"When a man's ways please the Lord, he makes even his enemies to be at peace with him."*

BAHA'I: *War is death while peace is life."*

SHINTO: *"Let the earth be free from trouble and men live at peace under the protection of the Divine."*

BUDDHISM: *"There is no happiness greater than peace."*

SIKHISM: *"Only in the name of the Lord do we find our peace."*

JAINISM: *"All men should live in peace with their fellows. This is the Lord's desire."*

ZOROASTRIANISM: *"I will sacrifice to peace, whose breath is friendly."*

Chapter Twenty-Two

The Healing of Emotions

"The healing of memories from a person's past can aid in achieving physical, emotional, and spiritual healing." ...Agnes Sanford*

"There are specific locations within our energy system for the sensations, emotions, thoughts, memories and other non-physical experiences that we report to our doctors and therapists. The study of the aura can be a bridge between traditional medicine and our psychological concerns." ...Barbara Ann Brennan

"If we approach our life and healing from the depths of ourselves, experience has within it the power to transform and heal." ...Richard Moss

Emotional pain is the major cause of human unhappiness and dissatisfaction. This is not surprising since happiness itself is an emotion. What is surprising is our inability to free ourselves of emotional pain. It is far easier for Therapeutic Prayer to heal physical illness than painful feelings. What can we do about persistent emotional pain involving anger, anxiety, fear, hurt, bitterness, grief, painful memories and similar emotions?

Today's professional treatment relies heavily upon drugs to alter destructive emotional states. Many people remain suspicious of this approach because most drugs do not heal painful emotions. These drugs work mostly by masking the symptoms rather than curing the cause. Yet, because most other approaches fail or are not used, using drugs remains the only approach that offers many the possibility of personal happiness.

Emotions cannot be changed by thought processes. Thinking is helpful in listing possible approaches and choosing those to explore. Thinking seldom resolves emotional issues. Our life energy's model for the human energy fields in chapter five shows why this is true. *Emotional life and feelings* reside in the second energy field. *Mental life and linear thinking* are found in the third energy field. Therefore, thinking has little effect upon the feelings. Thinking can repress painful feelings. Though forgotten, they remain as repressed energy, able to cause unhappiness and physical illness. Drugs work because they can affect the functioning of the second energy field.

The human energy fields model provides further understanding. It explains why spiritual approaches heal physical, emotional and mental conditions. These three levels of being are contained in the first three energy fields. The energy of Therapeutic Prayer can heal these under certain circumstances. More will be said on this later.

Beyond these three are four more human energy fields. The fourth and sixth fields deal with love. The information in chapter eight indicates that love is the most powerful healing and creative force in the universe.

Popular wisdom states, *"Love cures all."* The love in the fourth energy field is humanly understandable, involving love and the human emotion of love. Love in the sixth field expresses celestial or divine love. This love is God and permeates the universe. When we are able to tap into life energy, we are bringing the power of divine love into our energy fields. When healthy, these love energy fields have the power to restore the first three energy fields to health. Humanity has spent centuries trying to do this.

The fifth energy field is empowered by God's Spirit and God's Word. The Spirit and the Word are the basis of all the world's religions. When filled with the Spirit and the Word, this energy field complements the other energy fields. This is essential for human health and happiness.

The seventh energy field is the higher mind that integrates the spiritual and physical dimensions. When these outer four energy fields are healthy, they can maintain physical, emotional and mental health. When they function poorly, people are handicapped and lack the resources necessary for wholeness. The emotional pain in the second energy field cannot be healed unless we either reach into the second energy field with love energy or strengthen the outer four energy fields. This is why religion and the spiritual dimension are so crucial for human health and happiness.

SPIRITUAL THERAPIES FOR HEALING EMOTIONS

This understanding explains the crucial role of spiritual life for health and happiness. The purpose of Therapeutic Prayer is to restore all seven energy fields and make them healthy. This is possible because Therapeutic Prayer brings the transforming power of God into human life, enabling all the energy fields to glow with health. This understanding allows <u>PrayWell</u> to offer several alternatives to drug therapy.

Chapters fifteen, sixteen, and twenty offer Therapeutic Prayer for the self-healing of emotions. Chapter fifteen explores how a shift in consciousness can produce self-healing. Chapter twenty-five tells how to find emotional healing in healing services. Chapter twenty-six describes how the love and prayers of a support group restore emotional health. These are all solid approaches to emotional healing.

This chapter focuses on two new approaches for use with counseling or psychotherapy. Both approaches are so simple they can be used by either professional or untrained caregivers. Using Therapeutic Prayer, they can produce dramatic or permanent healing of emotional pain because they tackle its source.

THE LIMITS OF PSYCHOLOGY

For more than thirty years, my professional specialty has been counseling. In theological graduate school, I angered my clinical psychology professor by insisting on seeking spiritual foundations for counseling. He feared any spiritual approach to counseling must be judgmental, and thus, therapeutically destructive. He warned his students that pastors must never use prayer during counseling sessions. This caused me to be cautious, but I was still looking for spiritual foundations for pastoral counseling.

Experiences during my appointment in my first parish convinced me of the power of love and prayer during therapy. The enduring problem in all psychotherapy and counseling sessions is the failure of a client's new self-understanding to produce emotional healing. A troubled client may continue therapy for years without finding emotional health and personal happiness. The therapist may listen to a complete life history, concentrate on painful events, hear a client talk emotionally about his/her feelings, use various techniques to help the client achieve self-understanding and clarify goals -- and end by not helping heal a client's painful feelings or relationships. This failure to internalize insight explains why drug therapy has become such a necessary part of treatment. I believe we have better and more workable ways available for healing emotions and relationships -- spiritual paths. This has given rise to Transpersonal Psychology and the pastoral care movement of clergy.

Love. In my first year out of graduate school, Charles and Mae were referred to me by their vacationing therapist for marital counseling. They told of unhelpful sessions with various therapists during the past five years. When their therapist returned from vacation, I summed up our four sessions by saying, *"I don't think I can help you. I don't understand the dynamics of your relationship. Go back to your original therapist. He is far more qualified to help you."'*

Their answer startled and puzzled me. Charles said, *"Walt, you have helped us more in four weeks than all of our other therapists put together. We sense that you genuinely care about us. We have seen tears of love in your eyes as we shared our pain. You have lost sleep in your concern for us. Our happiness is important to you."*

This is not what my textbooks had led me to expect. Six sessions later, their personal pain and relationship had been healed. Charles and Mae were once more whole and happy. What caused this success story? Later, I understood that caring love and a spiritual approach to life were the major factors. (Now, I must add the fact that I was a healer who was unknowingly sharing life energy with them.)

Prayer. Harry and Ann lived in a hopeless situation. Ann had sought my help in leaving home with her four children because of Harry's physical abuse. Harry was a sullen, chronically unemployed alcoholic. Ann and the children moved into the apartment I found for them. Harry wanted a reconciliation and the couple met with me one afternoon for an emotionally laden three-hour counseling session. Harry and Ann openly expressed their feelings of anger, hurt, hopelessness and frustration as they talked about drunkenness, poverty, arguments, physical violence, marital rape and family gun battles.

We closed the marathon session by joining hands and sharing a Therapeutic Prayer. The prayer summarized the session and asked God to heal them. My evaluation of the session was that their relationship was hopeless and I had been of no help. You can imagine my surprise when they returned an hour later holding hands and gazing into each other's eyes with unmistakable love. What a story they told! Harry was not the same defeated person. He was glowing with life, whole.

Harry explained, *"During your prayer, I felt a load leave my shoulders. It was like I was possessed and a demon left me. I was free and happy. When we got into our car, Ann looked at me and said, 'Harry, you are different. You have changed!' It was true, Reverend. I am a changed man."*

The change was obvious, but I remained skeptical. Then, the miracle of prayer continued to unfold. They came to church for the first time that Sunday. I later baptized the whole family and they became members. Harry became gainfully employed. He never drank again. He became a model husband, father and citizen.

This was my first awareness of the power of God in prayer. I will always be thankful to Harry and Ann for receiving the power of God's Word and the Spirit. The Word was expressed in my love. The Spirit came during our prayer and entered into their agony. God makes all things new.

THERAPEUTIC PRAYER IN PSYCHOTHERAPY

Therapeutic Prayer enables people to internalize their understanding while healing emotions and relationships. I have seen this miracle unfold hundreds of times with individuals, couples and families during therapy that included Therapeutic Prayer. Therapeutic Prayer also enhances the healing of traumatic memories and fixated thoughts. By this process, transformation and healing occur at both the conscious and subconscious levels.

Therapeutic Prayer significantly improves the recovery of those experiencing the pains of divorce and grief. In support groups, Therapeutic Prayer creates a group energy field that intelligently acts to transform and empower all those encompassed within it. Chapter twenty-six provides detailed guidance for support groups.

Untrained caregivers can also successfully act as therapists with Therapeutic Prayer. Caution here is warranted. You must use counseling skills. Blaming, moralizing and advice-giving do not work. Empathetic listening is your best tool. You must let people express their deepest feelings of pain and pleasure. You must love people with a complete acceptance of whom they are.

Therapeutic Prayer is offered at the close of a session. The therapist begins by accurately summarizing the content of the session. This includes the client's expressed needs, hurts, hopes, relationships and ambiguities. The Therapeutic Prayer expresses realistic hopes and expectations and also has the power to create new and beneficial realities. Caring love is the only qualification for doing this.

The following prayer models are taken from actual case histories. In each case, my objective assessment was pessimistic. At another level, I was hopeful. Following both Therapeutic Prayers complete healing took place.

A Therapeutic Prayer for a Troubled Marriage

God, we thank you for Jim and Jane and for the love, companionship and commitment that led to their marriage. We thank you for all the happiness and fulfillment of this relationship. And yet, God, betrayal, anger and distrust have now divided Jim and Jane. Jane is thinking about divorce. Jim appears to be indifferent to Jane's pain. We do not yet know the future, but we ask you to bless both Jim and Jane in their time of need. Heal the inner hurt and confusion, open lines of communication and fill them with your

love, joy and peace. Provide them with a higher wisdom that the best solu-
tion for both of them will emerge. Thank you. Amen.

A Therapeutic Prayer for a Troubled Woman

God, we thank you for Kate. We thank you for your gift of life to Kate. We
thank you for her hopes and dreams. Kate has been struggling with life.
She is lonely. She is unhappy with her job. She is bitter about men. She is
depressed. God, we ask you to heal Kate. Fill her loneliness with life. Help
her to find fulfillment at work. Heal her bitterness. Remove her darkness
and fill her with your marvelous light. Kate is seeking meaning in her life.
Guide her in finding meaning. Kate wishes to be happy. Fill her with your
love, joy and peace. Provide for her needs and protect her from all harm.
We anticipate a miracle for Kate. Grant her new life. Thank you. Amen.

In these counseling sessions, the expression of feelings seemed to be the
most important element. Having made contact with their feelings in counseling, we remained in contact with the feeling energy field during our
Therapeutic Prayer. This enabled God to heal, transform and empower.

MY EXPERIENCE WITH RADIANT HEART THERAPY

Everything I know about the process of Radiant Heart Therapy I learned
from Cher Wendt, a Fort Wayne, Indiana psychologist. After a few hours of
learning from Dr. Wendt at a Montreal seminar, I traveled to the Boston
area to practice healing.

One of my clients was a retired engineer named John. John came to
me for physical healing, but he also mentioned chronic anxiety. Since
childhood, he had constantly lived with anxiety. I explained Radiant Heart
Therapy to John and he agreed to let me use it to heal him.

John shared no details about his anxiety. He just said he had it. I sat
beside John on a couch, placing my healing hand on the front of his chest
over his heart. The other hand I placed upon his back. I gave John these
instructions.

"John, feel your anxiety. Now, give a color to your anxiety. Do you have
it? John, I want you to choose a flower and place your anxiety in the flower
bud as the color you have chosen.

"Now, I want you to put the flower bud in your heart. Imagine that flower
in the color you have chosen, representing your anxiety. Let the flower
bloom and flow into my hand as you let go of it. I am holding my healing
hand over your heart to receive it. It is filled with God's love. Let the flower
merge with my hand. Let go of the anxiety.

"Let us pray. God, I receive John's anxiety into my hand. May he be
forever free of anxiety. Fill his heart with your love, joy and peace and
make John whole. Thank you. Amen."

It took fifteen minutes in all. Afterwards, John reported being anxiety-
free for the first time he could remember. Two weeks later, I received a
letter from John at my Ohio home telling me that he has remained anxiety-
free.

OPENING YOUR HEART IN LOVE

The heart chakra is where we store our emotions. We can close off our emotions to others by closing off the energy of our heart chakras. We can also open our love to others by opening our heart chakras. As in romantic poetry, the heart is indeed the seat of love, as well as all other emotions.

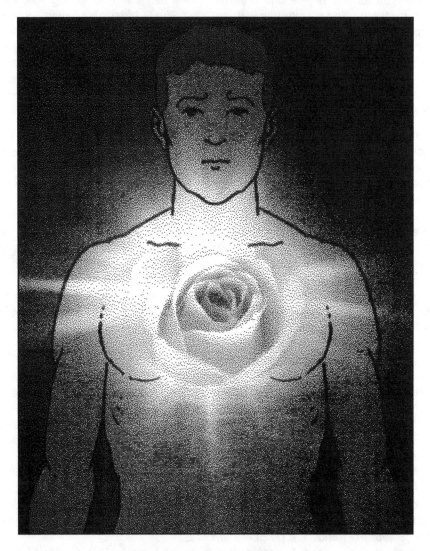

Figure 13. *Radiant Heart Therapy works because all one's emotions are accessible through the heart energy chakra. Emotions can be released through placing one's feelings in a flower and having a loving hand receive the painful memories and hurts.*

From the heart emerges the second energy field where we store our emotions. Knowing this, for years I have consciously opened my heart chakra to my counseling and healing clients. This enables me to feel their emotions and to send them healing love. This establishes emotional rapport with others. This permits healing interactions. I open my heart chakra by visualizing it and then willing it to open. Using Radiant Heart Therapy, I visualize my heart to be a red tulip bud that I open as a flower to the world.

DR. CHER WENDT'S RADIANT HEART THERAPY

Ten years ago, Fort Wayne, Indiana psychologist Cher Wendt came upon a mystery. Dr. Wendt was using Reiki healing therapy on a depressed woman. During the therapy, she leaned over the woman and hugged her. Afterwards, the woman remarked to Dr. Wendt, *"My heart is full."* Not only that, the woman's depression was gone.

Dr. Wendt was puzzled by what had occurred. What could have healed her patient of depression? It took four years of research for Wendt to find the answer. She discovered the woman was healed of depression because of the existence of energy chakras. In placing her heart upon the depressed woman's heart during her hug, Wendt had healed the woman's heart chakra and, thus, her depression.

For the past six years, Cher Wendt has worked from her heart; opening her heart chakra to patients. This is heart-to-heart healing of the emotions and physical body. She is also teaching others to open their heart chakras. She calls her new approach Radiant Heart Therapy.

Wendt's patients talk about the pain in their hearts. This is the pain of the *emotional* heart. Healing this pain through Radiant Heart Therapy is a process that is simple yet profoundly transforms people. It is so simple that one tends to think nothing is happening. A patient says, *"I am in pain. I am depressed. I feel an emptiness."* The cure is Radiant Heart Therapy.

Cher Wendt states that what used to take two years of psychotherapy now takes one to three sessions with Radiant Heart Therapy. She grins as she says, *"What I do now blows my mind!"*

THE PRACTICE OF RADIANT HEART THERAPY

Dr. Wendt places her hands on either side of the heart of a patient. She shares, *"I can **read** what is wrong with him. I ask a patient, 'Have you ever been badly hurt?' Many patients talk about such an instance."*

Wendt shares, *"I ask patients for the color of their feelings. The color does not matter. I ask them to place that color in the flower of their choice. I ask them place that flower in their heart and to radiate that color from their heart. I can feel it enter my hands. The patient will be sobbing. Then I will ask the patient to completely let go by giving the flower from his heart into my hands. This happened with a heart patient. Then I did ninety minutes of psychotherapy follow-up."*

A Cancer patient. A terminally ill cancer patient was undergoing nutritional therapy when he became Wendt's psychotherapy patient. His physician was using drugs to stimulate his immune system. In a preliminary interview, Wendt discovered he was unaware of his own spirituality. She began therapy by placing her hands on either side of his heart. He began sobbing. He told of his impending divorce. He told of the pain of it. He released his anger and poured out his hurt. He was shouting. He said his head was about to blow off. Then, he saw God in spontaneous imagery. The session went so fast, Wendt could not keep up. It was the only session he needed; two full hours. The melanoma soon disappeared.

Dr. Wendt works with many cancer patients. She has discovered cancer patients to be loving, giving people. They give with their hearts but are unable to receive love and energy from others. They are unable to love their own inner child. They are not energy-grounded. Her therapy with cancer patients is this:

1. Open your heart to receive.
2. Open your heart to the love of your inner child.
3. Enable yourself to become grounded in love.

A Sexual Abuse Case. Dr. Wendt states, *"When I suspect someone has been sexually abused, I attempt to touch a knee, just a brushing by. When the touch is avoided or when there is obvious pain, the person has been sexually abused. Most of the pain is in the lower part of the body."*

One of her sexual abuse patients was pregnant. She had never hugged people. Wendt went with the woman into delivery. She used hypnosis with her client throughout the labor. Then she got creative. She said, *"Open your heart chakra."* The woman did, for three hours. The delivery was perfect. This woman, who would let no one touch her, hugged her baby with immense bonding. She hugged all the nurses, a first for the patient. This is Radiant Heart Therapy.

RE-PARENTING THERAPY

Cher Wendt's Re-parenting Therapy grew out of Transactional Analysis. In Re-parenting Therapy, Dr. Wendt holds people in her arms. She rocks them while hugging them heart-to-heart, like a mother holding a sick child,

She held a hurt girl in her arms. She felt the energy of their hearts unite -- a parental bonding. She was not sure she wanted this deep a relationship, but she accepted the risks and commitments. It turned out well.

Healers need this. Dr. Wendt states that healers in particular need Radiant Heart Therapy and Re-Parenting Therapy because their hearts are constantly being drained by healing. During our seminar, Dr. Wendt invited a healer to lie down on the floor. Wendt placed her right hand on her patient's heart and recharged it with love. As usual, the consequences were immediate and dramatic, as the woman rose from the floor beaming, visibly altered.

Cher Wendt is writing a book. Its title is <u>Radiant Heart Therapy</u>.

CONCLUSION

Working on the heart chakra is the easiest way I know to heal a painful memory. It is easier than psychotherapy followed by Therapeutic Prayer. Both work.

In seeking to heal any physical disease or relational problem, first seek to heal the heart chakra of its pain. Often, this is all that is needed for complete physical or relational healing to occur.

Chapter Twenty-Three

Prayers for Absent Healing

"Long distance cell-to-cell or organism-to-organism communications may be accomplished by transmission and reception of electromagnetic signals through membrane receptors or enzymes." ...Tian Y. Tsong

"Reaching out to our fellow human beings requires a movement from hostility to hospitality." ...Henri J. Nouwen

"Ask, and it will be given you." ...Matthew 7:7

Randolph Byrd, MD, performed clinical studies[1] on the therapeutic effects of intercessory prayer at San Francisco General Medical Center from August 1982 through May 1983. Using a randomized double-blind protocol among coronary care patients, the study followed one hundred ninety-two patients receiving intercessory absent-prayer from a Christian prayer group outside the medical center. Two hundred one patients were used as an unprayed-for control group (though others may have prayed for them). At a statistical level of $p < .01$, the prayed-for patients required less frequent ventilatory assistance, antibiotics, and diuretics than the control group.

This is a rare medical journal report on the medical benefits of absent-prayer. It is significant because so few clinical studies of absent-prayer have been reported. Yet, absent-prayer is the most commonly used form of Therapeutic Prayer. It can be done quickly and privately within your own home. We must assume that absent-prayer works like touch-prayer. As you pray, you are transmitting an energy at plus or minus 7.83 hertz to the person needing it.

What enhances the effectiveness of absent-prayer? The traditional approach begins by having a loving concern, becoming one with the person and God, and utilizing some form of prayer for healing. Loving concern is expressed by emotions like love, anxiety, fear, faith and hope. The unity between the pray-er, prayee and God can be expressed both in the mind and in the words. These appear to attune the healing energy to the correct frequency.

During prayer, one's intentions are also important. The healing energy is information-bearing. There is a belief and some clinical evidence to indicate that the intentions of the pray-er are imparted into the information of the healing energy. Also, one must remember to send the message to the one to whom it is intended. Somehow, the universe has a means for identifying the one to whom you are sending the prayer. Sending the healing energy remains a must.

Emotions and mental pictures are thought to be beneficial resources that can be included in absent-prayer. There are several behavioral evidences for this.

Dream sleep has a strong impact through mental picture scenes and emotions, sometimes accompanied by spoken words.

The basis of premonitions appears to be the emotions associated with the ties of loving relationships accompanied by the emotions associated with pain, shock and death.

Parapsychology research has discovered that the sending of picture images is a far more reliable means for communicating mental telepathy information between persons than thoughts. The clairvoyant reality consists of mental pictures. Clairvoyants receive mental picture images of distant or future events.

Religious visions also involve intense motion picture-like vividness accompanied by words. All this evidence suggests that forming a mental image with emotional content during healing attempts would produce more consistent healing results.

We will also be using the methods gathered from the study of healers. In their work, healers either seek to transmit healing energy or to be one with God and the person.

LESHAN'S MENTALIST HEALING TECHNIQUE

Dr. Lawrence LeShan, using knowledge from his study of the paranormal universe, developed a rational healing style that I refer to as mentalist healing. In training, practitioners first spend three days learning to form complex mental images. The practice of mentalist healing uses twin mental images of any object -- with one image representing the healer and the other the healee. Once the twin mental images are formed, they are merged into one image. That is the complete LeShan mentalist healing technique.

I studied this technique for a week in Detroit. About ten of us sat in a circle and practiced this technique of absent healing on each other and then on people hundreds of miles away. In all cases, physical healings rapidly took place. My condition was a painful lower back produced by sitting on the floor for four days. As the rest of the group focus upon my healing, I was aware of nothing. The pain just quickly disappeared.

I speculate that Hindu and Buddhist healing use similar forms of mentalist healing. Mentalist healing works for those who are able to form clear mental pictures. A similar process is used in radionic healing. A picture or piece of tissue from the ill person is placed on the radionic device's sample tray, with a mentalist technique used to will healing. In a similar way, I knew a woman in Akron, Ohio who could heal any person's illness simply by looking at the person's picture and praying for healing.

A. STYLE ONE: INDIVIDUAL ABSENT-PRAYER

If possible, place a picture of the person before you. Your emotional concern for the person in crisis is probably motivating your prayer efforts. Let that emotional concern deepen with all the pain and anxiety it creates. Emotions are a helpful empowering element of prayer.

This next instruction will sound like a contradiction, but relax. Do not push, try hard or worry about results. Relax and depend upon God. Expect God to do the healing, not you. Remain in a state of miracle-readiness. Then, use the following prayer process. Feel free to use your own style.

A THERAPEUTIC ABSENT-PRAYER MODEL

I am upset. I am concerned for the life of _____. I ask that you use me as a channel for his/her healing. I have a faith, a hope and a knowing that you can intervene in this situation and make him/her well. Transform me into a channel for your healing light and love. Guide and use me as I pray for healing. I deeply care about this person and seek to help him/her become well. God, the Creator and Sustainer of all life, I know how your healing energy enhances the healing rate and regenerates tissue.

God, I ask you to heal _____ in body, mind, and spirit, and make him/her well. Remove the pain and discomfort. Enhance the healing rate. Restore and renew _____ completely. Protect him/her from all harm. Grant him an assurance that you are with him/her in this time of need -- filling him/her with your love, joy, peace and presence. Unite us and make us one with each other and you.

Before continuing, pause and be one with the person and God. Now, pray:

God, I ask that this healing begin now and continue until full health is restored. Thank you for the healing process that is already taking place. Enable me to be continually aware of your holy presence as I pray. Amen.

Continue to fill your mind with faith, hope, expectancy and love. If possible, welcome the white light of God into your mind. Focus on other parts of the person's identity: voice, personality and the experiences you have shared together. Now silently form a mental picture of the person in perfect health. This may be helped by looking at the person's picture. While doing so, repeatedly pray:

God, unite me as one with _____ and heal him/her and make him/her whole in body, mind and spirit. Amen.

While remaining in a spiritual state of consciousness, use the following healing modes:

1. Imagine the person as completely well and active -- smiling, walking, running, dancing, working, playing, joyous and whole.
2. Seek to form a oneness between God, the person and yourself -- the Healing Trinity.
3. Seek to transmit healing energy to the person. Fill yourself with love, faith and hope and imagine a beam of white light emerging from your heart, filled with these qualities, with the ray traveling to the person, filling him/her and transforming him/her into glowing health.
4. Form two identical images in your mind and merge them into one. One image is you. The other is the person. The images may be of two human twins merging or two animals or two buildings or two plants or trees. Keep forming twin images and merging them.

5. Pray for protection from all harm. This can be used with illness, for travel safety or any danger. Imagine a huge clear plastic globe encircling the person. And then pray,

God, heal him/her, provide for his/her needs and protect him/her from all harm. Come to his/her aid and make him/her well. Heal _____ in body, mind and spirit. Enable this to be. Thank you. Amen.

This whole prayer process can be repeated over and over again as you soak the person in prayer and love. Take periodic breaks. Then return to prayer. It is your choice how long you continue in prayer. I have continuously used this prayer process for five hours straight for the acutely or chronically ill. If others are present, invite them to do the same. Make copies. For medical emergencies of many days or weeks, provide each person involved with a copy of PrayWell.

B. *STYLE TWO: GROUP ABSENT-PRAYER*

The power of prayer is the square of the number of persons praying even when they are praying from different locations. During a medical emergency, it is both practical and preferable to gather persons together for group prayer. Five persons praying together is twenty-five energy units of prayer power and twenty persons represent four hundred energy units of prayer power. This causes an immense increase in the power of prayer to heal. With enough persons praying, complete healing of the person can occur following fifteen minutes of soaking prayer. To be sure, check on the status of the person every thirty minutes.

Someone must take the initiative for group prayer. Before suggesting it, have a quiet, private place in mind. In a hospital setting, there is the patient's room, a small waiting room and a chapel. Ask a staff person for a private place where the loved ones of the patient can gather for prayer. If no such place exists, consider gathering in an empty area of the waiting room.

Invite your loved ones to join you in prayer. You might say, *"I would like to pray. I have found a private place where we can all gather. Will you join me?"* If some choose not to go with you, do not argue. In their reluctance, they may not be suitable channels and make actually block the healing power of God. Let those who will, gather together.

Once gathered, volunteer, *"If it is all right with you, I would like to lead us in a group prayer for _____ ."* If they are unaware of PrayWell principles, do not go into detail. To do so can create confusion and disharmony. Before praying, you might make a brief statement, somewhat like this:

"I have been studying prayer. I have learned that when loved ones gather together and pray, they create an energy for healing that can greatly help a patient. The power of group prayer is immense, so each of us plays an important role. The energy of prayer increases a person's healing rate. Your concern, faith and hope are important in empowering our prayers. I am going to lead us in prayer and then offer guidance for our continuing prayer together. Are there any questions?"

A GROUP THERAPEUTIC ABSENT-PRAYER MODEL

Let us pray,   (Pause five seconds for a spiritual transition.)

God, we are thankful to be gathered here in prayer for _____. We are deeply concerned for him/her. Our hearts reach out in love to care for _____. We are thankful, God, that you are here with us. You are the source of all life and all wholeness. You make all things new. We thank you for your presence. Guide the doctors and nurses as they care. Protect _____ from all pain and harm and fill him/her with your peace.

God, we ask you to use us as channels for your healing power. Grant us faith, hope and love that this prayer might be empowered. Restore him/her to health. God, heal _____ in body, mind, and spirit and make him/her whole. Fill him/her with your love, joy and peace. We thank you for the healing that has already begun. We entrust _____ to your care and continue our prayers in your peace. Unite us as one with _____ that renewal may occur. Amen.

Then explain to the group, *"We are going to continue praying by repeating this prayer over and over together:"*

God, heal _____ in body, mind and spirit. Make us one with _____ that in our unity with him/her, s/he may find wholeness and newness. Enable this to be. (Use ten repetitions.)

Tell the group, *"Now I want you to imagine _____ being healthy and vibrant in your mind. See _____ actively living. smiling, walking, running, dancing, working, playing, joyous, and whole....*

"Seek to form a oneness between _____, yourself, and God. Merge into a unity -- the Healing Trinity. Let us pray:" Return and repeat the initial prayer.

When this first prayer process is completed, ask if anyone else would like to lead the group in prayer. Sing a familiar sacred song together or share in a prayer you all know. Check on the person's progress. If possible, join together again and repeat this prayer process. You might wish to make a copy of the absent-prayer model above available to each person.

C. *STYLE THREE: PRAYER CHAINS*

Prayer chains are the most common ongoing method for offering absent-healing prayer. Prayer chains can be found in organized religion, schools, workplaces, clubs, neighborhoods and self-help groups. When twenty-five persons in a prayer chain (squared, that is six hundred twenty-five energy units of prayer power) are daily praying for the sick, about sixty percent of persons whose illnesses are resistant to medical treatment will experience a complete alleviation of their symptoms. Prayer chains can be one of the most affective means for providing a steady supply of healing energy that yields consistent results.

Unfortunately, it must be added that most prayer chains are ineffective. This is because most participants are not prepared and do not know how to pray for healing. Rather than pray, they pause for a moment's sentiment of concern for the sick. This originates from the fact that few prayer chain organizers know anything significant about healing prayer. Nor do they attempt to discover why so few healing results are reported.

PAM'S HEALING THROUGH PRAYER CHAIN PRAYER

Shortly after teaching the church prayer chain Therapeutic Prayer, my secretary informed me at ten o'clock one morning, *"Pam's daughter is on the line."* Pam had been diagnosed with a ruptured disc and was in traction at the hospital.

I picked up the phone and Pam's daughter said, *"Rev. Weston, my mother is in immense pain. She has had all the pain medication permitted but she is still crying. You know how gutsy my mother is. She must be in bad shape. Will you start the Prayer Chain?"*

I started the Prayer Chain, prayed, and headed for St. Joseph's Hospital. As I entered the medical center, I was feeling tense about Pam's pain and my role in helping her. I cautiously entered her room about eleven o'clock, an hour after starting the Prayer Chain. And there stood poor Pam at the foot of her bed -- smiling at me.

After embracing, she said, *"Watch!"* I watched in amazement as she proceeded to bend her five-foot, nine-inch frame and touch her toes with both hands. She explained, *"The pain stopped a few minutes ago. I felt wonderful. I removed the weights, got out of bed and had just stood up when you came in."* She continued stretching and testing her body. *"As soon as the doctor gets here, I am going home. Thanks for starting the Prayer Chain."* Pam's back remained healthy for years afterwards.

GUIDANCE FOR OPERATING A PRAYER CHAIN

A prayer chain operates like this. Prayer requests are phoned to the leader. The leader has a list of captains who lead chains -- a list of people. The prayer requests are passed to each chain captain. The captain phones the first person on the chain list. Each caller phones the person below him on the list. Unanswered phones are skipped and one goes to the next person on the list. The last person on the chain calls the chain captain to signify completion. If the chain captain does not receive this phone call, the captain phones around to see where the chain has stopped. Each person phoned is given a list of persons who are ill or hurting. They are to pray daily for each person for a week.

As stated, prayers are seldom offered in most prayer chains. To change this, prayer chain participants need either a course in prayer or a list of prayers to use, along with detailed instructions. It can be speculated that most prayer chain participants view their responsibility as unimportant because they have a low regard for their role in the power of prayer. They do not view themselves as bringing the power of God into the life of hurting persons.

SUGGESTIONS FOR A SUCCESSFUL PRAYER CHAIN

Use both sides of a sheet of paper. On the front page, list the chain members, with phone numbers, along with instructions on how to function as a prayer chain. On the back page, give guidance for prayer and provide some sample healing prayers.

PRAYER GUIDANCE

A. God invariably uses human agents as channels for his healing power. God does nothing, but through prayer.

B. Scientific data indicates that a praying person is transmitting a healing energy at a specific frequency that acts intelligently to produce healing. It initiates healing which is resistant to medical treatment, speeds up normal healing by two to one hundred times, and regenerates tissue. Prayer must be offered daily to be effective because the healing energy diminishes as it is utilized in healing and must be replenished by prayer.

C. The power of prayer is the square of the number of persons praying. If all sixty persons on our prayer chain prayed daily, the power of their prayer is thirty-six hundred times more than one person praying. If ten persons do not pray, the power of our prayer chain is reduced by eleven hundred energy units of prayer power. Your work on the prayer chain is important. It can be more effective than an antibiotic and hasten the results of medical treatment.

D. The power of prayer is increased by your compassion, faith, hope and expectancy. Anticipate a miracle and it will occur in most of our efforts.

PRAYER CHAIN THERAPEUTIC PRAYER MODELS

1. A PRAYER FOR HEALING: *God, I praise and thank you for your creative and sustaining power. I feel inadequate in acting as your agent for healing and ask you to guide and transform me during this prayer. Fill me with faith, hope and concern, that this prayer might be empowered. Open me to the pain of human suffering that I might identify with those for whom I pray.*

God, I ask you to heal the following persons in body, mind, and spirit and make them whole: (name the persons _____). Fill these persons with your love, joy, peace and assurance. Make me one with others who are praying, with each of these persons and with you. Thank you for the healing that is taking place. Amen.

Now imagine God's healing power emerging from your heart as a white beam of light and traveling to the person(s) for whom you have prayed. With each person, imagine it entering, filling, and healing him/her. Then, while being aware of God, envision each person or name merging into oneness with you. While doing so, say,

Let us be one as the healing flows into and heals these persons. Thank you, God. Amen.

2. A PRAYER FOR GRIEF: *God, I thank you for your presence throughout (name the deceased) _____'s earthly journey and ask you to enable her/him to have a smooth transition into your spirit kingdom. I thank you for the love s/he shared through the years with family and friends. My heart goes out to all who grieve in their loss, especially for _____. May your presence fill and comfort each of these persons, healing their pain, sustaining with strength, guiding the present and providing for their needs. Lift our eyes beyond the shadows of this earth and enable us to see the light of Eternity, for you are with us in life, in death and in life beyond death. Grant each of us your peace. Amen.*

Now imagine the person(s) filled and comforted with God's love. Then unite in oneness with each person.

3. A PRAYER FOR INTERPERSONAL HARMONY: *God, I pray for all the persons involved in this situation: (name them ___). Fill them with your understanding and compassion. Provide peace for each of them with justice. Guide them into a newness of life. Bring healing to them in body, mind, and spirit. May they become one, just as you are one with us. Amen.*

Now imagine this oneness.

4. A PRAYER FOR EMOTIONAL WHOLENESS: *God, _____ is emotionally hurting. Remove her/his inner pain, provide for his/her needs and restore inner harmony. Fill him/her with your love, peace and joy, that s/he might become one with you, focused and made new. Amen.*

Now imagine this happening.

5. A PRAYER FOR MATERIAL NEEDS: *God, you are the source of all we need. Provide for the needs of_____. Provide the resources that are necessary. Bring people into their lives who can help. Thank you. Amen.*

Now imagine this happening.

6. A PRAYER FOR PROTECTION: *God, I ask you to protect _____ from all harm. Place him/her in a protective bubble of your white light and deliver him/her from all harm, keeping him/her safe.*

Now imagine this happening.

CONCLUSION

Other absent-healing efforts are but variations on these three styles. Be persistent. Check on results. Expect no acknowledgment that you played a role in someone's healing. Your only reward lies in helping someone. Thank God for any healing and wholeness that result.

Chapter Twenty-Four

The Practice of Touch-Healing

"When you have eliminated the impossible, whatever remains, however improbable, must be the truth." ...Arthur Conan Doyle

"True joy, peace, and happiness are found only in loving, knowing, and serving God and the neighbor with true humility, simplicity, compassion, meekness, patience, and obedience to Christ." ...St. Francis*

"God's power is real." ...Agnes Sanford*

The practice of absent-prayer is far more prevalent than touch-healing. Absent-prayer is convenient, fast and private. In contrast, touch-healing requires more time, effort, confidence, experience and interpersonal skills. In touch-prayer, one must expend the time and effort needed to visit the person, relate in a meaningful manner, receive the consent of the recipient, overcome natural resistance, touch in unfamiliar ways and offer a spoken prayer.

BARRIERS TO PRAYER

Once you have made the commitment, being competent in touch-healing spoken prayer is not your greatest obstacle. Presently, the most difficult task involves overcoming resistance and winning the cooperation of others. Therefore, we include guidance for approaching people about praying. In the midst of crisis, people are far more open to prayer. A hospital-based crisis lowers most people's resistance to joining you in prayer.

AN INTIMATE ACTIVITY

Because prayer is perceived to be an intimate activity, there is a direct correlation between the emotional closeness and relational appropriateness of those involved and the willingness of others to cooperate. The most acceptable people to offer prayers are an immediate family member, a close friend or someone in the caring professions.

In most situations, prayer must be preceded by a deepened relationship. One's first goal is to offer caring. Only after this has been successfully achieved is prayer normally appropriate. There are a few exceptions. With little interpersonal preparation, touch-prayer may be offered in a grieving group, before surgery, with persons who are too weak for conversation, with those in comas or sleeping and with those suffering trauma injuries.

Touch-prayer might be compared to a romantic kiss. When an American couple begins dating, it is considered inappropriate to kiss until the interpersonal relationship has reached mutually acceptable levels of comfort, emotional closeness and trust. Similar deep relational levels need to precede the intimacy of prayer. Once a trusting relationship has been established, I have never had anyone refuse my offer of prayer.

A PRIVATE ACTIVITY

Because of its intimate nature, prayer activity is best practiced amidst the most privacy possible. Uneasiness or embarrassment may result when prayer is practiced in the midst of strangers, around institutional staff or in public view. This social taboo is similar to the privacy demanded by most persons in the United States during the breast feeding of an infant. Just as the hunger need of infants may require public breast feeding, so may the demands of a crisis require personal praying in full public view.

A POSSIBLY DEMEANING ACTIVITY

In addition to being an intimate and private activity, prayer can also be perceived as a demeaning activity. Most persons can see the need of prayer for others, but many persons have trouble accepting prayer for themselves. The root of this issue appears to be pride. Accepting personal prayer may be perceived in the same light as a charity hand-out. Some may feel, *"I do not want a free meal or any charity gift. I want to recover through my own efforts."* This attitude derives from a basic human need to be self-reliant and independent. In a religious context, it translates as, *"I do not need God's help nor your forcing me into an uncomfortable, inferior role."* In this context, never ask to pray **for** someone, which is demeaning. Say something like, *"I would like to share a prayer **with** you,"* or *"Can we pray together?"* Relate to any prayer recipient with respect as an equal.

Refusal may also be rooted in other issues. It may involve a fear-denial reaction along the lines of, *"If I accept a prayer, then I am admitting that I am extremely bad off."* It may be rooted in rejecting the religious connotations of what you are offering, or it may be based upon a disbelief in or a hostility toward God, prayer, and especially spiritual healing.

OPENING PERSONS TO THE TRANSMISSION

If healing energy is transmitted and acts consistently and intelligently, why are some persons not healed?

First, people have the ability to block the reception of the healing energy. This ability is partly related to free will. Humans maintain considerable control over what enters their own energy fields, as well as how it is used. If a person does not want what you are offering, the healing energy is naturally rejected, blocked from entering or being utilized. My hands sense this resistance as a lack of a healing flow, like a coolness from touching a cool wall.

Some people are born socially private persons, naturally placing a protective shield around themselves. When trust relationships are built, they can voluntarily open their energy fields to healing. Blocking of healing energy may also occur due to a lack of relationship and trust, to the rejection of touch and prayer, to choosing to be ill, to being withdrawn, to being too exhausted to open oneself to receive what is being offered. Thus, understanding and voluntary cooperation are necessary in most healing encounters. However, my experience is that sleeping and comatose patients, because they offer little resistance, show consistently good healing results.

Second, some medical conditions require a threshold level of healing energy to build to a peak before a healing flow is sensed. Therefore, we must be cautious about drawing quick conclusions about personal resistance.

During the Chouhan-Weston Clinical Studies, my hands immediately felt the healing flow with both a healee with a head cold and one with chronic back pain. The videotape confirmed this. Each healee's energy aura quickly changed from a blue with a whitish fringe to white. The healing energy was being immediately utilized by the healee, building to a threshold level that would eventually produce complete healing. In the case of the head cold, it took only eighty-nine seconds to produce a stable, healthy energy field. My hands sensed that the healing was complete when the flow dramatically diminished. The healee was filled-up and needed no more energy. The healee sensed this as extremely painful heat throughout her body, jerking away from my hands because of the heat. Within an hour, all cold symptoms were gone.

It took longer for the healing of the woman with ten years of chronic back pain -- three daily ten-minute sessions. On the second and third days, she arrived with her energy aura still charged white from the previous day's prayer. In the midst of the third session, all symptoms disappeared. To restore her spine to health, the healing energy threshold had to be maintained for forty-eight hours.

My experience is that most bacterial and viral infections, as well as trauma injuries, heart damage and arthritis, produce no sense of resistance to the healing energy. Therefore, any sensed resistance is due to resistance by the healee. However, there are exceptions.

Cancer is different from most diseases. During the Chouhan-Weston Clinical Studies, my hands sensed that each cancer subject was not receiving the healing energy. My interpretation proved wrong. The videotape showed that the blue aura remained constant for eight to ten minutes, and then explosively and instantly changed, becoming bright white and three times larger. My hands sensed this moment of change. Early in the session, I could be heard on the audio portion of the videotape, stating that the subjects were not receiving the healing energy. At the moment of the explosion that transformed their energy field, I stated, *"Now, they are receiving the healing flow."*

My revised interpretation is that while the healing energy was building to a therapeutic threshold level, like water seeking to fill a reservoir, my hands could feel no energy movement flowing throughout the body. But, when the reservoir was filled and began overflowing to encompass the whole body, I could sense that flow. By that time, the restoring of the energy field was already complete and the body was using the healing energy flow to convert the cancerous cells to normal.

Other exceptions include those diseases affecting the central nervous system, like Lou Gehrig's Disease and multiple sclerosis and those with impaired brain-functioning like senility, Alzheimer's disease, benign tumor and brain trauma injuries. These block access to memory functions. With all of these, my hands sense no energy flow during the healing encounter. Can we conclude that the same process is taking place as with cancer? I do not know. Standard touch-healing prayer has healed multiple sclerosis and brain trauma injuries even without my sensing an energy flow. I have been unable to help victims of Lou Gehrig's Disease, senility and Alzheimer's disease. In all these cases, I have been unable to sense any energy fields with my hands. It is as though the energy fields have withdrawn within the body, or no longer exist.

My most recent approaches with these special conditions are encouraging. I now seek to restore the health of the energy fields first, working for five minutes about four inches from the skin, then another five minutes at the distance of an inch. My hands sense the restored energy fields. I follow this with standard touch-healing prayer. In all cases, this has accelerated the healing process.

GROUNDING HEALEES TO THE EARTH

Healers have consistently stated that a healer must be grounded to Mother Earth both mentally and spiritually. I now have evidence that such grounding must be literal grounding by wire to Earth.

Recently, I worked with a Canadian clairvoyant for two days. She receives referrals from doctors because she is able to diagnose illness by *reading* energy fields. As I practiced touch-healing prayer, she described the energy patterns involved. She *saw* my transmitted healing energy as green. The negative energies around diseased body areas she *saw* as red with some blues.

She stated that when a healee is not grounded to the earth, the negative energies decrease during healing but remain present following healing. This causes temporary healing results for a day or two but then the negative energies re-assert themselves, continuing the ill condition.

When a healee is grounded to the earth, the red and blue energies leave the healee permanently through the grounding wire. This was demonstrated to me time after time by the clairvoyant. The red energy clings to arthritic joints and to nerves in nerve diseases like multiple sclerosis and Lou Gehrig's Disease.

She had grounded her treatment table by placing a sheet of metal under the padding and running a ground wire from the metal to the ground in the electrical receptacle. If you know little about this, ask an electrician. People can also be grounded by direct contact with the Earth, or to concrete grounded to the earth, or by a wire running to a cold water pipe. I chose the latter, placing a computer static electricity grounding strap wrapped in metal foil around the healee's ankle, with the wire running to and clamped to a cold water pipe. I am still experimenting with the grounding of healees. So far, it has improved my results.

My hands now sense a healing flow in circumstances where I had previously felt blockage that required long and repeated sessions. Grounding has permitted me to heal arthritis in less treatment time. It has improved my effectiveness with cancer and the healing of painful memories and relationships. I look forward to learning more about this technique.

COMPASSIONATE LOVE ATTUNES THE ENERGY

Compassionate love grows out of relationship. Compassionate love not only empowers the healing energy, it also attunes it to the right frequency for a person's needs. Perfectly attuned energy moves through the barriers of negative emotions, blocking neurons and chemicals. It acts intelligently to initiate and enhance healing. Anyone can learn caring skills. Relational caring skills are natural for therapeutic personalities. Those in the helping professions are usually trained in caring skills. Family nurturing also improves caring skills.

Caring accumulates and attunes healing energy in a variety of ways. Anytime we sense another person's pains and hurts, including our own fear, anxiety and stress of concern, or have known their sacred identity, we have established an empathetic link that naturally attunes. Mutual affection or closeness attunes. Sharing the presence of God attunes. Faith, hope and expectancy facilitate attuning. Attuning naturally occurs in relationships that are experienced as mutually caring.

COMPLEMENTARY APPROACHES TO TOUCH-HEALING

I entered the field of spiritual healing as a young United Methodist parish pastor and spent a dozen years learning to practice healing within the context of my Christian tradition. Within Christianity, touch-healing is practiced through a simple touch on the head or the holding of hands, accompanied by prayer. The channel for healing has traditionally been viewed as passive, with God mysteriously doing everything. I can no longer accept that viewpoint. All the clinical evidence indicates that God and humans actively work together in the transmitting of an energy that heals. This understanding grew out of my apprenticeship as I learned to practice healing and became a journeyman healer within my religious tradition.

Wanting to know everything there is to know about healing, I spent the next dozen years learning to practice healing outside my religious heritage, using Eastern and secular healing styles. During this learning experience, I attended dozens of healing workshops led by teachers who each offered their own unique approaches and techniques. I experimented with each of these techniques. They all worked. But, my earlier approach using simple skin-touch and prayer worked equally as well in most situations.

This led me to the conclusion that techniques serve two purposes aside from healing. Techniques provide an acceptable explanation within which practitioners can comfortably function. Techniques also appear to serve the purpose of keeping the conscious mind occupied so that the subconscious healer within can quietly emerge and become involved in the healing encounter.

Two complementary healing approaches are touching the skin with the hands, and touching the surrounding energy fields with the hands. Both approaches work on the human energy fields. They transmit an energy with the hands that heals by transforming the human energy fields, which then heal the physical body. Scientific evidence indicates that these healing models are accurate.

As mentioned earlier, scientific data indicates that during skin-touch-healing, the healing energy is usually transmitted evenly throughout the energy fields. As reported in the last section, there are medical conditions that do not respond well to skin-touch-healing. Therefore, practitioners of touch-healing prayer would also find it helpful to learn to work on the human energy fields.

ENERGY ASSESSMENT AND HEALING

Those who practice energy field touch-healing use assessment techniques that explore the heat consistency of the human energy field with the hands, with a pendulum, with dousing rods or through muscle strength testing. Those most capable of assessing energy fields have developed their intuitive sensitivity.

Other assessment techniques seek to identify blocked energy centers (called chakras) whose blockage either contributes to illness or prevents the body's own natural self-healing process from occurring. Healing unblocks the chakras or restores their proper rotation. This involves cleansing the energy fields. This is achieved by moving the hands downwards over all skin areas or by whisking the energy field with the hands around the area of illness or injury.

A third step involves restoring the energy fields through hand motions similar to those used in cleansing them. For our purposes, skills in energy field assessment are not viewed as a high priority. Instructions will be directed toward energy field cleansing and recharging.

For those interested in professional training in energy field assessment, Barbara Ann Brennan's book, Hands of Light, is an excellent resource, as are some applied kinesiology courses. For those interested in healing techniques other than those taught in PrayWell, here are just a few of the options:

HEALING TECHNIQUES

1. Barbara Ann Brennan's books, Hands of Light and Light Emerging - The Journey of Personal Healing. The Barbara Ann Brennan School of Healing, P.O. Box 2005, East Hampton, NY 11937 Phone: 1-700-HEALERS; FAX 1-700-INLIGHT.

2. Dolores Krieger's book, Therapeutic Touch, or a Therapeutic Touch seminar. Therapeutic Touch academic credits can be earned at many nursing colleges. There are certified TT instructors in most cities. It is also taught by Krieger and her associates in New York City.

3. A Reiki workshop.
4. A Silva Method seminar.
5. A Lawrence LeShan healing seminar.
6. Training and accreditation in a spiritualist church.
7. John F. Thie's book, Touch for Health or a Touch for Health seminar involving a form of applied kinesiology.
8. My own PrayWell seminars.

This may sound disparaging, but from hindsight I now know that I did not need to attend dozens of healing workshops to learn skills. I have wanted to be sure that I was not missing something I needed to know. The true value of the work shops is actually in the building of my own confidence and in the fellowship I enjoyed with other healers.

CAUTIONS ABOUT PHYSICAL TOUCH

Many healers who work only in exterior energy fields warn against physical skin-touch during healing. They warn about the ineffectiveness of skin-touch and the danger of contracting a disease. My experience contradicts these warnings. Throughout thousands of healings, I have always made contact with the skin during touch-healing and have only been aware of the positive results. Objectively, I do not understand the logic of the caution. Whether touching the skin or working at one to four inches away, one is always in contact with six of the human energy fields. Touching the skin puts you in direct contact with the other, the first energy field, the physical energy field, but even at one inch away one can be in contact with this field.

TOUCH-HEALING APPROACHES

This is a summary of touch-healing approaches as covered in earlier chapters. We will be using all of them.

1 Some persons focus on transmitting healing energy with their hands.
2. Some sense a oneness with God and the person.
3. Some mentally visualize the intended results.
4. Some visualize twin objects and merge them into one, with one object representing the healer and the other the person.
5. Some use a combination of the above techniques.

The establishment of scientific and clinical data on the practice of spiritual healing is still extremely limited. Opinions rather than clinical facts pervade the field. With this disclaimer, we can consider the following data:

A few experienced healers have observed that some of these methods are inferior to others. For instance, some report that seeking to transmit healing energy provides only temporary healing, while seeking unity produces long-term healing. Experimental results in absent-prayer indicate that visualizing the intended results is less than half as effective as seeking unity or oneness. Yet, there are reasons to doubt these assessments.

Because no scientific experimental data is available on the effectiveness of various touch-prayer approaches, these reservations raise other questions. It is likely that people vary in their ability to use differing approaches. Each individual has specific abilities that may make one approach more effective for that person. Some people may also be more skilled at healing than others, causing good results that cannot be achieved by everyone.

Can one practice any healing technique without also inadvertently using other methods? In my own healing, I first sense a oneness with God and the person. This results in my sensing a healing flow in my hands. While still in this state of unity, I visualize the healing energy flowing to the area needing healing. By experimenting, you can discover which methods produce the best results for you.

WHAT TO DO DURING TOUCH-HEALING SPOKEN PRAYER

A. Purity of intent. Your only intent is to offer generous love and healing.

B. Daily healing. Offer touch-healing at least every other day, and more frequently with acute conditions. It is like administering an antibiotic that needs to be replenished to maintain a threshold of healing energy. As with an antibiotic, continue to apply for several days after the healing appears to be complete.

C. Empowerment. Your faith, hope, love, relationship and expectancy empower. So does confidence.

D. Welcoming help. When possible, invite others to join you to increase the power of the healing energy. When two or more people place their healing hands on top of each other, it increases the healing flow. Others can touch other parts of the body. Another way is to gather in a circle around the healee and hold hands while practicing spoken prayer. This bathes the healee in the healing group energy field, as would happen in a healing service.

E. Wash your hands before and after healing. Before healing it cleanses your energy and afterwards it stops the healing flow. This prevents your becoming drained.

F. Relate to the healee as a caring friend before praying.

G. Request permission to touch and to pray.

H. Enlist cooperation. In long-term healing, enlist the person's cooperation. Explain the healing process, or have the person read PrayWell. Have him repeat after you, *"I wish to be well. I accept the healing which is being offered me."* Then, during healing prayer, ask him to sense God's presence and to be one with God and yourself.

I. Opening and balancing/charging the energy fields. If your hands sense resistance to the healing flow (as if a wall were there) or if the person seems indifferent or hostile to healing efforts, first cleanse the human energy field and then balance and recharge it.

    To cleanse. Have the person stand or lie down. With the intention of cleansing, start at the head and move the flattened palms and fingers of both hands in sweeping motions downward over the entire body down to the feet from about one-half inch away.

    To begin healing. Repeat this procedure with the intention of imparting healing energy. This takes about three minutes. In some healing techniques, this is the complete healing procedure.

    Always use this technique as a necessary opening procedure on persons with neurological conditions like multiple sclerosis, Lou Gehrig's

Disease and stroke, with brain conditions that block memory functions and with cancer. Try grounding the healee to Earth.

J. Energy field brain work. With the neurological, brain and cancer conditions mentioned above, it is essential to proceed to the energy fields surrounding the head. Make repeated cleansing sweeps with your hands about four inches from the head, covering the whole head area. Then, balance and charge the brain energy fields in three steps, from four inches away, one inch away and touching. In each step, place your hands at the front and back, either side, and then on the nape of neck and top of the head for about one minute each. This whole procedure takes about ten minutes. Then proceed with touch-healing vocal prayer. Try grounding the healee to the Earth.

K. Touch contacts. When working with a newcomer to healing prayer, normally just hold one hand while lightly touching any other convenient part of the body. This has worked for me in thousands of healings. These further options are available according to the comfort level of the subject.

1. Take the healee's hand in yours and touch the top of the head with the other hand.
2. Touch the forehead and nape of neck.
3. Touch on either side of the area needing to be healed.
4. Cover every area of the torso, arms and legs with the flattened palms and fingers of both hands for fifteen seconds. This could take fifteen minutes.
5. With a partner: Have the partner hold an ankle in each hand while you perform the above four steps.

L. Healing styles. After offering the healing prayer, use any or all of these options:
1. Seek to form a spiritual oneness with the person. Before beginning, silently pray: **"God, make me one with _____ in body, mind, and spirit. Bless this unity that it might produce wholeness."**
2. Seek to transmit a healing energy with your hands by silently praying: **"God, use my hands to transmit your healing power."**
3. Mentally visualize the intended results, silently praying: **"God, enable _____ to be restored into your perfect genetic image."**
4. Visualize twin objects and merge them into one, with one object representing the healer and the other the person.
5. With hands in place, talk with the person in a conversational manner. The two most intimate and spiritual human interchanges are to touch and to talk. Doing this helps the attunement and utilization of the healing energy.

M. Calming. Energy field cleansing and charging as well as touch-healing prayer can also be used for the healing of emotions and memories during an emotional crisis or to restore interpersonal relationships. These uses are detailed in chapter twenty-two and in Part Four. Repeating the energy field cleansing and recharging above can more quickly accomplish this. A side-effect of all healing encounters is a sense of inner calmness that lasts about two days.

N. Praying. Begin your prayer by saying, *"Let us pray,"* then pause ten seconds before proceeding.

O. Practice. If possible, rehearse on someone before doing the real thing by going through the whole process alone.

TOUCH-HEALING PRAYER MODELS

1. <u>TOUCH-HEALING SPOKEN PRAYER ONE</u>. God, we thank you for your gift of life to _____ and your presence along her/his life's journey. We know that you are the Creator and Sustainer of all life and wish to bring wholeness to all persons. This person chooses the path that leads to wellness. Use my hands as a channel for your healing power. Heal _____ in body, mind, and spirit. Fill her/him with your love, joy and peace. We thank you for the healing that is taking place and that will continue until wellness is complete. Make us one with you and with each other. Amen.

2. <u>TOUCH-HEALING SPOKEN PRAYER TWO</u>. God, the Creator and Sustainer of all life, we thank you for bringing us together this day. We thank you for your sacred gift of life to _____. We thank you for all of her/his life experiences -- the struggles and failures, the pain and the hurt, the dreams and accomplishments, the love and the sharing -- for they have molded her/him into the person s/he is today. We know that you desire s/he be well and that you are far more willing to give than we are to receive. _____ chooses to accept your gift of life and opens herself/himself to your gift of health. Create in _____ a vision of a new day -- a day when s/he has been transformed and made whole.

God, I ask to be used as a channel of your healing power. My intention is for your healing energy to flow through me and be effectively utilized to make _____ well. God, heal _____ in body, mind and spirit and make her/him whole. Let this healing begin now and continue until wellness is achieved. Deepen our faith, our hope, our expectations, that your healing energy may be empowered. Attune us to _____'s needs and to her/his essence as a person. Grant her/him your love, joy and peace. We thank you for the healing that is taking place. We trust in you. Amen.

3. <u>TOUCH-HEALING SPOKEN PRAYER THREE</u>. God, heal _____ in body, mind and spirit and make her/him well. Amen.

4. <u>A SPOKEN PRAYER FOR THE HOSPITAL</u>. God, we are thankful for the doctors, nurses and other staff who are here to serve. Guide and sustain them as they care for _____. We accept their care in love and appreciation. Empower _____ with the ability to maintain control over his/her life and guide and sustain her/him until s/he is well.

Creator and Sustainer of all life, we ask you to fill _____ with your presence. Release his/her frustrations, fears and anger. Fill her/him with your love, joy and peace. _____, in God's name, be healed in body, mind and spirit and made whole. God, initiate the healing that is needed and let it continue until wellness results. Thank you for the healing which is taking place now. We accept it with deep appreciation. Amen.

5. A SPOKEN PRAYER BEFORE SURGERY. God, we thank you for the upcoming surgery that will permit _____'s body to heal itself. We thank you for the skills of each member of the surgical team. We trust them and securely place _____'s life in their hands. Guide them in the use of their skills as they successfully repair this body.

I pray that you will use me as a channel for healing. Let your healing energy flow into the surgical area, restore the organs in that area and fill them with life-giving oxygen. Enable all the cells of this body to fight for health as they communicate with each other. Protect this person from pain and bleeding during surgery and afterwards. Enable the surgical wound to heal quickly. Fill _____ with the calm of your presence. We rest in your care, knowing that you desire wholeness for _____. Amen.

TOUCH-HEALING FIRST AID

You may initially utilize touch-healing prayer for major medical emergencies. But remember that it can be used to supplement medical first aid treatment of minor medical trauma injuries, spinal conditions, osteoarthritis, benign breast lumps, bacterial and viral infections, headaches, sunburn, skin diseases, pain, toothaches and emotional pain. Practice will enable you to grow in competency and awareness.

A TOUCH-HEALING PRAYER SESSION MODEL

1. **Limit your earliest contacts to family and close friends.** Wash your hands before going to the healing encounter. Relate by being a friend. Focus upon the person's situation. Listen and sympathize. Avoid advice-giving.

2. After establishing relationship and trust, **request permission to offer touch-healing prayer.** Gaining access to people is the greatest challenge in touch-healing prayer. I do not know a best approach. Here is a suggested opener: *"I am concerned about you and would like to be helpful. There is evidence that prayer provides a significant energy for healing. May I pray with you?"* If the answer is in anyway positive, you can proceed.

3. **Enlist the healee's full cooperation.** Suggested question: *"Will you accept the power that God is offering through our prayer together?"*
Await the answer. This may be a time for assurances. Then make this statement: *"When we pray, God's healing power passes through the pray-er's hands. That energy of prayer is able to restore your depleted energy field and your physical body. This is a process that works like an antibiotic to make you well. Let us first work on your energy field. After the prayer, I am going to move my hands around your energy field."*

4. **Prayer and energy field work**. *"Let us pray."* Pause for five seconds and center yourself: *God, we thank you for your loving presence in our lives. May your loving presence be with us as we pray. I ask you to use me as a channel for _____'s healing. May your healing power flow through my hands. Thank you. Amen.*

If the healee is lying in bed, let him remain there. If not, ask the healee to stand. Pray: **"God, cleanse _____'s energy field."** Start at the head and move flattened palms and fingers of both hands in sweeping motions downward over the entire body to the feet from about one half inch away, from both front and back if the person is standing.

Then pray: **"God, restore and balance _____'s energy fields."** Now repeat this procedure with the intention of imparting healing energy.

5. **Energy field work**. Skip this unless it is for neurological, brain conditions, cancer or for emotional calming. Pray: **"God, continue to use me as a channel for your healing power. I let go and let you flow through me."** Make repeated cleansing sweeps with your hands about four inches from the head, covering the whole head area.

Then, balance/charge the brain energy fields in three steps: from four inches away, one inch away and touching. In each step place your hands at front and back, either side, and then on the nape of the neck and top of the head for about one minute each. Now tell the healee to be seated in a straight chair for *your* comfort. You must be in a comfortable position or your own body will ache. If the person is in bed, find a chair from which you can work comfortably.

6. **Touch contacts**. If the healee seemed uncomfortable with your energy field healing, back off a bit now by just holding one hand and gently touching some place else on the body. If the person is open to it, you have options. Touch on either side of the area needing to be healed. Or, hold one hand, touching the top of the head with the other. Or, touch the forehead and nape of neck. Or, cover every area of the torso, arms and legs with the flattened palms and fingers of both hands for fifteen seconds. After positioning your hands, offer a spoken prayer. A prayer model and inner dialogue are offered below.

7. **SPOKEN PRAYER AND INNER DIALOGUE DURING TOUCH-HEALING**. *"God, thank you for _____. Thank you for her/his birth and life, hopes and dreams. I am concerned for her/him. S/he wishes to be whole. Free the inner burden, the heaviness within her/him. Free her/him from the inner darkness and replace it with your marvelous love and light. Fill her/him with your peace and presence.*

"God, you are the creator and sustainer of all life. With you, all things are possible. Grant us faith and hope in your miracles of love. Heal _____ in body, mind and spirit. Recreate and renew every cell and organ of her/his body. Unite us with God, making us one in spirit. Thank you for the healing that is taking place. Amen."

A. <u>**Seek to form a spiritual oneness with the healee.**</u> Silently pray: *"God, make me one with _____ in body, mind, and spirit. Bless this unity that it might produce wholeness."* This is the healing trinity of God, you and the healee.

B. <u>**Become aware of your hands**</u>. Seek to transmit a healing energy with your hands while silently praying: *"God, use my hands to transmit your healing power."*

C. <u>**Mentally visualize the intended results,**</u> silently praying: *"God, enable _____ to be restored into your perfect genetic image."*

D. <u>**Visualize twin objects**</u> and merge them into one, with one object representing you and the other the healee.

E. With hands in place, <u>**talk with the healee in a conversational manner**</u>. The two most intimate and spiritual human interchanges are to touch and to talk. Doing this helps the attunement and utilization of the healing energy.

F. <u>**Concluding spoken prayer**</u>: *"God, fill _____ with your presence. Let this healing begin now and continue throughout the coming hours and days. Thank you for the healing that is now taking place. Amen."*

8. <u>**Afterward,**</u> thank the healee for praying with you. Ask if you can pray together again tomorrow. Be sure to stop the healing flow in your hands because it can deplete your personal energy. If possible, wash your hands, or clap your hands, or rub them vigorously together.

CHARGING MATERIALS WITH HEALING ENERGY

Water, cotton and wool cloth and surgical gauze can all be charged with healing energy. These have many practical applications. Healing-charged towels can be placed for long periods of time or continually on areas needing to be healed. Surgical gauze used for medical dressings can similarly be charged with healing energy. A gallon of water can be charged with healing energy and be ingested four times a day, two ounces at a time. The healing water then flows into every cell of the body, making it excellent for use in many diseases or for the healing of negative emotions.

The healing charge lasts up to two years, but dissipates in sunlight and extreme heat or with handling by others. You can charge your own medium by holding cotton dish towels or gauze dressings for ten minutes and water for twenty minutes. I usually charge materials immediately following a healing session because the healing flow is present and already attuned to the person. Ask the person to place the towel over the area needing healing as often as possible.

PRODUCING A TIME-RELEASE HEALING ENERGY CAPSULE

Several years ago, a French-Canadian healer showed me how to produce a time-release healing energy capsule. He offered a convincing demonstration of this, using me as the test subject. For all of my openness to new ideas, I initially rejected this procedure in my own practice of healing, seeing it as a unique skill that surely only this very talented psychic healer possessed. It was just too incredulous to believe that others could do it. I felt incapable of doing it, myself. Two years later, I began experimenting with time-release healing energy capsules with my own healing clients.

At the close of a touch-healing session, while your hands are still flowing with healing energy, cup your hands together and rotate them in opposite ways to produce an energy ball. Place that energy ball into the diaphragm of the healee with your healing hand with the expectation that it will release a constant supply of healing energy for a week. It will and does. It works for me. It may work for you.

CLINICAL STUDIES ARE THE NEXT STEP

This guidance is not the final word on the practice of touch-healing. It is the best we know at the present time. I envision the day when medical centers will routinely provide healers with opportunities for clinical studies. The studies will have to be carefully designed. Such studies could begin in the specific hospital units where conditions most responsive to healing exist. These include orthopedics, surgical units, trauma units, infant intensive care, coronary intensive care and the emergency room.

Negative thoughts, attitudes, beliefs and feelings short-circuit healing energy. One negative person can hinder the healing flow of any healer. Therefore, clinical studies must use a carefully chosen staff. The best design would hide the real purpose of the studies. A possible hidden design would be a "cover" explanation beginning in the pastoral care office. It might be called *The Calming Effects of Prayer upon Surgical Patients,* while its intentions would actually be for physical healing.

Once clinical results have been established, healers will need clinical studies for their own understanding and development. Healers have their own research priorities. For me these involve the energy frequencies and fields of specific diseases, changes in energy fields, the time needed to heal a specific condition, the best techniques, team-healing, the psychological condition of healees and the correlation of healer and healee personality types. All these issues will yield substantial results when explored in a clinically controlled setting.

Chapter Twenty-Five

Benefiting from Healing Services

"When minds are closed, they become impervious to reason."
...Jawaharlal Nehru

"So, faith, hope, love abide, these three; but the greatest of these is love." ...Corinthians 13:13

"Too much of a good thing is wonderful." ...Mae West

The public image produced by faith-healing services is a scandal for Christianity. No wonder most nations of the world established laws generations ago prohibiting spiritual healing. In the United States, all fifty states prohibit the professional practice of spiritual healing anywhere but in a church setting. It is probable that only constitutional protections of religious practices have kept faith-healing services from also being banned by law.

A few years ago, an American faith-healer was jailed in Germany for conducting a faith-healing service and released only when he agreed to leave the country. More recently an undercover policeman in Montreal, Quebec entrapped a healer who had offered his services. After the undercover policeman's third healing session, he offered a ten-dollar gift of appreciation. When the healer accepted the gift, he was jailed like a prostitute who offers her wares to a customer. The legal position is that professional healers are unscrupulous swindlers or scam artists, because they are offering no real benefits to their clients. The public image conjured by faith-healing services has helped to create this low opinion of healers. This has hampered the potential contributions of healers to all humanity.

Why all the fuss? The promised product, health, is seldom achieved. The magazine *Consumer Reports* would have to rate faith-healing product performance as extremely poor, and therefore, unacceptable, because less than one percent of those seeking healing in a faith-healing service are healed. Thus, most faith-healing services are guilty of fraudulent advertising claims. Or, are they? It is all in one's perspective.

The cure of illnesses resistant to medical treatment has not been the primary goal of most faith-healing services. For the sponsors, the primary goal of faith-healing services is religious, to increase the faith of the participants in the power of God. Few faith-healing ministries permit medical documentation of healings on the grounds that this would hurt the faith of believers. None keeps statistics on percentages healed. So, faith-healing remains a religious expression rather than the healing opportunity that the chronically and terminally ill are seeking.

Faith-healing services also promote the inaccurate public impression that healing occurs because of religious faith, and that healing is an instant magical act of God. These two images do not reflect the experimental scientific evidence. This is not to imply that faith-healers are dishonest. A few spectacular healings do take place. Most faith-healers would like their product performance record to be better. The statistical fact is that only one in six hundred to twelve hundred healings are instant healings. The steady message that one healing encounter will bring about a cure constitutes false advertising, fraud and irresponsibility.

If offering practical healing results is not their purpose, faith-healers need to advertise that fact to be ethical. It is sad to observe a hundred wheelchair-bound people, most of them children, present for cures, knowing they have only one chance in a thousand of being helped.

INCREASING THE HEALING RATE

How can faith-healers increase their healing rate? By going beyond the religious belief that God will somehow magically heal to becoming aware of the scientific data on how healing rates can be immensely improved. From PrayWell's perspective, the primary purpose of any attempt to offer spiritual healing is to bring about wellness or wholeness in the body, mind, spirit and relationships of each hurting person. To raise expectations falsely is wrong. To ignore the fact that healing is a process taking place over a period of many sessions is tragic. Scientific evidence requires a huge change in the way that spiritual healing is currently understood and practiced. Not to make changes in practice consistent with the evidence becomes both irresponsible and unethical.

For instance, when my mother, Hazel, broke her hip in July 1990, the physician predicted that normal healing would take ten weeks for an eighty-four-year-old woman. The clinical evidence indicated that if I wished to be truly helpful in assisting the medical treatment, I needed to offer her touch-healing prayer every other day. I did. To do otherwise would have been to act like Don Quixote, jousting uselessly at windmills. To see her only once a week would have been a waste of my time and a tragic abuse of her hope. I have had personal experiences of broken bones healing in a day or a week as a result of only one healing encounter. But I did not have the assurance of weekly x-rays in assessing the progress of the healing. The results from her first x-rays thirty-one days after her hip was set and pinned showed a complete healing of her hip. How long prior to that her hip had healed, we have no way of knowing.

Until spiritual healing has the full cooperation of health care professionals who will check the continuing progress of a condition, the conscientious healer must overdose healees with healing energy. Bernard Grad's experimental laboratory healer, Oskar Estebany, regularly cured overactive thyroid glands but he required the healees to receive five sessions of healing a week for six weeks. That is like taking thirty sessions of radiation treatment, but without any side-effects. Most acute, life-threatening and chronic illnesses currently must be treated in this cautious way.

SCIENTIFIC FACTORS BENEFITING HEALING SERVICES

Responsible healing ministries need to utilize the factors that research has shown to produce consistent healing results.

First, they must be able to create a powerful healing group energy field. The purpose is to enable everyone to have access to huge quantities of healing energy. This can be done by a healer who can act as a charismatic catalyst for this process, or through ritual.

Present evidence indicates that all healing services should be led by persons who represent the ENFJ personality type of Myers-Briggs Type Indicator, or who generate a constant 7.83-8.00 hertz energy. Rituals creating a coherent healing group energy field include group prayers and litanies, sacred songs, rituals and symbols.

The second factor involves the quality of the healing energy, the healing frequency. This is created by the combined individual knowledge, beliefs and intentions of each participant, which attunes the group energy field to the healing frequency. This information is contained within the healing energy created by religious ritual and the emotion of love. These then act intelligently to transform energy fields and produce health.

The factors creating a quality healing group energy field include the intentions and charismatic qualities of the leader, the expectations of the participants, religious rituals and symbols, compassion, faith, hope and trust, the religious maturity of the participants and a knowledge of how healing energy works. Only a few of these factors are necessary. Maximizing the number of factors present should increase healing results.

Cynical scoffers. The most negative factor in any healing encounter involves the presence of cynical scoffers. Cynical scoffers untune the healing energy frequency and diminish the power of group energy fields. All evidence indicates they are the major factor inhibiting healing results. The issue of cynical scoffers must be addressed in the earliest part of the healing service, or even before the service begins.

My style would involve a direct and loving encounter with all the cynical scoffers. Such an encounter would truthfully admit their potential negative influence on group energy field coherence and the healing frequency. Because they are rationally minded, I would then seek to rationally win their support by verbally drawing a scientific picture of what can occur with their cooperation. Because most cynical scoffers have never experienced a healing encounter, I would invited them to come forward to experience touch-healing prayer. Most of them would accept this invitation. I would then trust in sacred touch to transform them and alter their beliefs.

The third factor is to ensure that the ill actually receive the healing energy. Most healers have the ability to attune the healing energy to a few people, resulting in a few healings. The failure to attune to everyone produces the noted poor results. This is the greatest issue in spiritual healing.

Attunement is related to the state of at-one-ment, or emotional-mental-spiritual unity. This can be accomplished by many methods. Expressions of compassionate, non-judgmental, inclusive love permit the healees to know that they are loved, accepted and part of the whole. Personal involvement of the potential healees in sacred rituals and songs that speak to their needs is crucial. The same sacred rituals plus words from the healer lifting up the sacred worth of every person present are also important factors. Healers at their best are able to attune clairvoyantly to either the personality or the disease of the healee.

For at-one-ment or unity to occur, healing services need to avoid alienating the ill by their approach. The inclusion of political and moral issues repels many healees and this prevents their openness to healing. The lashing-out-with-a-smile at people and groups who are different is an expression of anger that restricts unity and compassion. The inclusion of rigid theological beliefs that are not necessary for healing to take place also alienates some, preventing many healings.

In a healing service consisting of like-minded participants, religious conversion can lead to some healing. My observation is that the conversion energy frequency is different from the healing frequency, though not necessarily so. This is true because all energy is information bearing and acts intelligently upon the basis of that information. If conversion information is equated with health and wholeness by both healer and healee, then healing can occur.

The fourth factor involves enabling the healees to receive and to utilize the healing energy effectively for their own healing. This calls for the conscious or unconscious opening of the healee's energy fields to the healing energy. This may be accomplished by opening the seven energy chakras as described in chapter twenty-two by taking the healing energy present and visualizing it entering body and going where it is needed.

Part of healing is an act of will, of wanting to become well. Becoming passive and yielding to God may help. This can happen with the simple prayer, *"God, I want to be well. I open myself to and freely accept this healing energy into my energy fields. Heal me in body, mind and spirit."* More healings might occur by providing personal prayers affirming this statement.

No research data is available in this area. This is the area where more clinical research is needed through the study of human energy field interactions with healing energy. Faith-healing ministries could also explore this, using in-depth interviews with healees to discover correlations between prayer-use and healing results.

A fifth factor is the need for all responsible healing ministries to bathe the ill in healing energy over an extended period of time. The healing energy is used up as it works and thus needs to be systematically replenished for healing to be completed. This can be accomplished through several means. Healing services can be offered at least three times a week. Individual touch-healing prayer sessions can be provided daily. Small touch-healing prayer groups can meet daily to work directly with the ill. My experience is that this is the best way to produce healing. The easiest way would be for all participants in a healing service to offer daily absent-prayer for healees. Some individuals may hold the limiting belief that the healer is the only one who can offer healing. To overcome their reservations, a healer can assure everyone that his healing gifts will be present in their prayers and actions.

In my healing work, I ask to see my clients at least three times a week. If this is not possible, I charge up a cotton dishtowel and a gallon of water with healing energy for clients to use between sessions. Clearly, we are talking about a significant time investment for practitioners of spiritual healing. Someone must pay for this time investment, unless the healer has an independent income. If Estebany had charged for thirty sessions at fifty dollars each, it comes out to fifteen hundred dollars -- a small long-term investment to produce a thyroid gland that operates normally.

Finally, providing wellness counseling or a wellness support group helps people deal with the emotional issues created by their conditions, and fosters their investigation of the mind-body connection. Wellness counseling can be provided by a healer. Wellness support can be provided by a touch-healing prayer group. Combining these functions is an efficient use of time and effort.

STYLES OF HEALING SERVICES

Healing services vary in style and most of these styles produce healing results. Within a local parish, the liturgical Christian traditions (Roman Catholic, Episcopal, Lutheran) are based upon formal liturgy that uses powerful rituals to provide divine power and unity. Of these, the Eucharist is the most powerful.

Perhaps because of my own informal religious tradition and a background in counseling and small-group work, I am an advocate of small, intimate healing services of twenty-five to two hundred people. In this setting, up to twenty percent can receive healings at any given service. This occurs due to many factors. Smallness permits inclusiveness, personal caring, a sharing of hurts and healings and an easier attuning of the healing group energy field.

If healing is the primary purpose, then healing ministries must offer specific aids responsibly. Prospective healees should be informed that healing is a process and that one-time attendees are not likely to achieve complete health. Ongoing attendance is a must. A participant in healer Kathryn Kuhlmann's services reported attending her forty-seventh service before healing occurred. Accountability calls for individual wellness counseling and healing sessions. Potential healees need to be given self-healing prayer directions as well as guidance for inviting loved ones to offer daily touch and absent prayer.

DESIGN FOR A SMALL HEALING SERVICE

1. **Plan a means for achieving close interpersonal encounters.** Everyone needs to experience individual love and caring. Healing services with more than twenty-five persons need to create ways to join people together into smaller groups. Support groups using prayer need to be broken down into groups of no more than eight or ten.

2. **Keep it informal and personal.** Welcome participants in a way that gives everyone an individual opportunity to be personally known. Have

each person introduce herself, tell why she has come, and share what is happening in her life. This may be a sharing of a personal hurt, and later on, a sharing of how God is healing her.

3. **Share your intentions at the beginning,** giving a detailed overview of what will follow. This should include short-and long- term goals.

4. **Sing sacred songs,** providing everyone with the tunes and words.

5. **Offer a prayer,** asking for God to be present in love and power.

6. **Ask people to share their healing needs.** Give them time to tell their stories.

7. **Ask people to share stories** of their recent healings.

8. **Briefly talk about healing** and explain how you are going to do it in this setting.

9. **Invite people to come forward** and either sit in a chair facing the congregation or kneel. If there are a number of clear channels for healing, use an equal number of chairs. Invite any loved ones present to come up along with the person to be healed. Give them the opportunity to place their hands on the healee. Offer individual prayers for those being healed.

NEGATIVE CHANNELS

Some persons may be smiling and cooperative, and yet act as negative channels for healing, doing more harm than good. These persons are filled with negativity, fear, anger, anxiety, inadequacy, sadness or egotism. It is wise to caution people. *"If you are filled with anger or other strong negative feelings, please do not take part in the healing."* These persons can usually be sensed ahead of time and gently excluded. This may sound cruel and exclusionary, but this intentional leadership is necessary.

Negative channels differ from cynical scoffers. Their intentions are usually good. They have come, wanting to offer healing. Offer the healing of emotions through Radiant Heart Therapy early in the practice of healing. If the practice of healing restores them to emotional health, they can safely be invited to assist in healing. This is both a loving and helpful approach

A DESIGN FOR A CONTEMPORARY HEALING SERVICE

1. **Begin with comedy**, using humor dealing with God, healing and illess. The goal is to create laughter, relaxation, and group unity.

2. **Sing songs,** using familiar tunes with song sheets available.

3. **Invoke God in prayer**. Use a pray-along prayer, with the leader saying each phrase and the congregation repeating it.

4. **Use symbols and rituals** evoking faith, love and hope in God, who seeks to renew everyone with his healing energy.

5. **Employ a ritual of introduction**. Ask everyone to talk to two people, introducing themselves and stating why they are present.

6. **Include a short talk** explaining spiritual healing with stories of healings.

7. **Sing a sacred song.**

8. **Share a healing story** from a person who has experienced healing in the past.

9. **Celebrate with an offering** or a ritual of sharing and commitment.

10. **Make available prayers to be used during healing.** Provide written copies of prayers for everyone and ask them to pray continuously throughout the healing time. Some prayer models for use during the service:

A. <u>A PRAYER FOR EVERYONE</u>: *God, come to our aid. Just as you created the universe, the planet Earth and all that is upon it, renew your creation here. Recreate each of us and make us perfect, even as you are perfect. We offer you our brokenness. Recreate and restore us, making us whole. We accept your power and presence in our midst. May your love, joy and peace fill us and make us new. God, come to our aid. Thank you. Amen.*

B. <u>A PRAYER FOR ONESELF</u>: *God, I have come anticipating miracles of love. I believe that healings will occur. Transform me that I might be a willing channel for your healing power. Fill this place with your power and love. Make us one with you and with each other. Thank you. Amen.*

C. <u>A PRAYER FOR OTHERS</u>: *God, I pray for your miracles of healing to occur all about me. I pray for persons who are hurting and ill. Enable them to be whole. I pray especially for ___. Heal them and make them whole in body, mind and spirit. Thank you. Amen.*

D. <u>A PRAYER FOR SELF-ATTUNING</u>. *God, I sense your presence and power all about me. I open myself to you. I let go of the darkness of the past and open myself to your marvelous light. Fill me to overflowing with your healing presence. I wish to be healed and accept the healing you offer. I need these healings _____ (name them). Please heal me and make me whole in body, mind and spirit. I seek to be one with you. I accept you into my life. Thank you for the healing that is beginning now and will continue until I am well. Make me one with you and fill me with your love, joy and peace. Thank you. Amen.*

E. <u>A PRAYER FOR ATTUNING TO GOD</u>. *God, I wish to be healed. I believe that nothing is too wonderful to be true. Enable a miracle to begin in me this day. I choose to be healthy and happy. Make me new and youthful as you restore every cell and energy field in my body. I open my painful memories to your touch. I forgive everyone who has ever hurt me, and I release the pain. I forgive myself for the pain I have caused myself and others. Please heal my past. I open my fears, angers, resentments, hurts and inadequacies to your touch. I release them to your care.*

Help me attune to your healing flow. I open myself to your presence and invite you to dwell within me. Enable me to be one with you. Flow throughout my being and wherever you touch, renew and restore me. Help me to get in touch with my sacred nature that I may be empowered and glow with your presence. Fill me with your love, joy and peace that I might be healed. I open my physical body to your touch. Wherever I am ill or out of balance, I ask that you restore me. I accept this healing. Let me be one with you and everyone present. Fill me with the unity of your Spirit and recreate your right spirit with-in me. I remain open to your love. Thank you. Let this be.

In some settings, a kneeling rail may be appropriate, but most services favor setting up chairs before the first row of seats facing the gathering. At first, only one chair may be needed. As the series of services continue, new persons who have become channels of healing will emerge. Invite them to take part. Provide in-service training for them. Keep adding healing chairs. Invite persons to come forward informally as chairs open.

If God's Spirit is powerfully present in the healing group energy field, people will not need to be touched for healing. An attuning healer can provide attuning of individuals or groups, or the healing of specific illnesses. Participants can also learn to attune themselves.

To build everyone's trust in the healing possibility, encourage people to share any healings immediately. Encourage people who sense healing after returning to their seats to come forward and share this with the leader. Have a microphone ready for an interview to share the witness being given.

12. **Pray for each other**. After the healing time, ask everyone to share in healing one another. Ask those who seek healing to raise a hand. This is to be done only by those who sense holiness and wholeness. Ask persons to gather around these healees, laying on hands and praying for healing simply by saying: **"In God's name be healed and made whole in body, mind and spirit. Thank you. Amen."**

13. **Give out postcards** to report later results or list a phone number to call to report. These reports can be used in several ways. The reporter can be asked to fill out *"Validation of a Healing"* record, including medical verification, for an ongoing *Registry of Healing Validations.* This registry provides a record of the evidence of the validity of that healing service for all consumers who might inquire. It would provide that healing ministry with patterns of conditions likely to be healed. It could also be used in a *National Registry of Validated Healings.* The reporter can also be asked to provide a verbal or reportable witness for a future service.

14. **Close with a sharing of love,** a song and a sending forth. Those who are seeking healing need to be encouraged to remain afterwards to make appointments for wellness counseling, prayer groups or individual healing sessions. Those who serve as channels of healing need to remain afterwards to meet with persons who have questions, comments and concerns. Refreshments may be served.

Chapter Twenty-Six

Therapeutic Prayer for Support Groups

[Including "A Course in Prayer"]

"Inward holiness is the true regulator of the outward life." ...Madame Guyon*

"Spiritual religion is based upon personal experience of the One who sustains our highest ideals, and is nourished by a mood of worship." ...D. Elton Trueblood*

"Essential though it is, reason cannot provide the answers we seek; on the contrary, the human desire for truth exposes the limitations of mathematics, science, and philosophy." ...Blaise Pascal

The impressive consequences of being bathed in healing group energy fields show that their use is ideal for support groups. Healing group energy fields are a revolutionary new tool for enhancing personal transformation and wholeness. When applied to existing effective support groups, the results will be nothing less than phenomenal.

My data indicates that when touch- and absent-healing prayer have been practiced in various prayer groups over a five-session period of time, 75% of participants reported physical healings, 83% reported emotional healings, 87% reported interpersonal healings and 95% reported experiencing the ongoing presence and peace of God. This percentage has been consistent among more than six hundred test subjects used in four urban communities, showing that the concepts provided in PrayWell are not just theory. They have been practically applied through seventeen years of field work with test groups. Self-help and other support groups can anticipate similar results.

Millions of Americans participate in support groups. They do this because they are hurting and have sought out proven help. Most support groups are for specialized hurts caused by alcohol, drugs, grief, divorce, rape, physical or sexual abuse, mental illness, cancer, multiple sclerosis, arthritis, etc. When persons love and care for each other in support groups, it enables participants to cope with their burdens and to begin traveling on the path leading back to wholeness.

There is another reason for the proven therapeutic effect These groups are already quietly creating and maintaining a group healing energy field through the love they share. This healing energy can be sensed throughout the meeting-room, as it produces an inner sense of calmness and well-being. If that weak group healing energy field could be strengthened intentionally, it would increase the effectiveness of the group immensely. It could have the spiritual power of a healing service. This spiritual power is capable of quickly transforming the inner nature of persons, producing wholeness. The best way to strengthen a group healing energy field is through the power of individual spoken prayer.

THERAPEUTIC PRAYER IS RELIGIOUSLY NEUTRAL

Some self-help groups follow the Twelve-Step Program established by Alcoholics Anonymous. Twelve-Step programs acknowledge dependence upon the Supreme Being and the need to surrender to this power-beyond-ourselves to become whole. They often engage in group prayers for healing by led one person. This approach does not have the power of individuals praying aloud for each other's specific needs. Nor does this make use of the forceful, intentional style of healing prayer that provides the best results. Therapeutic Prayer is a new style of prayer that is religiously neutral and thus appropriate for any therapeutic group. By using it, individual therapeutic pray-ers would increase the energy available for personal healing and wholeness. Adding individual touch-prayers to the above provides the most efficient means for transmitting healing energy.

Remember, the healing energy is information-bearing. The core information is produced by the intent of the group and empowered by love and prayer. The healing group energy field also contains God's creative-sustaining life purpose. The energy is additionally enhanced by the information making up the purpose, process and wisdom of the group. This information acts intelligently to transform, heal and empower participants.

The Twelve Steps of Alcoholics Anonymous have been appropriately altered in order to become the basis for many other types of support groups. The twelve steps of this spiritual wisdom can also be altered to fit the therapeutic needs of classrooms, communities and nations. They provide the purpose or Word for individual Therapeutic Prayers that might be included for the transformative process.

THE TWELVE STEPS OF ALCOHOLICS ANONYMOUS

1. We admitted we were powerless over alcohol -- that our lives had become unmanageable.
2. We came to believe that a Power greater than ourselves could restore us to sanity.
3. We made a decision to turn our will and our lives over to the care of God as we understood him.
4. We made a searching and fearless moral inventory of ourselves.
5. We admitted to God, to ourselves, and to another human being, the exact nature of our wrongs.
6. We were entirely ready to have God remove all these defects of character.
7. We humbly asked Him to remove our shortcomings.
8. We made a list of all persons we had harmed, and became willing to make amends to them all.
9. We made direct amends to such people wherever possible, except when to do so would injure them or others.

10. We continued to take personal inventory and, when we were wrong, promptly admitted it.
11. We sought through prayer and meditation to improve our conscious contact with God as we understood Him, praying only for knowledge of His will for us and the power to carry that out.
12. Having had a spiritual awakening as the result of these steps, we try to carry our message to alcoholics, and to practice these principles in all our affairs.

AN OVERVIEW OF THE GROUP DESIGN

Integrating individual spoken prayer into a support group requires breaking down the total group into smaller working units. Individuals work with a partner, in a small group of eight, and in the total group. In each context, each person is being coached in the skills of spoken prayer as a tool for healing. Weekly, individuals practice touch-healing with the partner, each person in the small group and the total group. Daily absent-prayer is offered for the specific needs of those in the small group. This permits a steady flow of healing energy for wholeness.

The first step is for each participant to choose a partner. Such partners should not be relatives or close friends; that way potential barriers to sharing hurts are eliminated. The partners are first asked to share hurts that need to be healed. They learn to pray with each other. They share their needs with the small group of eight and practice touch-healing weekly. When participants are ready, the same process occurs in the total group.

At both group levels, participants are asked to tell about healings that have taken place. At the beginning of the meeting, individuals describe healings that have been experienced since the last session. At the close of each session, healings that occurred during the session are shared. This reporting of results increases belief, faith, hope, trust and anticipation among the participants. It also fixates the improved conditions.

There are several reasons for forming smaller units within the larger one.

First, it is emotionally safer and educationally more effective to learn the new skills of spoken prayer and touch-healing first with one person and then in a small group. This especially benefits introverted and shy persons. Bypassing this process by having one person offer prayer for the total group will not produce high-level healing results. For maximum results, each person must learn the necessary skills individually. This adds to the total group energy and produces the skills necessary for absent-prayer.

Second, it permits the healing energy to be attuned to individual personal needs.

Third, it creates a far more powerful and information-laden group healing energy field.

Adding healing prayer to existing support groups will probably require major revisions of the group's format for about six sessions. Once the process is learned, inclusion will take about half an hour per session. This design meets the needs of a newly-created support group. It can also be used for the purpose of teaching individuals to pray. Asking participants to read <u>PrayWell</u> will save hours of group presentation time as well as providing a more complete picture of spiritual healing.

The results of using the Therapeutic Prayer process unfold gradually over a period of time. Inner calming will be noticed by most persons within a week. A few will make dramatic improvements in the first week or two. Most will need a full five or six weeks for a complete and permanent alleviation of all physical, mental, emotional, spiritual and interpersonal symptoms.

A few will become symptom-free but their conditions will not be cured. Without the continuous reception of healing energy, they will revert to lesser levels of wellness. They will require regular immersion in healing energy for years, or possibly a lifetime. For them, the healing energy acts as insulin does for diabetics, needed in daily doses to maintain a healthy energy field. This approach reflects the experience of members of Alcoholics Anonymous, who rely upon the support and energy of group meetings throughout a lifetime.

The following design for *A Course In Prayer* can be used in support groups, prayer groups, healing groups, community groups or by any four, eight or more persons who might wish to gather to take advantage of its beneficial effects. Use your own methods for promoting the use of *A Course In Prayer.*

A COURSE IN PRAYER

Session One

A. **Beginning.** Provide name tags, sheets of paper and pencils. Use movable chairs. One person needs to time activities and remind everyone when it is time to move on to the next activity.

B. **Welcome and an explanation** (5 minutes).

C. **Presentation One** on <u>PrayWell</u>. Summary (10 min.); full details (45 minutes).

D. **Pairing one**: Choose a person with whom to work. This is not your permanent partner. Face each other. **Assignment**: Talk about a personal experience in which prayer played a major roll (each talk 3 minutes - 6 minutes total).

E. **Pairing two.** Choose another person with whom to work. This is not your permanent partner. Face each other. **Assignment:** Discuss how you think prayer works and what is occurring in the healing encounter (6 minutes for pair). Then discuss this in the large group (10 minutes).

F. **Choose a permanent prayer partner**. Do **not** choose family or close friends for these reasons: There is deeper sharing of hurts among strangers. It prevents the existing pattern of one person dominating interaction. You are more likely to maintain daily prayer disciplines. Absent-prayer efforts become more realistic.

Interview your partner. Get acquainted. Tell your partner who you are. Your partner may ask questions. If the group operates in privacy, use only first names and feel free to limit information that would reveal your identity. Make notes. You'll need this data later to introduce your partner to your group of eight (each talks 3 minutes - 6 minutes total).

G. **Choose another twosome.** With your partner, choose another two-some. Say hello to each other by first name. Sit in a circle. **Assignment**: Discuss what brings you happiness (2 minutes each - 8 minutes total).

H. **Choose your prayer circle.** Your foursome joins with another four-some. Sit in a circle. This is your Prayer Circle with whom you will be working.

Assignment: Introduce your prayer partner to your circle members. Include not only what you have been told, but also what you have observed. After each introduction, circle members can ask their own questions. Use a full sheet of paper to write down each name, spacing between each for eight names (2 minutes each - 10 minutes total).

Example: *"My prayer partner is Tom. Tom is married with three grown children. Tom is in sales. Tom tends a garden in the summer and bowls in two winter leagues. He is very outgoing and easy to talk to. He is a bit skeptical about what we are attempting to do but he would like to believe in the predicted results. Tom is a recovering alcoholic and he has been in AA for ten months."*

J. **Affirming by name.** This builds group cohesiveness and establishes good feelings. Each person states, **"My name is _____."** Then everyone in the circle responds in unison, **"Your name is _____."** Proceed around the circle (2 minutes).

K. **Alone with prayer partner. Purpose**: To share a major hurt that needs to be healed, so that prayer can be offered.
* Healing needs are confidential information to be shared only in one's own circle. Later, it is a person's own decision whether to share his/her needs and prayer results with others in the total group.
* Focus upon your personal needs and no one else's.
* If you wish to be healed, please be honest about your needs. Once a man gave his need as having to deal with his uncontrollable anger. His anger was healed, but he complained at the last session that his back still hurt. He had never mentioned this. Prayer at that session healed his back.
* Nothing is impossible. We have no laboratory data indicating any limitations upon the effects of God's healing energy. Situations given for possible healings include physical conditions or illness, painful memories and emotions, interpersonal alienation, addictions, compulsions and phobias, mental illness, detrimental personality traits, criminal and delinquent behavior, sexual dysfunctions, job needs, school motivation and mental concentration. Make written notes on your partner's responses.

Questions to your partner.
   1. Tell me about yourself.
   2. What brings you happiness and satisfaction?
   3. What brings joy to your life?
   4. Where are you struggling in your life?
   5. Does any personal condition hamper your life? What is it?
   6. Do you have pain in any part of your body? Please explain.

Example of need. *"I have painful arthritis in both knees and my right shoulder. My daughter and I do not get along. I am struggling with a weight problem.*

Clarification. Help your partner clarify his/her needs. Write them down. Accept only the needs of your partner, not a loved one of your partner. Others may be included at a later time.

Rephrasing for prayer. Now rephrase needs in a positive way. What end results are desired?

Return to the larger group. Write down and understand your homework assignment that prepares you for Week Two.

HOMEWORK ASSIGNMENT FOR WEEK TWO

1. **Read these chapters in <u>PrayWell</u>:** _____

2. **Offer absent-prayer daily for your prayer partner**. Set apart a specific time of day for praying for your prayer partner. Begin tomorrow. Most persons forget it for a few days. If you do, then begin when you remember. But be reminded, your prayers have an effect that is not present when you do not pray.

   Daily prayer model for your use during the week: *"God, I thank you for my prayer partner. I hold ____ in your love and light."*

   Then imagine a picture of your prayer partner held in the midst of God's love and white light. Alter the following model for your prayer partner's needs.

   "God, I pray for ___ knees and right shoulder. May he and his daughter once again love and respect each other. Help ____ lose weight. Thank you for the healing that is taking place. Amen."

3. **Find two persons to pray with during the week**. Use a prayer you know from your own religious tradition. Christians might use the Lord's Prayer. If you look at the wording, you will discover that the Lord's Prayer is a non-religious prayer which people of other faiths might feel comfortable in using.

   Approach each person, saying something like, *"I am taking a course in prayer and need your help for my homework assignment. I am learning to pray out loud. Will you let me hold your hand and be silent while I pray? I might goof up because I have never done this before so please bear with me."*

   This may be one of the scariest moments of your life. Stage fright is normal. Many persons forget well-known prayers. Laugh at your own mistakes. You are learning, no matter how you do. When you have done it twice, you will feel a sense of accomplishment. This is the toughest assignment you will have.

The Lord's Prayer: *Our Father, who art in heaven, hallowed be thy name. Thy kingdom come, thy will be done on earth as it is in heaven. Give us this day our daily bread. And forgive us our trespasses as we forgive those who trespass against us. And lead us not into temptation but deliver us from evil. For thine is the kingdom and the power and the glory, forever. Amen.*

4. **Contact your prayer partner** once in midweek. Ask how s/he is doing.

Session Two

A. **Welcome** (5 minutes).

B. **Presentation Two on PrayWell**. Summary (10 minutes); full details (45 minutes).

C. **Be seated in your Prayer Circle**. Is everyone present? Fill in for missing prayer partners with newcomers. Form new circles with newcomers (3 minutes).

D. **Homework report**. With your prayer partner, discuss your homework experiences. How many days did you pray for your prayer partner? How do you feel about that experience? Did you sense that you were being prayed for? Did you pray with two people? How did you do? Was it helpful (7 minutes)? Then discuss this with your Prayer Circle (5 minutes).

E. **Give your Prayer Circle a name**. Discuss names. Reach a consensus. Write the name down (10 minutes). Share your circle name with the total group (3 minutes).

F. **With Prayer Partner**. Have your prayer needs remained the same? Would you like to alter them? If so, in what way (5 minutes)?

G. **Write a prayer addressing your partner's needs** (30 minutes). Use information from last week.
   1. Address God and praise him as the source of all wholeness.
   2. Acknowledge the person's sacredness and preciousness.
   3. Acknowledge the hurt. Sympathize with your partner's situation. State this clearly. This might involve fear, hurt, pain, sacrifice.
   4. State your intentions by clearly expressing the needed positive results.
   5. Offer a healing blessing.
   6. Offer a spiritual blessing.
   7. Thank God for the wholeness which is taking place.

The following prayer example is lengthy for three reasons. It explores the whole range of possibilities in healing prayer. As a learning tool, it provides you with maximum complexity. It places you in prayer long enough to yield healing results. This example is an expression of the author's personality, experience and beliefs. You are free to alter this style to express your unique self while keeping the directive forceful style of healing prayer.

A PERSONAL TOUCH-PRAYER MODEL

1. Address and praise God: *God, we praise you for your creative and sustaining presence in the universe. We thank you for your love that is the basis of all life. We know that you are far more willing to give than we are to receive. Enable us humbly and joyously to accept all your gifts. Be with us as we pray.*

2. Affirm the person's relationship with God: *We thank you for your gift of life to _____, for your presence along his life's journey, for the struggles and the celebrations that have molded him into the person he is today, and for sustaining him along the way.*

3. Affirm the person's uniqueness: *We thank you for ____ and for the love he so generously shares.*

4. Acknowledge the hurt: *God, _____ has hurts that need to be healed. He finds the clashes with his daughter to be painful. He is frustrated by his inability to lose weight. His knees and shoulder hurt.*

5. Clearly state your intentions: *God, I ask you to use me as a channel for healing. Let _____ be made whole. He wishes to live life to its fullest -- to be able to enjoy family life, to work and play, to express joy and happiness, to offer love and caring to others and to be whole.*

6. Offer a healing blessing: *God, heal _____'s arthritis, enabling him to be pain-free and have full joint movement as you restore his body. Remove the barriers between ____ and his daughter that they might grow closer and share affection. Free ____ from the barriers that keep him from losing weight. As he diets. enable the pounds to drop accordingly. Heal him in body, mind and spirit, making him whole.*

7. Offer a spiritual blessing: *God, fill _____ with your love and light, that he might rejoice in the journey. Bless him that he might become a blessing to others.*

8. Thank God for the wholeness that is taking place: *Thank you, God, for your love that is restoring ____ and making him whole. May your presence abide with ____ now and forever. Amen.*

Write your prayer, and then go back and rewrite it with more clarity and forcefulness. Read the prayer four times to yourself so that it comes naturally to you.

H. **Touch prayer with your partner** (12 minutes). Each partner takes a turn. Remember, touch is the most efficient means of transmitting healing energy. Have your partner be seated. Decide how you wish to touch. Some options: Sitting and holding partner's hands, standing behind and placing your hands upon partner's shoulders, or standing at partner's side and placing hands on forehead and nape of neck. All styles work.

Offer the prayer. Say, **"Let us pray."** Pause. Attempt to be one with God and your partner. Then, begin your prayer. You may read it. When you have finished, touch your partner and gently attempt to transmit healing energy. Do not force it. Be almost passive in withdrawing yourself and permitting the energy to flow through you. While doing so, pray silently or aloud, **"God, heal _____ in body, mind and spirit."** Visualize the intentional healing results; perfect health where needed.

I. **Prayer Circle sharing** (10 minutes). Let each person share briefly how they felt about praying and receiving prayer.

J. **Share your needs in your Prayer Circle** (15 minutes). Each person shares her/his prayer needs with circle members. Write down each of the prayer requests under the proper name.

HOMEWORK ASSIGNMENT FOR WEEK THREE

1. **Finish reading PrayWell**

2. **Pray with one person during the week.** Possible words used in approaching a person: *"I am taking a course in prayer through PrayWell. I need your help in learning to pray. Will you let me write a prayer for you? This will help me learn to pray. This involves interviewing you about your needs, preparing the prayer and then returning to pray aloud with you."* Write the prayer, using the form above.

Return to the person, saying something like, *"I have written this prayer for you. Because I am new at this, I may need to read it. May I hold your hand while I pray with you?"*

Have your written prayer before you. By this time, you will be familiar with what you have written and will probably not need to look at your written prayer. You may be tense. That is normal in any new venture. Remember, pausing in the midst of prayer is normal. It comes through as the thoughtfulness it is.

Say, *"Let us pray."* Pause for several moments of inner quiet and centering upon God. Ask God's guidance for your prayer. Then offer the prayer. Afterwards, thank your companion for letting you pray.

There is rarely a negative reaction to a personal prayer. If you sense one, explore it. Say, *"I sense that I may have touched a tender nerve; I may have said something during the prayer that upset you. Will you help me to understand what happened?"* This will be a learning experience. Two sources of negative reactions come to mind. The person believes you have used the prayer to manipulate or control him. Or the person is not ready to recognize his or her hurts and the need to be healed.

3. **Daily pray for members of your Prayer Circle.** Set aside the same time each day. Daily seek to use the same quiet, private location, which then becomes sacred space. Prepare for prayer by releasing feelings of being rushed, by stretching, by deep breathing and inner quieting. Regard this intercessory or absent-prayer time as an exciting adventure. Anticipate the blessings your prayers are bringing others.

Absent-prayer for several persons need not be detailed. The following model will help you begin. You will soon develop your own style. Place the list of prayer needs before you. Center yourself in God's presence.

A DAILY ABSENT-PRAYER MODEL

God, thank you for the precious gift of life. Please guide me as I pray. Use me as a channel for healing. I care about these people and ask you to bless them. I pray for the following persons to receive your wholeness. Heal them in body, mind, and spirit.

I pray for _____. Heal his arthritis and restore his body. Remove the barriers that exists between ____ and his daughter and build bonds of understanding and affection. Remove all barriers to _____ losing weight. Heal him in body, mind, and spirit, making him whole.

I pray for ____. (Continue with specific requests throughout your circle. Then close.) *God, thank you for the healing that is taking place in these persons. Make me one with you and each person for whom I have prayed. Bless me that I might become a blessing to others. Amen.*

This long prayer form is a learning tool. It teaches you patience about prayer. It makes you aware of specific personal pain. It names your intent. With practice, all of these qualities can be included in a much briefer form.

4. Contact your prayer partner once in midweek.

Session Three

A. **Welcome** (5 minutes).

B. **Presentation Three on PrayWell.** Summary (10 minutes); full details (45 minutes).

C. **Total group sharing** (10 minutes). Gather into prayer circles and share in the total group. Ask, *"How many of you prayed at least four days this week. How are you doing with prayer?"*

D. **Prayer partners** (10 minutes) Share how prayer is affecting your life.

E. **Prayer Circle praying** (30 minutes). Circle members will pray with each person in the circle. Place a chair in the middle of the circle on which the prayee sits. The prayer partner touches the prayee however he chooses. He offers the first prayer for the prayee. Then each circle member offers a brief prayer for the prayee. You may remain seated or rise and touch the prayee while praying. **Some brief prayer models:**
"God, heal ____ and make him whole."
"God, bless ____ with your love, joy, and peace. I hold him in your presence."
"God, I am feeling deep love for _____. I rejoice in the healing that is coming with your presence among us."
"God, I praise and thank you for the love present among us. Enable it to heal _____ in body, mind, and spirit."
"Make us one with you, one with each other, and one with ourselves."

"Thank you for the healing that is taking place."

F. **Expanding Prayer Circle requests** (10 minutes). Add other prayer requests about family and friends of circle members. Write these down and add them to your absent-prayer list.

G. **Total group** (10 minutes). Has anyone experienced? Please tell about it.

HOMEWORK ASSIGNMENT FOR WEEK FOUR

1. **Finish reading <u>PrayWell</u>.**

2. **Pray with one hurting person during the week.** Make an appointment to visit someone who is hurting because of illness, grief, divorce, loneliness, etc. Have a friendly visit. Care in normal ways. Avoid advice-giving. If s/he mention her/his hurt, listen sympathetically.

Before leaving say this: *"I am just learning to pray. I would like to have a prayer with you if you don't mind my stumbling a bit."*

Naturally take his hand. Say, *"Let us pray."* Pause for several moments of inner quiet and centering on God. Offer the prayer, including only information or observations that you observed. You have offered a service and are acting as an equal.

3. **Continue daily absent-prayer.** Use the same approach as you did last week with detailed prayers for your circle. With the additional prayer requests, you need not be specific. As you pray for these, simply say,

"God, I pray for you to heal the following persons in body, mind, and spirit: _____." If you choose, you can add the intentions for each through visualization or holding their names in God's light.

4. **Contact your prayer partner** once in midweek.

Session Four

A. **Welcome** (5 minutes).

B. **Group discussion** of <u>PrayWell</u> (20 minutes).

C. **Prayer Partner** (10 minutes). With prayer partner, discuss your homework experiences. How many days did you pray for circle members and added persons? How do you feel about that experience? Did you sense being prayed for? Did you pray with a hurting person? How did you do? Was it helpful (7 minutes)? Then discuss these with your Prayer Circle.

D. **Prayer Circle** (15 minutes). Individually share any healings that have occurred in your life since beginning the Course in Prayer.

F. **Total Group Soaking Prayer** (60 minutes). A microphone may be helpful. Gather the larger group in a circle or in concentric circles. Place seven chairs in a circle within the larger circle, with the eighth chair in the center. One prayer circle begins by sitting one member in the center chair. The prayer partner offers touch-healing prayer for the prayee in the center chair. Then those who choose may offer prayers. Pray-ers may either sit in place or stand and touch prayee. After each person in a prayer circle has received prayer, another circle replaces them. This continues through all circles.

G. **Total Group sharing of healings experienced** (15 minutes).

HOMEWORK ASSIGNMENT WEEK FIVE

1. **Pray with a loved one during week**. In the normal course of the week, as you relate with family and friends, seek an appropriate opportunity to offer a prayer. This could be before a shared meal, at bedtime, following the expression of a hurt, or just to celebrate life together. Guidance can be found in the next chapter.

2. **Continue daily absent-prayer.**

3. **Contact prayer partner** once in midweek.

Session Five

A. **Welcome** (5 minutes)

B. **Group discussion** of PrayWell (20 minutes).

C. **Prayer Partner** (10 minutes). Discuss your relationship, experiences, and healings during *A Course in Prayer.*

D. **Prayer Circle** (15 minutes). Discuss your relationship, experiences, and healings during *A Course in Prayer.*

E. **Written evaluation of the five sessions.**

F. **Total Group Soaking Prayer** (60 minutes). Same procedure as last week

G. **Total group sharing of healings experienced** (15 minutes).

H. **Future options discussed** (10 minutes).

1. **Existing support group**. Discuss a continuing relationship with your prayer partner, prayer circle and the total group.

2. **Newly created support or prayer group**. Invite others to join you. Expand your activities by developing prayer within your family, adding prayers to schools, workplace and community, and sponsoring other courses in prayer.

3. **Integrate new persons** by going through *A Course of Prayer* in a new group of four, six, or eight, or by merging them into an existing circle with tutoring in *A Course in Prayer.*

PRAYWELL

THERAPEUTIC PRAYERS FOR RENEWAL

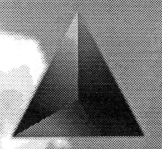

PART FOUR

THE ENERGY OF PRAYER RESTORES GOD'S PURPOSE TO CHAOS

The universe is running down. Natural disasters occur at random through out our planet, killing millions of people every year. Random accidents kill millions each year. Crops fail because of various weather conditions and millions of people starve. As one Christian hymn states, *"Death and decay, all around I see."*

The social order is collapsing into chaos. Acts of violence are soaring throughout the world. Dysfunctional marriages and families abound. Alcohol and drug dependencies have reached plague-like proportions. AIDS is the leading killer of young men in the United States and immune disorders are skyrocketing in number as our polluted environment causes our bodies to decay.

"Death and decay, all around I see; O Thou, who changeth not, abide with me." Why would we need to have God abide with us? Because in eternally not changing, God's energy provides a blueprint for divine purpose and unity that you can depend upon to restore your life and the life of Earth.

The scientific case for the use of the energy in prayer has been stated. Prayer produces the optimum conditions for life. Prayer enables the Creative Force to continue renewing all life on Earth. Prayer stops entropy -- chaos -- the running down of the physical Creation by reprogramming chaos with divine purpose. When chaos is controlled by the intentions of prayer, good things happen to people and to our planet. And the energy of God's good purposes overcome the evils of the world.

Prayer concentrates life energy through the intentions of the pray-er. Prayer transforms, renews and empowers individuals and groups. Groups empower prayer by the square of the number of people involved. In prayer, the Word and the Spirit work together to transform and make all the physical creation new.

Prayer can restore the loving energy of dysfunctional people, marriages, families, communities and nations. Prayer can bring order to chaos by restoring good purpose to the basic fabric of all energy and matter on Earth. God makes all things new. Group prayer, God and life energy can produce a Golden Age for all humanity.

One example is clear. All relationships tend to lose their good energy with the passage of time. The love and passion of a marriage tend to deteriorate from the wedding day onward. The only action that restores the original love and passion is Therapeutic Prayer. This is explained in the next chapter.

Part Four provides practical tools for renewal. It does this through the Word of God as expressed in words and the Spirit of God. The Spirit gives the Word life, making the Word come alive and act creatively and intelligently. The Word and the Spirit combine through the simple act of prayer.

May your marvelous adventure into prayer bring you joy and renewal.

Chapter Twenty-Seven

Therapeutic Prayers for Personal Renewal

"We seek happiness but cannot find it apart from a faithful relation to God." ...Blaise Pascal*

"Love alone is capable of uniting living beings in such a way as to complete and fulfill them. For it alone takes them and joins them by what is deepest in themselves." ...Teilhard de Chardin

"Love is patient and kind; love is not jealous or boastful; it is not arrogant or rude. Love does not insist on its own way; it is not irritable or resentful; it does not rejoice at wrong, but rejoices in the right." ...I Corinthians 13:4-6

When my wife and I began praying aloud daily for each other's needs, the beneficial results began immediately. The quality and depth of our relationship noticeably improved. The rough edges disappeared. Bickering, irritations and blaming ended. Intimacy levels deepened, with the quality and quantity of personal sharing improving dramatically. We resolved our disagreements more easily. Our love, companionship, passion and commitment achieved new heights. These wonderful results have continued for ten years.

This should come as no surprise to those who have read the research data. A side-effect of healing prayer is an inner sense of calmness, accompanied by the presence of God. This side-effect amazingly increases personal happiness and satisfaction in ways never before dreamed. With God's presence and peace, dramatic transformations begin. Painful memories are healed. Negative emotions disappear. Troubled relationships dramatically improve. The forceful, intentional style of Therapeutic Prayer produces these effects consistently and intensely.

This chapter utilizes our knowledge of prayer in seeking to restore health and happiness to individuals, marriages and families. The intentionally directed energy in prayer produces dramatic transformations in individuals and between family members -- transformations that appear miraculous in nature. The Apostle Paul said, *"Christ makes all things new."* Nowhere is this statement more true than in this context.

God's presence in prayer enhances the quality and satisfaction of human life. Religiously speaking, God's presence transforms and renews, making one whole in body, mind and spirit. Scientifically speaking, God's presence restores and strengthens the human energy fields, causing mental, emotional, physical and interpersonal wholeness. Prayer reprograms chaos with purpose.

Praying together enhances personal relationships. This results for several reasons. When two or more persons gather in prayer, God's power (or the healing energy) is the square of the number gathered. Their individual energy fields combine and form a group energy field that is filled with God's presence and with the intentions expressed in prayer. After repeated Therapeutic Prayer sessions, this energy permeates all the physical objects of each room, bathing anyone who enters with this information-bearing, intelligently-acting energy. One has created sacred space or a holy place in one's home. The energy works to create optimum health and high quality personal relationships.

In addition to enhanced personal and family relationships, God's presence also produces an inner calmness. It heals frayed nerves and negative emotions. It reconciles persons and deepens relationships by lowering dividing barriers and building trust. Responsibility naturally develops in individuals and families. A calm pervades the home. There is an increase in personal energy and purpose.

Those struggling with stressful situations or moral issues sense a sustaining and guiding Presence. Those praying together become more understanding and accepting. They draw emotionally closer and naturally support each other in love. Over a period of time, a healing of compulsive, obsessive and addictive behaviors may occur. In times of crisis, prayer restores strength and wisdom.

The content expressed in prayers also acts intelligently to produce prayer results. When caring thoughts and words are expressed in prayer, they are empowered. Affirmations make us feel better, but affirmations expressed in prayer are spiritually empowered. They transform us and change the reality around us. This process usually takes place over a period of time, but it can also occur suddenly.

We have discovered something new. Therapeutic prayers can change people far more effectively than a counseling session. Having said this, I must add that many troubled relationships still need the help of a counselor in addition to therapeutic prayer.

A PERSONAL EXPERIENCE IN PRAYER

An example from my own personal experience may prove helpful. During the early years of marriage, my personal prayer life was private. When our children were at home, we did have table grace before the evening meal. During special holy seasons we daily shared family devotions after dinner. But the children never fully appreciated this and it brought little satisfaction to any of us. This experience probably parallels that of many families with good intentions. In hindsight, I now realize that my traditional approach to family prayer was unworkable. At that time, I held no understanding of the significance of healing prayer.

All this changed following my participation in a prayer conference where former Roman Catholic priest Francis MacNutt convincingly persuaded me of the value of sharing spoken prayer in a family setting. (See Francis MacNutt, Prayers That Heal, Ave Marie Press.)

MacNutt teaches a concept that is so simple and yet so profound. He states, *"Pray for one another's needs."* I was electrified by his simple statement. It hit me like divine revelation. He went on to state that a survey of the one hundred thousand people annually attending his prayer workshops indicates that only one couple in a hundred has ever prayed aloud together for each other's needs. That statistic includes clergy couples, my wife and myself included.

MacNutt has devoted his entire professional life to the ministry of spiritual healing. I have, too. But he had made a connection I had not. As a pastor, I had prayed for the needs of the ill, the dying, the grieving and other hurting persons, but not for my own family's needs nor my own. My family prayers had been vague, with no focus. Once stated, the fact was so obvious: God's prayer healings apply to everyday living.

Using prayer to focus upon both human needs and divine guidance would make prayer more fulfilling. God's presence would deepen family relationships and produce greater satisfaction and wholeness. There is an energy in prayer that enhances all life, including family life. Whether he knew it or not, what MacNutt was advocating was the style of praying involved in healing prayer.

When I returned home from that conference, my wife eagerly embraced my suggestion of daily prayer for each other's needs. It fulfilled a deep mutual yearning. We were both experienced vocal pray-ers so we did not have to learn the mechanics. Like millions of couples, our nightly bedtime ritual had been to hug, peck kiss, say *"Goodnight!"* and then turn over to sleep. A simple additional ritual produced a miraculous change in our overall lives. We added vocal prayer addressing our needs and those of other family members.

We first did a full body embrace (touched) and then vocally prayed for our needs and the needs of others. Then came the first surprise. We were provided with a graphic demonstration of the existence of the seven major energy vortices, the chakras. From that first night on, we felt heat emanating from all the torso chakras during our prayers.

Surprise number two dramatically emerged. The beneficial results began immediately the next morning. The quality and depth of our relationship noticeably improved. The rough edges disappeared. Bickering, irritations and blaming ended. Intimacy levels deepened with the quality and quantity of personal sharing improving dramatically. We resolved our disagreements more easily. As veterans of the marriage enrichment movement, we suddenly integrated what we had learned, and began to utilize it constructively. Our love, companionship, passion and commitment achieved new heights. Our souls were energy linked -- the two of us one spirit.

That did not mean that everything remained blissful in this new Eden, and that we have lived happily ever after. Several years into our prayers, we experienced a fall from grace. A crisis came upon us with the suddenness and fury of a raging tornado. Maybe we became too confident of the strength of our relationship and our loyalty to each other. Conflicting demands were made, rage and bewildering distrust divided us and our prayers together ended -- a victim of the games of marital warfare.

The first mutual agreement of our eventual reconciliation was to restore our daily prayers. In shame, we stood, our souls naked before God, and prayed for the chance to re-enter paradise. Vocal prayer once more opened the gates to us. Prayer healed our hurts. Praying together pro-

duces healthy human energy fields, creates a bonding of unity and facilitates understanding, reconciliation, healing and growth in relationships.

THERAPEUTIC PRAYERS

Therapeutic Prayers express caring. They are religiously neutral or universal. Because of their universal nature, persons of all religious beliefs
can use them. This also means that families whose members come from
diverse religious traditions and differing beliefs can use them without fear of
conflict or embarrassment.

PREPARING FOR YOUR PRAYER JOURNEY

This chapter provides prayer models for individuals, children, youth, families, couples, singles, senior citizens, college students and military personnel. These prayer models are meant for temporary use until persons learn
their own style of praying. They have been provided to overcome the
mental and emotional barriers to praying together vocally. These barriers
include not knowing how to pray with others, not having the needed words
for prayer, taboos against vocal prayer with others, resistance to family
members who seek to initiate such prayer and disbelief in the possibility of
a satisfactory experience. These prayer models are divided into specific
sections: table graces, daily prayers for various persons, special occasion
prayers and crisis prayers.

Pray vocally. When praying with others, everyone is encouraged to
pray vocally. This addresses an essential issue of group prayer -- wandering
minds. When everyone is praying, all are focused and all are contributing
to the energy and intention of the prayer. Provide copies of the prayer for
each person. When you are ready to develop your own prayers, consider
making copies of your prayers so that everyone can pray them aloud with
you.

Pray-along prayer. An alternative to group prayer is pray-along prayers. With these, the prayer leader voices the prayer in brief phrases that
are repeated by everyone phrase by phrase. This style is especially recommended when praying with children who do not yet read, with persons
who may be illiterate, with the sightless and with persons who may be too
weak to read.

I first learned of pray-along prayer while praying with hurting people.
They wanted to join me in saying a prayer or a scripture passage. Most often, we prayed the Lord's Prayer. I would say a phrase and they would repeat it. These were far more rewarding experiences than my saying the
prayer for both of us.

Re-use prayers. If you find a specific prayer that meets your needs,
feel comfortable in memorizing it and using it regularly. My father has used
the same meaningful table grace for more than sixty-five years. My wife
and I use about three-fourths of the same phrases in our daily evening
prayer. Most religions effectively utilize rituals and prayers that have been
repeated over and over by believers throughout the centuries.

Use your own tradition. In a similar context, when praying with others
of your own religious tradition, you are encouraged to add your own meaningful names for God and any traditional prayer openings, closings and

rituals. When praying with persons from other faith traditions, if possible, discuss your mutual sensitivities prior to prayer. Using the provided prayer models should provide an acceptable religious neutrality.

Begin praying alone. If you wish to involve your loved ones in prayer, it would be helpful to first begin your own prayer journey alone. You can pray alone any time and any place you choose. I pray, not because God needs my prayers, nor to be religious, but simply because prayer enables God to help me in practical ways. In other word, my prayers are therapeutic prayers that restore me. I pray before each meal, whether alone or with others, in both private and public places. I pray mornings alone, asking God to guide and bless what is before me during the day. I pray at bedtime with my wife. I also offer other prayers throughout the day.

Pray regularly. I do not save prayer for just the most important issues or occasions. I pray alone before meeting with a person, that it may go well, or before beginning to write on my word processor, to be more creative, or for guidance. I pray with the ill and the hurting. When approaching an area where car parking spaces are rare, I pray for an open space. You have complete control over your choice of time, place and appropriateness.

REQUESTING COOPERATION

Praying with loved ones can be difficult. That is one of the reasons for church prayer groups. Many loved ones have no interest in praying. In seeking cooperation, you must first receive their consent. Begin by saying something like, *"I have a growing need for prayer. I have come to understand that prayer provides an energy for living that enriches everyone involved. Would you join me in prayer for a week to see if praying together is workable for us? Then we can evaluate whether we choose to proceed. I have found a book that provides guidance."*

If the answer is *no*, drop it. Do not plot or manipulate to get what you desire. If one or more persons agree, then let those who agree participate. At mealtimes, let those who decline just watch passively. If at least one other is cooperating, then ask any others to help by being silent while praying aloud. If you wish to pray only before meals, silently pray on your own. Do not ask others to do anything different. Let them talk or begin eating while you pray silently.

REACHING AGREEMENTS

After receiving the cooperation of others, you must reach agreements on when and where to pray. It will be up to you to offer a plan. Suggest a prayer before each meal you eat together plus one other prayer in the morning or at bedtime. Negotiate. The location of mealtime prayers is normally at the table. Try to agree upon one specific location for the other prayer. As a spouse or parent, receiving the cooperation of others is fairly easy. Achieving this in other relationships could take more time.

YOUR ROLE AS LEADER

You are the leader. Since you have initiated prayer, you remain responsible for providing leadership in most situations. People need leaders in prayer. Once a leader appears who seems to know more about prayer than they do, most persons welcome the leadership and are pleased to take part. Many people have wanted to do something like this with loved ones for a long time but did not know how to begin. You will need to remind others of the prayer agreement. You will need to provide the setting. Others may not be as enthusiastic as you. That is to be expected. Be content that they have agreed to try. To influence their full involvement, use either unison prayer, with each person having a copy, or pray-along prayer, with you saying a phrase and them repeating it. Ask for silence. Expand leadership to others.

Hold hands. When praying with others, joining hands increases the impact. It is the best way of sharing spiritual energy. You will have to initiate the joining hands. When praying alone with your spouse at bedtime, begin by holding hands.

Spouses embrace. When you no longer need to read a prayer with your spouse, you can pray while embracing in bed. The reason for this is not romantic. A full body embrace places the chakra energy vortices opposite each other. During prayer, they become more energetic and an exchange of energy occurs that balances the body's energy, encourages wellness and links the couple as one, as in the wedding ceremony. In this case, the two become one through uniting personal energy fields.

BEGINNING

Begin a prayer by saying, *"Let us pray."* Then pause for about five seconds of silence. If necessary at first, try a practice run, saying the prayer for practice and then repeating it in a more unified way. After the prayer, it is appropriate to talk about how it was received. Do this by saying, *"Because we are new at this, I would find it helpful to hear your reactions to the prayer."* This permits helpful feedback. It also enables people to react negatively by grumbling about their discomfort in doing a new thing. Do not let negative comments hurt or stop you. Accept them graciously by listening with kindness. If necessary, gently insist that they continue for the week as agreed. These are normal leadership functions.

EVALUATION AND PLANNING

When the week is over, set aside a half-hour of time when no one is rushed to evaluate and plan for the future. As the leader, you might find these questions helpful. They can be given out ahead of time or asked at the meeting. What personal effects did our prayers together have upon your life? Did the prayers bring us closer together? Did you sense more love, peace, happiness and cooperation among us? Did you feel more alive and focused? How did the prayers affect the rest of your life; was there a carryover? Would you like to continue? How would you like us to continue? Would any of you like to take turns with me in leading prayers?

PRAYER MODELS

A. TABLE GRACES

If you choose, join hands. There is an alternative that I use in private or while alone in restaurants. During prayer, most people emit God's healing love energy with their hands. This energy can energize the food we eat, making it more nutritionally alive. Therefore, an alternative is to place the palms of your hands above the food that you are about to eat while praying.

Note the pause dots between phrases. These are phrase pauses where you can break if you use pray-along prayer. The large variety of table graces is offered because meals are the most likely times that persons will offer a prayer. If prayer is not a regular part of your life, the special occasion prayers provide opportunities for introducing prayer to your loved ones. Make an open invitation for others to add their prayers after any prayer.

1. Breakfast. God...thank you for this new day...with all the wonders and opportunities it offers. Please fill us/me with your peace...surround us/me with your love...and protect us/me from all harm. Open us/me to newness...guide us/me...and provide all that we/I need. May only good flow to us/me...and flow through us/me...that all we/I do this day...might be a blessing to your whole creation. We/I pray for the following special persons and needs: _____. Bless this food...and enable it to nourish us/me fully. Amen.

2. Lunch. God...we/I thank you for this food before us/me. We/I trust in your care...and rely upon your love. Refresh us/me...as we/I pause to eat. Amen.

3. Dinner. God...the giver and sustainer of all life...remove our/my tiredness...and fill us/me with life anew. We/I thank you for this food...and those who have provided it. Surround us/me in your presence...and make us/me one...with all whom we/I love. May your joy fill our/my heart(s)...as we/I enjoy the remainder of this day. Amen.

4. With children in the home. God...we are so separated...much of the time. We thank you...for gathering us together...as a family...in your love. Help us let go of our hurts. We release them to your care...and accept your healing. Thank you...for making each of us...special and important. Fill us with your love...and help us to love and care for each other. Provide for our needs. May your peace...fill our hearts...and make us strong. We thank you for this food. May it nourish our bodies. Amen.

5. For a couple. God...we thank you for another day together. We let all that hurts and divides us go...trusting in your renewing presence...to restore us. We reaffirm our mutual love and passion...our companionship and commitment...to each other. We trust in your care...and ask you to guide us...and provide for our needs. We thank you for this food...and for you...the Source of all...life, goodness, and love. Amen.

6. For single adults. God, fill me and sustain me with your love. Guide, sustain and protect me this day. I thank you for this food. Bless it that it might nourish my body. Keep me well and make me whole. Thank you. Amen.

7. For a student. Thank you, Divine Creator, for the wonder and beauty of your creation. Bless this food and those who have provided it. Renew me in body, mind and spirit. Calm me within, provide me with energy, and enable me to grow. Thank you for my life and for the opportunities stretching before me. Amen.

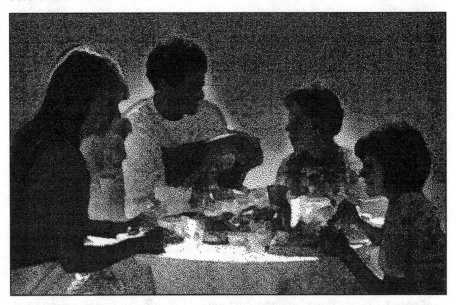

Figure 14. Prayer bathes this family in the life energy of their sacred group energy field that produces love, peace and harmony in their midst.

8. For military personnel. Sustainer and Protector, I continue to place my life in your hands. Enable me to remain capable and whole as I serve my nation. Bless this food and those who have provided it. Thank you. Amen.

9. Birthday. God, we/I thank you...for the special joy...of celebrating _____'s birthday today. We/I thank you for the richness of the years...for her/his uniqueness and specialness...as a person...for the joyful memories...of the times we have shared together...and for her/his dreams and hopes. May this day mark...the beginning of a great new year...and of more happiness and fulfillment. Bless _____ this day and fill him/her with your love. Bless this food as we proceed...with this celebration of life. Amen.

10. Wedding Anniversary. God, today is special. This is our _____ wedding anniversary. We remember the hard times...and the good times...and rejoice in our life together. We renew our vows...of love and loyalty. Deepen our love and passion...our friendship and commitment...that the coming years...will continue to be...rich and rewarding. We thank you...for the loved ones...who have brought joy to our life. We thank you...for bringing us together...sustaining us...and uniting us as one. Bless this food...and all the celebrations...we share this day. Amen.

11. Moving away of loved ones. God...we feel both joy and sadness...as we gather for this meal. We are happy that _____ is/are with us. But we also feel a sense of loss...as _____ move away. May this be a special time...of remembering and closeness. Maintain the bond...of friendship and love between us. Guide _____ safely to _____(name of community). May happiness and fulfillment...continue to bless her/him/them. May our hearts remain with them...though parted by distance. Bless this food before us...and enable this meal together...to be a time of celebration. Amen.

12. Special celebration. God...we are happy...as we share this meal. For it gives us the opportunity...to celebrate _____'s grades/graduation /promotion/raise/award/achievement/win/trophy. We rejoice in his/her happiness...in the faith and hope...struggle and hard work...and deep satisfaction for us all. Thank you for this food. We share it together...in appreciation. Amen.

13. Grief in death of a loved one. God...we gather in sadness...in memory of _____. We celebrate her/his life....her/his entrance into the afterlife...and the love we shared with _____. Comfort us in our grief...and grant us your peace. Bless this food before us. Enable us to enjoy one another...as we share this meal. Amen.

B.	PRAYERS FOR INDIVIDUALS

14. Morning. Thank you, God, for this day you have given me. Feed my soul with your holy Presence, guiding and empowering me in this day's events. May I approach each moment as a gift, an opportunity to serve you. Keep my mind free to think, my body whole and complete, my emotions healed of negative feelings like anxiety, anger, tension and insecurity, and fill me with your love, joy and peace. I now pray for the following concerns and persons: _____. Bless me this day that I might become a blessing to others. Make me an instrument for your peace. Amen.

15. Evening: Dear God, I thank you for the events of this day. Some were tedious, tiring and downright painful, and some were joyous and lifegiving. Forgive me for those times I was unwilling to love with understanding and compassion. I forgive all persons toward whom I feel anger, resentment and frustration. Heal my inner being with your love and presence, that I might become whole in body, mind and spirit. May I seek not so much to be loved as to love. I pray for the following concerns and persons: _____. I place myself in your hands. Be present with me while I sleep, that I may be secure and awaken refreshed in the morning. Amen.

C.	**EVENING, BEDTIME OR ANYTIME PRAYERS**

16. Pre-school child 1. God...I love you.   Thank you...for Mommy/Daddy/_____. Thank you...for the happiness I had today. Now help me sleep. Keep me safe. Let me wake up in the morning...feeling rested and strong. Amen.

17. Pre-school child 2. God...you made everything. Thank you. I am now ready to sleep. Help me to relax and grow sleepy. Keep me safe. May tomorrow be happy and fun. Amen.

18. Pre-school child: illness. God, I know you want me...to be well. So take away my sickness. Help me to feel better. Let me wake in the morning...happy and strong. Good night, God. I love you. Amen.

19. School-age child: general. God, thank you for the beauty and life all around me.   Thank you for Mom/Dad/_____, for my friends _____, and for my teachers. Bless them and protect them from all harm. Help me to know that I am special and deeply loved. I have these special concerns I wish to pray for: _____.   I ask you to heal my hurts and fill me with your love and peace. Guide and sustain me tomorrow. Grant me a good night's sleep and help me to wake up in the morning feeling happy and ready to live. Amen.

20. School-age child: troubled. God, I have had a bad day. I am hurting. I forgive everyone who hurt me today. I give away my anger and fear. I accept the fact that some days are bad. Please heal my hurt. Help me to understand life. I accept myself for who I am -- special, sacred and precious. Help me be loving and caring towards everyone. I am now ready to sleep. Fill me with your love and peace. Strengthen and guide me tomorrow. May I awaken rested and happy. Amen.

21. School-age child: illness. God, I feel terrible. I want to be well. Please take away my hurt and my pain. I forgive anyone who has hurt me. I forgive myself for any hurt I have caused others. I give you all my worries. I know you want me to be well, so I accept your gift of health. Make me well in body, mind and spirit. Fill me with your love and peace. Thank you. Amen.

22. Youth: general. God, thank you for this wonderful universe in which I live and for the beauty of this small planet, Earth.   Thank you for Mom/Dad/_____, for my friends, _____, and for my teachers. Bless them and protect them from all harm. I also pray for persons everywhere who are hurting. Enable our planet to be a good place for everyone to live. I commit myself to building a better world where there is peace and justice for all. Guide and direct me in developing the special abilities that bring me happiness, satisfaction and self-confidence and contribute to my own welfare as well as the welfare of others. Help me to do well in school and to have the friends and social life I need. Enable me to let go of my hurts and fears, and be filled with your love and peace. As I cooperate with others, help me to remain free and able to make my own responsible decisions. I have these special concerns for which I pray: _____.

Grant me a good night's sleep and help me to awaken in the morning feeling full of energy. Guide and sustain me throughout tomorrow and protect me from all harm. Thank you. Amen.

23. Youth: hurting. God, help me in this time when I am hurting. Difficult as it is, I forgive everyone who has contributed to my hurt. I forgive myself for contributing to the hurt. Heal any hurt, fear or anger within me. I release these to your care. Fill me with your love, joy and peace. Enable me to be calm and to think clearly. Help me to understand what has happened and to learn from these experiences. I place myself in your care. Renew me and create a right spirit within me. Guide and sustain me as I continue to work through these issues. Provide for my needs and protect me from all harm. I feel your life coursing through my veins. Thank you. Amen.

24. Youth: illness. (Place your hands upon the area needing healed.) Divine Physician, I turn to you because I want to be well. May your healing power flow through my hands and renew every cell in my body. Remove my pain and discomfort. Fill me with your peace, presence and love. Enable me to recover quickly and feel good once again. Unite me with you that we might be one. Fill me with faith and hope, for you make all things new. I rest in your care. Amen.

25. Family 1. God...thank you for making us a family. We love each other...but sometimes living together is difficult. Help us to care for each other...and to live in respect and harmony. Heal our hurts...unite us as one...provide for our needs...and protect us from all harm. Help us to sleep well tonight...and awaken in the morning feeling good. Thank you. Amen.

26. Family 2. Divine Creator and Sustainer...thank you for your gift of life...for another day. We rejoice in the love and support...we share with each other. We ask you to provide for our needs...and protect us from all harm. We forgive each other...and let go the memories of past hurts. Heal our hurts and our tiredness. Unite us as one...and yet...provide us with the private space we need...to be our own selves. May your love and light surround us...and fill our home. May only good flow to us...and through us...now... and in the coming day. Amen.

27. Family 3. God, we thank you for your presence...which guides, strengthens, and sustains us. Remove any tensions existing between us... and allow us to understand and respect each other deeply. Hold us together in love and hope. Provide for our needs as a family. We have these special concerns: _____. Thank you for hearing our prayer. Amen.

28. Couple 1. God...we thank you for this day. We pray for our family, for (name them)____. Fill them with your love and light...provide for their needs...and protect them from all harm. We pray for _____. Heal them and make them whole...in body, mind and spirit. We pray for ourselves, God. We place our concerns in your hands. Provide for our needs...and unite us as one as we share life together. Grant us your peace...and refresh us while we sleep. Guide and sustain us...in all that is before us. Thank you. Amen.

29. Couple 2. God, we thank you for this day...with all its work...joys and challenges. We praise you for being with us...offering us the gift of life. Grant us your peace...as we end this day...and offer us wholeness in body, mind and spirit. Deepen our unity with each other...and with you. We pray for the following concerns: _____. Be with us, God...as we sleep... protecting and nurturing us...and restoring us into the image of your perfect creation. Amen.

30. Couple: harmony. God, we are frazzled right now. We are out of harmony with each other. Open us to loving and understanding each other. Take away the pain and hurt...each of us is feeling. Enable us to understand that each of us is unique...in our style of being human. Help us to accept each other as we are. We forgive each other for all the hurts of the past...and seek to begin again in harmony. Help us be aware of...and bring justice...to each other. Fill our home with your love...that we might love each other as you love us. Thank you for the peace, joy and love...that you are forming within and between us. Amen.

31. Couple: healing hurts. God, we thank you...for our love...for each other. But we are hurting. We are so frustrated. I confess...that I have not loved...as I wish to be loved. Forgive me for seeking...only what I want...while ignoring the needs of my spouse. I give up my resentments...my hurts...my fears...my nasty games. Forgive me, God...for inflicting pain upon my spouse...whom I dearly love. Enable me to share my feelings...and my needs... honestly and openly with my spouse. Enable us to understand each other...and to resolve our differences. Heal our separateness...renew our trust...and bring us mutual justice. Hold us in your abiding love...and grant us your peace. Amen.

32. Couple: joy. Divine Creator, we thank you...for the beauty around us...and for the joy we feel...for each other. We celebrate the look of love...the tender touch...those things we do...for each other daily...as expressions of our love. I have joy...in the special thoughtfulness...my partner expresses...by words and actions...and in the sacrifices...my spouse makes for me. Enable me to be aware of the special ways...my spouse loves me. And make me thankful...for each moment of our marriage. Grant us your love, joy and peace...that we might always rejoice...and be glad. Amen.

33. Couple: deepening love. God, thank you...for joining us together...in the rich bond of marriage. We remember...the faith, hope and love...of our wedding day. We rejoice...in our struggles and celebrations. We keep before us the sacred wisdom: *"Love is patient and kind. Love is not rude. Love does not...insist on its own way. It is not irritable nor resentful. Love rejoices in the right. Love bears all things...believes all things...hopes all things...endures all things."* God, fill our souls...with your love...that we might always...cherish and honor each other...in gracious love. Amen.

34. Couple: morning. God, who has joined us together...in the sacred bonds of marriage...strengthen our understanding...our closeness...and our compassion for each other. Heal us of any negative feelings...that separate us...and renew the depths of our love. Be with us...as we carry through our separate responsibilities this day. Protect us from all harm...and offer us opportunities for serving you. And now we pray for these concerns: _____. Thank you for letting us...share this day with you. Amen.

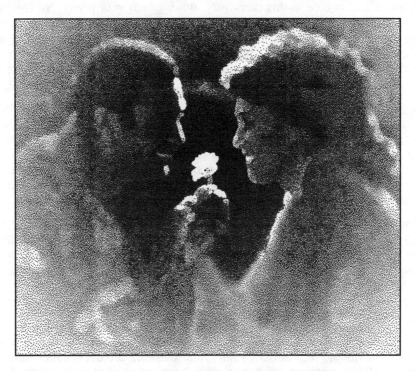

Figure 15. *Couple exchange energy and balance their energy fields through Therapeutic Prayer, enriching their love, peace and harmony.*

35. Couple: passion. Divine Creator...who created us male and female for each other...who made us sensuously attracted to each other...who gave us sexual desire...that we might celebrate and enjoy...the preciousness of our sacred love...and who wishes us to be ever renewed...and united as one. Help us to recall our history...as a couple...the trials and the struggles...the joys and the celebrations...the preciousness of our oneness and intimacy. Heal anything that denies our unity...and help us to share a fresh awareness...of each other's sacred wroth...that our passion for each other... will ever be fresh and meaningful. Create in us the capacity...to celebrate our love freely and spontaneously. Fill our lives...with your loving and holy presence. Amen.

36. Couple: reconciliation. God, whose love has united us...in the sacred bonds of marriage...we confess that we have not loved each other...as we ought to have loved. We are filled with anger and hurt...with frustration and mistrust...with misunderstanding and separation. Forgive us for our pride... for seeking only what we want...and ignoring the needs of each other. Make us aware of mutual justice...and the means for reconciliation. Heal all the negative feelings...making us feel so miserable...and grant us newness and joy with each other. In your love and light we trust. Amen.

37. Couple: conception. God...the creator and giver of all life...we wish to celebrate...the depth and sacredness of our love...by conceiving a child. We relax and rejoice in this possibility, flowing with your love. We ask you grant us...the gift of conception. We also ask that...you make our child whole and perfect...at conception. We promise to live healthy lives...for our unborn child...and to share...the abundance of your love...in raising our child. In calmness, we rejoice in our hope. Bless us, God, that we might be blessed as a family. Thank you. Amen.

38. Couple: pregnancy. God...we are joyful...in your gift of conception. Thank you for blessing us...with this child. Please deepen our love...and help us to support each other...throughout this pregnancy. We promise to live healthy lives...for the sake of our unborn child.   We ask you to bless the mother...with good health and happiness...and to protect her...from all complications. Keep our unborn child...whole and safe. Enable the birth... to be a joyful experience. We entrust our lives to your care. Amen.

(Pray with your unborn baby. Remember, during prayer, hands emit a healing energy. Both the expectant mother and father may place their hands on the abdominal area daily, praying, *God, bring wholeness and health to our child. Thank you. Amen.* Then, with hands still in place, seek to be one with God, each other and the unborn baby. After birth, placing your hands in the same process on the baby's head, at least once daily, enhances health, development and intelligence.)

39. Couple: birth of a child. God...we thank you for the birth of this child. We are so happy. Fill our child with your love and protect him/her from all harm.   We appreciate all those who have supported and assisted us throughout pregnancy and delivery. Now, God, bless us that we might be the best of parents. Fill us with the love, knowledge and wisdom necessary for raising this child. Provide for our many needs. May mother and child both remain healthy and grow stronger with each passing day. Thank you. Amen.

40. Grandparents 1. God, we thank you...for all the blessings of this day. We thank you for our children, *(name them)* ____, and their families. Fill them with your love and light...provide for their needs...and protect them from all harm. We pray especially for _____. Bring healing and wholeness to them...in body, mind, and spirit. We pray for ourselves. Provide us with meaning and challenge each day.   We entrust ourselves to your care. Grant us wholeness and renewal as we sleep. Thank you. Amen.

41. Grandparents 2. God, we thank you...for the richness of the years. We treasure the memories of earlier days...with our children as they were growing up. We thank you for the joys of sharing continuing love...with our children, their spouses and our grandchildren. Bless our children and their families...and hold them in your care. We pray for our own needs. Continue to bless us with health, happiness and financial resources. We continue to rely upon your sustaining love and guidance. Grant us your peace and renew us as we sleep. Thank you. Amen.

42. Single parent 1. God, thank you for helping me through another day. I am tired and weary. Grant me your peace and renew me in body, mind and spirit. I place all my concerns in your hands. Guide and protect my family and provide for our needs. Grant me the strength, confidence and wisdom needed to be a good parent. Bless my children. Fill them with your love and light. Help me to love them and provide the support and love they need. Enable me to be a happy, fulfilled, appreciative person. Grant me a good night's sleep and enable me to awaken rested in the morning with a smile of hope and satisfaction upon my face. Thank you. Amen.

43. Single parent 2. God, thank you for the gift of life and for these children you have entrusted to my care. It is an enormous responsibility to raise children, but I gladly do it because I love them dearly. Provide me with the strength, wisdom and resources to be the best parent I know how to be. God, I pray for my children. Fill them with your love and light, sustain and guide them through each day and protect them from all harm. Help them to grow and to be whole and responsible persons. May your love fill our home. Thank you for being present with us. Renew us as we sleep and help us walk in your light throughout tomorrow. Amen.

44. Single adult 1. God, the giver of life, I place myself in your hands. Fill me with your ongoing peace and presence. Provide for my needs and protect me from all harm. Fill me with hope and satisfaction. I pray for my loved ones that you might bless them, also. Restore me as I sleep. May tomorrow bring me fulfilling challenges and continuing happiness. Thank you. Amen.

45. Single adult 2. God, sometimes I feel so vulnerable and alone. At other times it feels so wonderful to be free to completely plan my own life. I place my concerns and needs in your hands. Sustain, strengthen and guide me. Provide for my needs and protect me from all harm. Especially, bring people into my life to fulfill my social needs. I place myself in your presence. Fill me with your love and peace. Be with me as I pray for these special needs and persons: _____. Thank you. Amen.

46. College student. God, I thank you for the many opportunities I have to grow and to become. Life stands before me and I want to know all I can about your universe. Satisfy my curiosity, bring me joy in learning and satisfaction in all my classes. Keep me clear-headed in class, in study and in exams, enabling my education to bear fruit. Provide for my needs for money, for social life, for friends, for inner security, for sleep and energy and for the fulfillment of my hopes and dreams. I pray for peace with justice for all the world's people and for the ecological restoration of the planet Earth. Be with me as I pray for these special needs and persons: _____. Grant me your calmness and your presence. I accept the wholeness you offer. Thank you for being with me in prayer. Amen.

47. Military personnel. God, thank you for the beauty and wonders of this day. Sometimes I am happy, enthusiastic and challenged, while at other times I feel sadness, boredom, loneliness and a sense of great futility. Enable me to understand and appreciate what my military service is all about as I serve my nation. Enable me to have satisfying relationships with the persons with whom I work and live. God, guide and sustain me throughout the day, protecting me from all harm and providing for my needs. Be with me as I pray for these special needs and persons: _____. Thank you. Amen.

D.	SPECIAL PRAYERS

48. Protection during travel. God, _____ is taking a trip and we/I are/am concerned for _____'s welfare. We/I ask you to protect her/him/them from all harm. Please place a protective bubble around _____ that no harm can come to her/him/them. Thank you. Amen. *(Then visualize the person(s) enclosed in a clear protective bubble.)*

My daughter's prayer protection. *I used a similar protection prayer one night in my home when I had a premonition that my teenage daughter was in danger. A few minutes after my prayer, she walked in the door and reported that, indeed, she had been in danger. While she was driving home on a four-lane highway, an approaching car had entered her lane, coming directly at her. A head-on collision was inevitable. She and her girlfriend thought they were about to die, but instead of the inevitable collision, the approaching car had harmlessly passed completely through their car, resulting in no damage whatsoever.*

I have heard several stories of similar prayer protection in potential vehicular accidents. Some of my friends say that this occurrence was impossible and warn me that telling this story damages my credibility. I stand by the actuality of this miraculous event in which God changed the laws of physical reality.

49. Blessing a new residence. God, we are thankful...for our new home. We ask you to cleanse it...and prepare it for our presence. May this place where we live...be filled with your love, light, and peace. May only good flow to it and through it. May all who enter...know its warmth and love. May this be a safe and secure place...to live...to play...to work...to love...to share...to relax. Protect our home from all harm...and bless it with your presence...that it might form...a sacred space for our lives. Thank you. Amen.

Then enter each room, raise your arm and hand up in front of you, sweeping the room with it, while commanding, "Be filled with God's love, light and peace."

50. For someone's competence. *In her late-thirty's my wife was in college studying to become a registered nurse. She would panic during exams, her mind losing access to the information she had studied so thoroughly. I began praying for her from wherever I was when she was taking exams. I would visualize her sitting calmly with the exam in front of her and would visually encircle her in God's love and light, praying,*

"God, surround _____ in your love and light and grant her your peace. May her mind be creative and flow with all she knows. Thank you. Amen."

My wife began excelling in subjects that had previously caused her problems. Similarly worded prayers can be offered for a smooth flow of competence in other situations.

51. Personal crisis. God, I am upset. I ask that you enable me to cope. I trust in your care. I place this crisis in your hands. *(Visualize God receiving the crisis.)* Surround it in your love and peace. I release my anxiety and accept your peace. Enable something good to emerge from what has happened by redeeming the situation. God, grant me an inner calm...and provide for my needs...protecting me from all harm. Thank you. Amen.
(Then sit or lie down while using this calming exercise. Breathe deeply for ten minutes. While inhaling, silently say "peace" as you inhale. On each exhalation, let the peace flow throughout your body. The peace is God's peace entering you.

52. In conflict with others. God, I am upset with _____. I open myself to your presence in this conflict. Fill me with your presence and understanding. I also ask you to surround _____ in your love and light. *(Visualize this.)* May only fairness, harmony and wisdom flow from what has happened. Bless us in this time of pain and hurt. Thank you. Amen.

53. Employment. God, I need employment to provide for my financial needs. Please provide for me with a job fulfilling all my needs. Guide me to places and to persons who can help me. I need this employment by _____. Enable this to be. Thank you.

54. Student in crisis. God, I sense the walls of life closing in about me. I do want to complete my education. Please provide what I need to continue in school. Bless me so that I may grow and become what you intend. Thank you. Amen.

55. Protection from danger. God, We/I are/am concerned for _____. We/I ask you to protect her/him/them/us from all harm. Please place a protective bubble around ____ that no harm can come to her/him/them/us. Thank you. Amen.

(Then visualize the person(s) enclosed in a clear protective bubble.)

56. Your own safety in the midst of danger. *Cry out:* **God, come to my aid and save me! Thank you.** *(It is best to call out using your own personal name for God)*

57. Accepting God into your life. God, I am so thankful for your sustaining presence in my life. At this time, I invite you into my life forever. Fill me with your presence, love and peace. Transform me and make me into a new person. I commit my life to your guidance and your service. Bless me that I might become a blessing to you. Thank you. Amen.

E.	**SELF-HEALING IN TIMES OF CRISIS**

58. Physical health: God, the creator, sustainer, and healer of all life, I do not want to be ill. I choose life and wholeness. Heal me in body, mind and spirit and make me well. *(Now pause and seek to be one with God and yourself.)* Use my hands that your healing power may flow into me. *(Place your hands on an appropriate area of your body.)* Thank you, God, for the healing that is taking place. Amen.

59. Emotional wholeness. God, I am emotionally troubled. I am trapped and cannot let go. I ask you to release me from this condition. I forgive all persons who have ever hurt me. I forgive myself. I let go of my anger, hurt, fear and anxiety. I entrust myself to your care. Provide for my needs and protect me from all harm. Fill me with your love, joy and peace. I accept your power to transform and empower me. Thank you for the calmness that is coming over me. Amen.

(Now sit or lie down. Close your eyes and take three deep breaths. Then slowly repeat over and over again, **"Love, joy and peace."** *Try to rid your mind of all other thoughts and feelings. Just push them gently aside. Do this for fifteen minutes.)*

60. Grief upon losing a loved one. God, the creator and sustainer of all life, I thank you for your gift of life to _____ and for the fullness of the years we shared. I entrust him/her to your loving care and thank you for his/her transition into your heavenly kingdom where s/he is being restored and made whole.

And yet, God, I am hurting terribly. The pain of my loss is almost too intense. There is a huge emptiness within me. It does not seem fair. I miss him/her immensely. Many emotions threaten to overwhelm me. I feel anger that this has happened. I feel uneasy about unfinished business. I feel so alone and vulnerable. My life is now completely different. Adjusting and coping is so difficult.

God, I need your support and presence as never before. I ask you to dwell with me and help fill the huge emptiness within. Please comfort and strengthen me and grant me your peace. Remove my weariness and make me whole. God, guide me this day. Help me to handle my daily tasks. Guide and sustain me, and protect me from all harm. Enable me to reach the place where I can reminisce about the love and life we shared together without breaking into tears. Heal my wounds this day and enable me to have faith and hope in your goodness. Please provide for my needs until life returns in all its fullness and joy. Thank you. Amen.

(Now sit or lie down. Close your eyes. Take three deep breaths. Then slowly repeat over and over again, **"You are my strength and my salvation,"** *for 15 minutes.)*

61. For the shock of a sudden death: God, I am numb. It seems like an endless nightmare, like a dream from which I will awaken. I have never been so shaken. The pain continues to roll over and through me. I am badly hurting and do not know if I can handle this. Strengthen me in this terrible time of crisis and grant me your peace.

God, bless _____*(naming the deceased)* and grant her/him calmness in the midst of her/his shock. I know that s/he is alive and aware on the other side. Enable her/him to be aware of that s/he has made the transition into the next life. Heal the shock of death. Grant her/him help in finding the Light which leads to your Kingdom. Thank you.

God, provide for my needs during this tragedy. Guide and sustain me. Increase my faith in your love. Enable me to cope with all that is before me. Help me to survive. I rest in your calming peace and presence. Thank you. Amen.

62. Interpersonal harmony: God, I am upset, frustrated and confused. I feel a gulf between _____ and myself. I have mixed feelings: wanting to maintain distance and yet wanting to have harmony between us again. Open us to our own higher wisdom. Enable us to draw back and look from a distance, that we might discern the truth and fairness of what is happening. Fill us both with your love, compassion and peace. Protect us both from all harm. Thank you. Amen.

MORE PRAYERS FOR CRISES ELSEWHERE

In chapter twenty, I have provided prayers for a variety of crises: an overwhelmed mother or father; marital betrayal, separation and divorce; loss of a job; a victim of violence; an auto accident; a house fire -- a total of sixty-two more prayers.

F.	*ABSENT-PRAYER*

63. For illness. God, I am concerned for _____. Heal _____ in body, mind, and spirit and make her/him whole. Thank you. Amen.

(Now seek to be one with God and with the ill person, holding the three of you in a oneness or a sense of unity in God's love, peace and health. See her/him as well and happy. Visualize her/him performing a task s/he enjoys. Do this for five minutes at a time.)

64. For grief. God, I am concerned for _____. Comfort _____ in her/his grief and grant her/him your peace. Thank you. Amen.

(Now seek to be one with God and one with the grieving person, holding the three of you in a sense of unity in God's love and peace. Do this for five minutes at a time. This is an important prayer, because you are providing God's power for a grieving person. Grief tends to block one's access to God presence, so the prayers of others can be vital in fostering healing.

65. For other needs. God, I am concerned for _____. Provide for her/his need and grant him/her your wholeness. Thank you. Amen.

(Now seek to be one with God and one with the person, holding the three of you in a oneness or unity of God's love, peace and wholeness. Do this for five minutes at a time.)

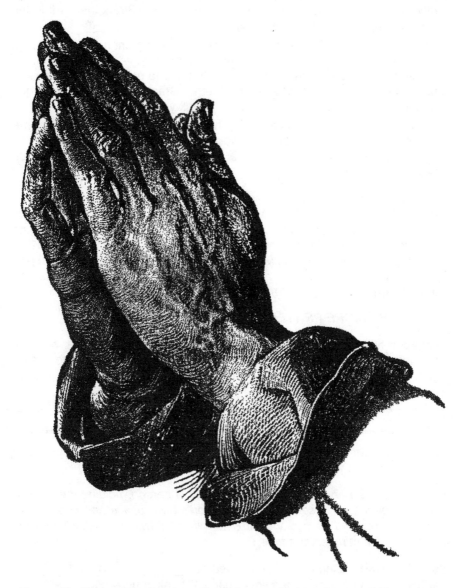

Figure 16. *The praying hands posture places palm to palm, completing an energy circuit. This permits divine energy to circulate and balance your energy fields. It also permits you to focus on prayer.*

G.	*FAMILY FIRST AID*

Most persons only turn to God in emergencies, but touch-healing prayer transmits a healing energy aiding all medical conditions. This should be used to supplement traditional first aid and medical care.

66. Daily healing prayer. With infants, toddlers, children, and youth, parents can enhance the overall sense of wholeness and health by daily prayer. Daily, place one hand on the nape of the neck and the other on the forehead. If both parents are present, the second parent places hands on front and back of the heart area. The healing energy will help children remain calm. It stops colic, diaper rash and sleep disturbances. It enhances wholesome parent-child bonding. The evidence is that it increases the growth of brain capability which is known as intelligence. Your prayer can be simple. *"God, bring healing and wholeness to _____ and fill him/her with your love, joy and peace. Amen."*

Other loved ones can offer this healing energy to each other in the same manner. When family members are able to gather in a circle and join hands, the same prayer can be offered for each person in the circle, with specific prayers for special needs. This creates a sacred group energy field that binds persons together as a loving family, diminishes irritations and squabbling, enables everyone to become more focused and purposeful, and equips each to face developmental stages and crises more effectively.

One caution. The act of praying can be a very powerful instrument for manipulation and control. Be cautious about hampering free will. Do **not** use prayer as a means for making everyone do one person's will or providing one person's answer for another's life. Example: Do **not** say, *"God, help Susie keep her room clean."* **Do** say, *"God, enable Susie to cope with living in our family."* When an accepting love is offered, it brings out the best in everyone. Trust people to find their own solutions.

67. Cuts, bruises, rashes, acne, inner hurting, etc. While touching the area hurting, pray for God to heal it. Do this twice daily for about five minutes each time. *"God, use me as a channel for healing. Heal _____ and make him/her whole in body, mind and spirit. Thank you. Amen."*

68. Acute Illnesses. Pursue normal medical care or a proven alternative. Then pray for healing in body, mind and spirit. Additional touching can be done by holding hands, holding the person on one's lap or sitting and embracing the individual against the chest. Once the prayer for healing is offered and the healing energy begins to flow, the energy will continue to flow as you just touch. You can talk, watch television or even sleep while transmitting. Apply four times a day. See chapter twenty-four for complete details.

Consider transmitting the healing energy to a cotton dish towel or a container of water. This can be done while praying with a family member. For charging, maintain touch for about half an hour. The effects of such procedure last indefinitely. Drape the towel over the person or wrap it around an arm or leg, or place under clothing. Give two ounces of charged water four times a day. In very acute situations, give the water hourly.

GUIDANCE FOR CREATING YOUR OWN PRAYERS

As you begin offering your own prayers, caution should be observed. Prayers need to be affirming. Your loved ones will resent tactics that promote your own view and diminish theirs, resulting in their refusal to continue praying with you. Trust that God is acting intelligently and creatively in the midst of prayer to bring about individual and relational wholeness and guidance.

Effective prayer requires a purity of intent. Seek the best for others. Be still, free of all ulterior motives and struggles, and allow God to act. Honestly state your own personal needs, ask for God's help and affirm God's power to create wholeness. Express concern for all others by asking God to bless them as you become one with them in peace. Effective prayers cannot offer advice, tell someone to do something, moralize or argue about what someone ought to do. Nor does effective prayer seek to warn or threaten, criticize or blame, lecture or instruct, control or manipulate or discuss or analyze.

GUIDELINES FOR PRAYING

The previous prayer models have been based upon the following guidelines. As you graduate from the prayer models and form your own prayers, you might consider these guidelines for yourself.

I. Quiet your inner self and seek a oneness with God.

2. Have a faith and hope that anticipates God's presence and blessings.

3. Let your prayer be based upon the highest wisdom of your religious beliefs.

4. Let your prayer express pure inner motives or intentions, wanting the best for the person(s) for whom you are praying.

5. Let your prayer honestly express the emotions, needs and concerns of person(s) for whom you are praying.

6. Let your prayer accept and respect the unique personal sacredness andfreedom of the person(s) involved. Trust each person to be capable of making his/her own personal decisions.

7. Let your prayer express loving compassion for the person(s) for or with whom you are praying.

8. Let your prayer seek God's blessing for the person(s) for whom you are praying.

9. Let your prayer seek a oneness with the person(s) for whom you are praying.

10. Let your prayer contribute to your own wholeness as well as to the wholeness of the person(s) for whom you are praying.

11. Let your prayer express what you would want others to express should they be praying for you under similar circumstances.

Chapter Twenty-Eight

Family Rituals of Affirmation

"The spiritual life is a reaching out to our innermost self, our fellow human beings, and our God." ...Henri J. Nouwen*

"What happens when we pray is that we allow ourselves to be known as persons before God; in prayer we unveil before God." ...C.S.Lewis*

"Genuine religion is found in an inner experience of the Divine." ...Dag Hammarskjold*

This chapter continues the quest for renewal and happiness through rituals affirming family members. Persons of all ages need to hear words from loved ones that accept, affirm, support and appreciate them. If these are not forthcoming within the family, people can spend a lifetime feeling inadequate, unloved, unhappy and angry. Mental states like this produce dysfunctional individuals, marriages and families, resulting in conflict, unhappiness and destructive actions. Spiritual rituals and prayer are used because the evidence indicates they provide an energy that heals painful memories and emotions, builds trust and intimacy, restores relationships and enhances family satisfaction and happiness.

Acceptance and Affirmation. Psychology teaches us that in order for persons of all ages to be whole and happy, their inner emotional needs must become satisfied. Every person has the need to possess self-worth and to know that s/he is valued by others. All have the need to give and to receive love. We need to be accepted, respected and appreciated. Every person needs a place to express her or his hurts and struggles, hopes and dreams. This is not theory. People hold a deep yearning for relationships offering these qualities.

Every time I hear the following old story, I wince at the immense pain implicit in it. A couple was celebrating their fiftieth wedding anniversary. The wife took her husband's hand in hers, looked him in the eye, and said, *"Henry, I love you. It has been a long time since I have heard that from you. Do you still love me?"*

Without pausing, Henry replied, *"Woman, I never need to say that again. I told you I loved you on our wedding day and, if I ever change my mind, I will let you know."*

In real life, people of all ages need to hear words of love, appreciation, acceptance and affirmation on a regular basis. Happiness, satisfaction, love and intimacy die quickly without these words. Motivation for learning to express these feelings begins with the awareness of just how rewarding such statements are for all involved. For some people these words are not easy to offer because the families they grew up in did not practice these ways of sharing.

I did not grow up learning how to hug family members. By the time we children grew up, my mother had learned to reach out in affection to us. Mom would stand just inside the door, waiting to hug and kiss us as soon as any us of entered her home. It took time and effort for me to extend a similar affectionate hug to my brothers and sisters.

My father and I had always a good relationship. But our only physical contact was to shake hands in greeting and departing. Finally, in my forties, it dawned upon me that I could not remember ever hugging my father. I experienced a growing yearning to do so before he died. It took me six months to work up the courage to offer this simple expression of love. Finally, it happened.

I found my father in the backyard working in his flower garden. I approached him feeling tense about this new thing I was about to do. He greeted me with, *"Hello, son,"* and extended his hand for our customary handshake.

I said, *"Dad, would you mind if we hugged today?"* We embraced. It was a powerful experience for both of us. Tears were running down our cheeks by the time our prolonged embrace was finished. It has been over a decade now that I have been able to enjoy hugging my father. It remains a powerful and tender expression of love for both of us.

Through the years, my parents, brothers and sisters have learned to say, *"I love you."* This has grown more important to our whole family with the deaths of two brothers and a brother-in-law.

My wife and I began expressing appreciation and affirmation of each other even before our wedding. It seemed like a natural extension of our love. We still thank each other for the little things we do for each other. We often compliment each other for achievements and affirm our relationship with the words, *"I love you."*

This affirming and affectionate style naturally extended to our children and then to our grandchildren. Nevertheless, I discovered that I had left some loved ones out. During a recent period of family tension, I wrote an affirming letter to one of my son-in-laws, closing with the statement, *"I love you like a son."*

Later, he told me, *"Walt, I needed to hear that. I was not sure how you regarded me. Thanks. I love you, too."*

The thought of establishing new family rituals can produce tension in most people. The family rituals of affirmation that you are about to practice are just extensions of the love and support you already share. These are forceful expressions of love, acceptance, support and understanding. They can also be used outside a family setting with any group of people who choose to care intentionally.

Getting Started. Someone needs to encourage family rituals of affirmation. If you are already sharing daily prayers, these rituals are a natural addition to your spiritual journey. You can simply say, *"I have found something else we can do together. It looks like it would be helpful for all of us. Would you be willing to give it a try? It is only once a week and we could do it on _____ (state a time)."*

If you are not praying with each other, you might approach family members during a meal together, saying, *"I have run across something that I think would be helpful for all of us. It is a way of expressing our love and appreciation for each other. Would you be willing to try it with me? It will only take about fifteen minutes. We could try it on _____(state a time)."*

FIRST FAMILY RITUAL OF AFFIRMATION

A family can meet weekly for the following ritual of affirmation. Be seated around a table, in chairs or on the floor in some approximation of a circle. The same person can lead each session or each family member can take a turn at leadership. Even toddlers can take part, if only to receive affirmations. Pray-along prayer is used, meaning one person says a phrase and everyone repeats it. Three dots (...) mark the division of sentences into pray-along phrases. This first ritual involves three affirmations, 1, 2 and 3 with an A and B section in each.

Opening Unison Family Affirmation: In unison or pray-along led by the leader. *God...we have gathered as a family...to affirm one another. We forgive each other...for any pain we have experienced...and ask the forgiveness of any family member...we have hurt. We promise to accept...and to respect each other. We affirm our love and support...for each other. We are thankful to be family. Amen.*

1. AFFIRMING STRUGGLES. Each person states where he or she is struggling in his or her life, with all family members offering affirmation.

Examples: *"Boredom at school," "being lonely and having no friends," "the pimples on my face which make me look ugly," "my fear of failure," "my failure to make the team," "the family budget," "getting a job,"* and *"my anger towards _____."* Here is the ritual:

1a. Statement of Personal Struggles. A person says:

"I am struggling with _____."

1b. The Ritual of Affirmation. The family in unison responds:

"_____, we unconditionally love and support you, just as you are, in all of your sacred preciousness."

2. AFFIRMING PERSONAL FOCUS. Each person states his/her present major life focus, with all family members offering affirmation.

Examples of focuses: *"Get a 'B' in my science class," "increase my job enjoyment," "deepen my relationship with _____," "control my temper and learn patience," "save enough money to _____,"* and *"be better at _____."* Here is the ritual:

2a. Statement of Personal Focus. A person says:

"The present major focus of my life is to _____."

2b. The Ritual of Affirmation. Family in unison responds:

"_____, we unconditionally love and support you in your focus."

3. AFFIRMING UNIQUE TRAITS. Each family member is affirmed by all others as each individually addresses the person by name and states a quality they value in him.

Examples of qualities: *"Your gentle smile," "your sense of humor," "the way you worked to achieve _____," "the way you handled _____," and "your understanding when I _____."* Here is the ritual:

3a. The Ritual of Affirmation. Go around the circle, focusing on one person at a time so that each family member can individually offer affirmation. Address the person by name and say:

"_____**, a *valued quality I see in you and appreciate is* _____."**

Closing Affirming Prayer. In unison or pray-along led by leader. *God... we thank you for this time together. May your love fill our whole family...with joy and peace. Bring healing and wholeness...to each of us individually...and to all of us...as a family. Strengthen us in our struggles... guide us in our focuses...and strengthen those qualities in us...which are blessings to others. May only good come to us...and flow through us. Bless us that we might be blessings to each other. Thank you. Amen.*

SECOND FAMILY RITUAL OF AFFIRMATION

The purpose of this family ritual is to acknowledge and understand the connection between our behavior and the emotional reactions of others, using the whole range of positive and negative emotions. This may be done weekly or as often as needed. Seat family members together in an approximate circle.

Sharing Actions that Bring Out the Worst in Others. The purpose of this particular exercise is to help cope with the irritations produced by family interactions. Using first person messages beginning with "I," each person states the specific words or actions of a loved one that produce the worst feelings or responses within him/herself.

One person begins by looking a chosen family member in the eye and making a statement. Persons may pass their turns. When all have had an opportunity, a second or third turn may be taken, but these must be addressed to someone other than the person(s) already addressed. Do not argue with a statement nor deny its truth. **Do not get violent.** The stated truth is the truth as experienced by the person making the initial statement. This process heals the wounds and restores the loving relationships of everyone.

Opening Unison Family Prayer: *God...our feelings have the power...to make us either...happy or unhappy. Our most real selves involve our feelings...which are often kept secret within us. We have gathered as family...to relate our words and actions...with each other...to our emotional responses. We seek to free ourselves...of inner pain...to affirm our affection...to deepen understanding...and create a bond of unity. We affirm our love and support...for each other. We are thankful to be family. Amen.*

The Ritual of Affirmation

4A. Statement. Person 'A' states, addressing a loved one by name:

"_____, *when you say (or do)* _____, *it brings out the worst in me, because I feel* _____."

4B. Response. The addressed person 'B', responds:

"_____, *I heard that when I say (or do)_____, you feel _____. Is there a way that I can say (or do) _____ that will bring out the best in you?*"

4A. Statement. Person 'A' answers:

"_____, *if you said (or did) it this way _____, it is more likely to bring out the best in me.*"

4B. Response. Person 'B' agrees:

"_____, *I have heard your answer and will honestly consider making this change.*"

4C. Group Affirmation. The whole group affirms both persons:

"_____, *we unconditionally love and support you, just as you are, in all your sacred preciousness.*"

The Ritual of Affirmation

The purpose of this particular exercise is to use first person messages to affirm those words or actions that build relationship. This is achieved by stating the specific words or actions of a loved one that produce closeness, trust, and affection. One person begins by looking another person of his choice in the eye and making a statement. There is no passing. All persons must make a statement. When all have had an opportunity, passing becomes an option and a second or third turn may be taken.

5A. Statement. Person 'A' states, addressing by name:

"_____, *when you say (or do) _____, it brings out the best in me, because I feel _____.*"

5B. Group Response. The whole group affirms:

"_____, *we rejoice in and affirm this bond of affection.*"

Closing Group Affirming Prayer. *God, we thank you for this time together. May your love fill our whole family...with joy and peace. Bring healing and wholeness to each of us individually...and to us as a family. Strengthen us...as we interact with each other...that our loving words and actions...may be shared honestly and wisely. Amen.*

THIRD FAMILY RITUAL OF AFFIRMATION

The purpose of this third family ritual is to help a family member work through a hurt from the past or present. It can be a hurt, a failure, a disappointment, a betrayal or a confession or a mistake. The affirmation ritual can be requested by the hurting person. It can, also, be compassionately suggested to the hurting person, who has the freedom to say, *"I am not ready for that."*

Gather in a circle. The speaker tells his or her story from a personal view-point, including feelings experienced at the time of the event. Example: *"I went to physical education class today. We were playing basketball. The teacher told me I was too awkward to play. He told me to sit and watch. I was crushed and embarrassed. I felt I was treated unfairly. I do not want to go back there ever again."*

One listener needs to take the responsibility of patiently drawing out the teller's story, including emotions. Should the teller not mention feelings, the active listener can gently intervene with questions like, *"What were you feeling at that moment?"* or *"What are you feeling right now?"*

The power to heal is present in the total unconditional acceptance of the teller's pain by loving people. As you listen, realize that this is the teller's story, the teller's truth. It is the teller's perception, interpretation and response. Do **not** correct, argue with, object to, moralize, blame, criticize, warn, threaten, advise, be impatient, lecture or instruct the teller. By telling the story and receiving your compassion, the teller will discover for himself all the truths you would like to offer.

Give the teller your full attention. If the teller becomes emotional, for example, if he begins to cry, do not touch or intervene with words. Any such intervention eases the impact of necessary pain, demeans the teller, and short-circuits the potential for healing. Receive the story as if you were hearing it for the first time.

Opening Affirmative Prayer. *God, we have gathered here...to offer support to _____. We accept and respect the depth of his/her hurt. We affirm the sacred worth of _____. We promise to listen compassionately and to respond in love and affirmation. Be with us, God, for this renewing process. Thank you. Amen.*

The Ritual of Affirmation

5a. The Story as Told by the Teller. An active listener helps to draw the story out and to focus upon the expression of the feelings involved.

5b. Group Ritual of Affirmation. After the story is completed, the group addresses the teller by name and states:

"_____, we unconditionally love and support you in your hurt."

Closing Prayer. Close in a circle around the teller so that each person can touch the teller during the prayer. *"God, heal the hurt. Restore newness of life to _____. Make him/her whole in body, mind and spirit. Thank you. Amen.*

Chapter Twenty-Nine
Rites of Passage

"And could you keep your heart in wonder at the daily miracles of your life, your pain would not seem less wondrous than your joy. And you would accept the seasons of your heart, even as you have accepted the seasons that pass over the fields, and you would watch with serenity through the window of your grief." ...Kahlil Gibran

"Cultivation of a compassion for others is needed to combat natural tendencies toward selfishness that block the flow of God's love." ...John Woolman*

"For whatever is born of God overcomes the world; and this is the victory that overcomes the world, our faith." ...John 1:5b

Missing from modern humanity are the rites of passage of primitive cultures. In primitive tribes, a youth became an adult male through a rigid testing of his masculine hunting and survival skills -- a rite of passage. This was followed by an initiation into the secret knowledge that only the men of the tribe knew. This bestowed status and power upon young men that they carried throughout life into old age. Young women experienced initiations appropriate for their defined roles.

For many centuries, no such rites of passage have existed for civilized humanity. Today, both males and females spend a lifetime of frustration searching for identity, belonging, competence, confidence and power -- all of which primitive tribes bestowed upon their young during puberty through rites of passage.

Mircea Eliade[1] writes, *"The various kinds of initiation rites can be classified in two categories; first, puberty rites, by virtue of which adolescents gain access to the sacred, to knowledge and to sexuality -- by which, in short, they become <u>human beings</u>; second, specialized initiations, which certain individuals undergo in order to transcend their human condition and become protégés of the Supernatural Beings or even their equals."*

Tribal roles and responsibilities are simple by modern standards. They are also extremely rigid with few deviations from the norm permitted. We have no exact equivalent nor can we create one. Yet, rites of passage are necessary for everyone. All youth seek their own rite of passage. If they do not, they spend a lifetime in misery. Previous generations had a simpler initiation into adulthood. They could follow in a parent's footsteps, continuing the roles of their parents.

Today, secular rites of passage include graduation from secondary school, military service, continuing education, working at a good job, marriage or parenthood. If none of these happens, then youth use other means for meeting their needs.

While most youth will for a time explore escapist adult behaviors -- alcohol, drugs, sex, fast driving, etc. -- those who cannot find a respectable rite of passage will pursue such activities to extremes. They may also join street gangs, display more violent behavior, and become non-productive members of society. Spiritually, they are lost -- and lost, first and foremost, to themselves.

ALL AGES NEED RITES OF PASSAGE

Just as people need to be affirmed, they need rituals to put events into perspective. As a society, we are not good at attaching meaning to events. We go through various stages of development and achievement with little understanding of what these mean. Our loved ones seldom talk about the meaning of events.

HEALTHY LIFESTYLE RITES OF PASSAGE

Making changes to a healthier lifestyle is difficult. Last January, I made the decision to resume walking daily and working out every other day. For six weeks, I thought about it every evening and forgot about it the next morning, until after I was dressed for the day. Finally, I asked my wife to remind me the next morning, and placed a note to myself on the kitchen table. This worked. It would have felt even better to have had support and affirmation for my efforts. So, the Healthy Lifestyle Rites of Passage are meant to encourage changes in your lifestyle.

MEDALS OF HONOR

Some events call for medals of achievement, as in the military. Use them sparingly to recognize unusual merit.

USING THESE RITES

Only you can decide the helpfulness of these rites of passage. Not every situation can be covered. These are models for your own created rites. You decide on the helpfulness of the results. Many of the rites used for younger people can be used by all ages.

These can be used informally, without the knowledge of family members, as words of support and affirmation. They can also be formally used by letting everyone know of their availability. Many can best be used during a meal when all family members are present.

RITES OF PASSAGE FOR EARLY CHILDHOOD

1. Potty training. "____, I know it has been difficult. I am proud of you. You will no longer be uncomfortable in wet diapers. Now you can go anyplace and proudly use the toilet."

2. Walking. "____, I am happy to see you walking so well. Now, we can walk many places together and enjoy each other more."

3. Talking in sentences. "____, I am happy you are talking so well. Now we can enjoy talking to each other. You can ask me questions and I can tell you about the world. You will have so much fun talking to everyone you meet."

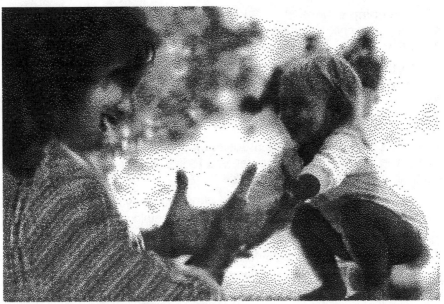

Figure 17. Mother and daughter exchange life energy during potty training.

4. Completely dressing yourself. "____, I am so proud of you for taking care of yourself so well, but please talk to me before changing outfits."

5. Tying shoes. "____, I am so happy you can put on your own shoes. When you do it, it saves me a lot of time."

6. Alphabet. "____, I am so happy you know the alphabet. Soon you will be reading books."

7. Telling time. "____, I am so happy you can tell the time. Now you know when it is time to get up and when your television programs are on."

8. For eating healthy foods. "____, I like the way you eat healthy foods. They make you feel good and give you more energy."

9. For washing hands and face. "____, when you wash your hands and face, you look so nice. It also keeps you healthier, because washing kills the germs that cause sickness."

10. For being warm and affectionate. "____, I feel so good when you love me like this. It makes me love you even more. Thank you."

11. For struggling with an illness. "____, I know how awful you must feel. None of us likes to be sick. I am going to love you back to health."

12. For returning to full health. "____, it is good to see you well again. I am so happy for you. Now, I do not have to worry so much about you."

13. First night away from family. "____, this is going to be fun. You are growing up. I will miss you. Enjoy yourself."

14. Beginning school. "____, I am happy you are so grown up that you are going to school. You are going to learn so many new things and make many new friends. You are going to enjoy school."

15. Birthday. "____, happy birthday. Birthdays are always special days. This means that you have lived ___ years. Each year you learn more about how to be happy and helpful."

RITES OF PASSAGE FOR SCHOOL CHILDREN

16. For competency in a school subject. "____, I am proud of you. Everything you learn well prepares you to live life more fully. What you learn will help you throughout your life."

17. For service to the school. "____, I am happy you are helping out at the school. It shows your appreciation for their helping you learn."

18. For service to your community. "____, I am proud of you for helping out our community. We all have responsibility for contributing to the good of this community that we appreciate so much."

19. For an orderly and clean bedroom. "____ I am proud of the way you take care of your bedroom. It shows that you are maturing. The way you take care of things here at home mirrors how you will live other parts of your life. A messy bedroom means that you are not organized in other areas of your life."

20. For playing harmoniously. "____, I like the way you cooperate so well with other children. Learning how to get along with others is an important lesson of life."

21. For generosity in caring for others. "____, I like the way you support people. I am proud of the way you give of yourself in caring for others. This is a quality I respect in my children."

22. Thinking clearly and acting responsibly. "____, I like the way you acted so responsibly. I feel so much better as a parent when you do things like that."

23. For making a responsible decision amidst social pressure. "____, I am proud of the way you held up and did the right thing under a lot a pressure from others. Being responsible will not always make you popular. It will build your character and integrity, preparing you for a responsible adulthood."

24. For the meaning of failure and suffering. "____, I know it hurts. It should not have to be, but everyone experiences this sort of thing at times. We learn and grow through bad experiences. Because I love you, this hurts me, too. Regardless of what has happened, I know that you are a wonderful person. Remember that."

25. For persistence in learning a new skill. "____, it takes determination and courage to learn something new. I am proud that you set a goal, struggled to learn and now know how to do this. You have picked up a new skill that will bless your life for years to come. In the process, you have grown more mature."

26. For productive use of time. "____, I like the way you use your time so constructively. Everything you learn and do contributes to your present and future, making life more satisfying."

27. For a grade report. "____, thank you for sharing your grades with me. I am proud of the way you are trying. How well you do in school determines your future potential at school and in any future vocational plans."

28. For promotion to the next grade. "____, I am proud of you for completing another year of school. This is another important step in your life."

29. For graduation. "____, this is very happy time for us. I am proud that you have reached this achievement in your life. Congratulations."

RITES OF PASSAGE FOR YOUTH

30. For choosing not to smoke, drink, do drugs. "____, I am happy you made that decision. This is an addictive behavior that can take away your free will and enslave you. Choosing to be chemically free keeps you in control of your own life. It will bless your life for years to come. I am delighted with your decision."

31. For first date. "____, dating is fun, but it is a privilege granted by me and carries with it certain responsibilities. I expect you to be where you have told me you are going to be. I expect you to behave responsibly. You are not to use alcohol or drugs. You are not to park in a seclude spot. You are not to kiss on the first date. If you are going to be late getting home, I expect you to phone me. I know you are growing up and I want you to enjoy yourself. Nevertheless, if you behave irresponsibly, I will ground you and not permit you to date until I know I can count on you to behave yourself."

32. For working in a paying job. "____, I think working will teach you valuable skills. I expect you to work hard and earn your pay. I expect you to save a certain amount of your pay and to spend the rest carefully. And, remember, school comes first. If your school performance drops, you will quit your job. I am proud of your determination to work and to earn extra money."

33. For driver's license. "____, a driver's license is a symbol of adult responsibility. To drive is to take life and death into your own hands. You will only drive the car after you have asked for my permission. I expect you to drive safely, obeying all laws. You are not to drink or use drugs and drive. If you do, leave the car parked and phone me at any time and with no lectures I will pick you up to bring you safely home. Above all, I want to you to return home safe and alive. I expect you to be where you have told me you will be. You are not to drive all over the county taking your friends wherever they want to go. You are responsible for the care of the car. I expect you to replace the gas you use and to keep the car clean. Enjoy this new privilege, but be aware that I am prepared to ground you for irresponsible actions."

RITES OF PASSAGE FOR ADULTS

34. First full-time job. "____, I am happy for you. This is just one more step in your adult life."

35. Leaving home for college. "____, I am overjoyed that you have this opportunity for higher education. Learn, grow and become. This is a vital foundation for the rest of your life. I am proud of you."

36. Entering military service. "____, I am overjoyed that you have this opportunity to serve our nation. Learn, grow and become. This is a vital foundation for the rest of your life. I am proud of you."

37. Leaving home for the last time. "____, I have mixed feelings. I am happy that you are moving on into a life of independent adulthood. I am sad that you will no longer be here for me to enjoy. May God bless, guide, and protect you."

38. Vocational choice. "____, you are beginning a vocation. No one knows if this is the one for you. I support you in this new adventure. May God guide and sustain you."

39. Vocational achievement. "____, I am so happy for you. Congratulations. May this be first of many joyful reports. I hold you in my prayers."

40. Changing vocations. "____, you are beginning a new vocation that may bless you for years to come. I support you in this new venture and my love goes with you."

41. Engagement. "____, I am happy for you. I hope this leads to a joyous wedding and many years of fulfilling marriage."

42. Wedding. "____, I am so happy for you both. I wish you happiness and fulfillment as you begin a new family. I will always be your family. May God bless you and your new spouse."

YOUR OWN FAMILY RITES

43. Wedding anniversary. "____, I rejoice in this past year of marriage. I celebrate our love and happiness. May our love, friendship, passion and commitment grow stronger in the coming year. May we bless each other with mutual support, acceptance and affection."

44. Pregnancy. "____, how wonderful. We are going to have a baby. May God's peace abide with us as we share this pregnancy together. God, bless our unborn child, that s/he might be born healthy and whole."

45. Childbirth. "____, God has blessed us. May we be a blessing to our child. God, nurture our baby, provide for her/his needs and protect her/him from all harm."

46. Parenthood. "God, you have blessed us with this child. Provide us with the wisdom and maturity we need to be our best. Bless our child with health and wholeness. Thank you."

47. Moving to a new residence. "____, this is another step in our life. We say good-bye to this home that has been our haven of safety and love. God, bless us as we move into our new home. Provide for our needs and help us to make the necessary adjustments."

48. Balancing career and parenthood. "____, this is a difficult and challenging time in our lives. This is what you have chosen and need to do. This calls for everyone in the family to cooperate and support one another. God bless us as we begin this new style as a family. Guide and sustain us day by day."

49. Going back to school with career and parenthood. "____, we are happy you have this opportunity to return to school. We support you as your family. It will be difficult for all of us but this is a vital foundation for the rest of your life. We are proud of you."

50. Struggling with life. "____, life has been difficult. God, fill us with your love and light. Strengthen us for the hurting on this part of the journey. We live in hope and seek your light to guide us."

51. Mid-life crisis. "____, we have lost our way. Life is not turning out as we expected. We are disillusioned. God, help us to get through this. We know that life will once again be good. We seek a clear mind and guidance into a better future. Fulfill our needs."

52. A new beginning. "____, it is scary to move in a new direction. It is also exciting. God, bless us on this new venture. Lead us into the light of this new dream."

53. Grandparenthood. "____, we are grandparents. This is a new stage of our life. We rejoice in this new opportunity as a family. May we be worthy for the task. God, bless our new grandchild and his/her parents. Guide and sustain them all."

54. Chronic illness. "____, I know this is a difficult time in your life. Your life has become so limited. Adjusting is difficult. I will support you and help you to live life to its fullest. I will help you use Therapeutic Prayer, as we seek to renew you in body, mind and spirit."

55. Retirement. "____, it is time to retire. It seems like just yesterday you began working. You have enjoyed the challenge of working day after day, year after year. Retirement brings us feelings of both sadness and relief. Now we enter a new stage of our lives that may be just as long and satisfying as our work years. May God bless us in this new and joyous journey."

HEALTHY LIFESTYLE RITES OF PASSAGE

56. For regular exercise. "_____, I am proud of your commitment to a regular exercise program. I encourage you in your efforts and will support you in every possible way."

57. Regular exercise for three months. "_____, I am proud of your persistence in exercising regularly. You are looking better and appear to have far more energy. I encourage you in your efforts and will continue supporting you in every possible way.

58. For a healthy diet. "_____, I am proud of your commitment to a healthier diet, low in cholesterol, fats, sugar and salt and high in carbohydrates, fruits and vegetables. I encourage you in your efforts and will support you in every possible way in your new healthy lifestyle."

59. A healthy diet for three months. "_____, I am proud of you for maintaining your healthy new diet. I know this has been a difficult lifestyle change. I encourage you in your efforts and will support you in every possible way in your new healthy lifestyle."

60. For weight loss. "_____, I am proud of you for your commitment to lose weight through regular exercise and a new diet low in cholesterol, fats, sugar and salt and high in carbohydrates, fruits and vegetables. I encourage you in your efforts and will support you in every possible way in your new healthy lifestyle."

61 Weight loss for three months. "_____, I am proud of you for maintaining your healthy new lifestyle. Your weight loss is obvious and you look great. I also note your new energy and self-image. I know this has been a difficult lifestyle change. I encourage you in your efforts and will support you in every possible way in your new healthy lifestyle."

62. Quitting smoking. "_____, I am happy about your decision to quit smoking. I recognize this is a challenging task as you strive for a healthier lifestyle. I encourage you in your efforts and will support you in every possible way. May God strengthen you, remove your withdrawal symptoms and smooth your way.

63. Quitting smoking for a month. "_____, I am overjoyed that you have been nicotine-free for a whole month. You have done well. I congratulate you on your healthy new lifestyle. May God grant you peace and continue renewing every cell in your body that you might enjoy excellent health."

64. Alcohol or drug free. "_____, I am happy about your decision to be alcohol (or drug) free. I recognize this is a difficult task. I encourage you in your efforts and will support you in every way. May God strengthen you and remove your withdrawal symptoms."

65. Alcohol or drug free for a month. "_____, I am overjoyed that you have been alcohol (or drug) free for a whole month. You have done well. I congratulate you on your healthy new lifestyle. May God grant you peace and continue renewing every cell in your body that you might enjoy excellent health."

66. Stress reduction. "____, I am proud of your commitment to lower your stress levels. I support you in your program plans. May God guide and sustain you and grant you peace."

67. Stress reduction for three months. "____, I am overjoyed that you have lowered the stress factors in your life. You have done well. I congratulate you on your healthy new lifestyle. May God grant you peace and continue renewing every cell in your body that you might enjoy excellent health."

68. Healing a hurt. "____, I am proud of your decision to heal your hurts. I encourage you in your efforts and will support you in every possible way. May God empower your efforts, fill you with love and heal your hurts."

69. Hurt healed. "____, I am overjoyed that you have healed your hurt and feel free to move happily on with your life. You have done well. I congratulate you on your new inner wholeness. May God grant you peace and continue renewing your soul."

70. Facing a serious illness. "___, I am proud of your decision to fight for your health. You have chosen to take charge of your life and explore all means for getting well. Have the courage and wisdom to explore alternative health care. Seek happiness and satisfaction in all areas of your life. Fill yourself with a new zest for living and find joy in each day. I encourage you in your efforts and will support you with my love and prayers. May God guide and sustain you. May God heal you in body, mind and spirit."

71. Progress in finding health. "___, I am overjoyed that you are making progress on your road back to health. I encourage you to continue your journey and will support you with my love and prayers. May God continue restoring your health."

MEDALS OF HONOR

Medals may be handwritten, typed or computer-generated on paper, or may be made of any substance or shape.

72. Medal of Honor. For extraordinary heroism against great odds.

73. Distinguished Service Medal. For outstanding service to loved ones.

74. Legion of Merit. For providing outstanding support during difficult times.

75. Purple Heart. For enduring unwanted suffering with courage and grace.

76. Medal of Valor. For courage displayed while doing your best.

77. Good Conduct Medal. For responsible living in the midst of great pressure.

PRAYER in the World's Great Religions

CHRISTIANITY: *"Therefore I tell you, whatever you ask in prayer, believe that you will receive it, and you will."*

ISLAM: *"Never, Lord, have I prayed to You with ill success."*

BUDDHISM: *"There is no meditation apart from wisdom, and no wisdom apart from meditation. Those in whom wisdom and meditation meet are not far from Heaven."*

HINDUISM: *"I make prayer my inmost friend."*

JUDAISM: *"Pray to the Lord our God that He may show us the way to go and the thing we should do."*

SHINTO: *"If the poorest of mankind come for worship, I will surely grant their heart's desire."*

CONFUSIONISM: *"...cultivate the virtues of reverence. When a man is devoted to this virtue, he may pray to Heaven."*

Chapter Thirty

Prayers for Renewing the Community

"The present task is to help create the fundamental conditions that will reestablish living contact with God, who alone can give meaning and purpose to life." ...Alfred Delp

"God is able to subdue all evil, but God calls on humankind to cooperate in this task and strengthens those who do so." ...Martin Luther King, Jr.*

"Whoever loves God loves all persons without regard to whether they are just or unjust." ...Saint Maximus the Confessor*

Would you be willing to cooperate in dramatically changing the quality of life in your community? What if you could participate in making your community crime-free from the comfort of your home? What if you could increase the quality of the safety and education of your neighborhood schools by offering Therapeutic Prayer for ten minutes a day? Would you be willing to help fill your community with the spirit of love, caring and calm?

These goals are possible if people cooperate in bathing a community in God's love by forming a huge therapeutic sacred group energy field. In chapters seven, eight, ten, twenty-five and twenty-six, the benefits of sacred group energy fields were explored. People bathed in such a group energy field would slowly but surely be transformed by the information present. Would your community do it?

The power of prayer is the square of the number of persons praying. One thousand people praying is one hundred thousand units of prayer power. Ten thousand people praying is ten million units of prayer power. One million people praying is one trillion units of prayer power. *What a powerful and helpful therapeutic sacred group energy field they could form!* Any community could use Therapeutic Prayer for transforming people into kinder, gentler, more responsible and caring humans. A nation with fifty million praying people would form a therapeutic sacred group energy field of 5,000,000, 000,000,000 units of prayer power.

For centuries, leaders rooted in the religious community have proclaimed that the source of our human problem is the absence of God from our homes, schools, institutions and communities. Science has now proven this truth. God transforms and makes all things new. God creates the optimum conditions for human life. God heals the body, mind, spirit and relationships. God is the source of all love, compassion and responsibility.

THE DEVELOPMENT OF SECULAR HUMANITY

Every year humans become more isolated from each other. Every year our planet becomes more violent. Every year human unhappiness seems to grow. Every year marriages and families seem to struggle more to survive as safe, nurturing shelters for people. Every year more people fill our cities. Every year humanity becomes less aware of God. Every year humans become more secular. These trends grow stronger with each passing year.

Before the 1960s, God seemed to be present in every aspect of community life in the United States. While I was growing up, my public school teachers read the Bible and offered prayer at the beginning of each school day. My scoutmaster offered prayer at Boy Scout meetings. Many families practiced devotional prayer and table graces. At every community gathering, prayer invocations were offered. Many businesses and industries began the day with prayer. But through the years, we have seen prayer being systematically excluded from almost all areas of American life. This is true in many other nations, as well.

Many events account for these changes. The United States Supreme Court barred all prayer and other religious expressions in public schools. This meant that children who did not participate in organized religion had little awareness of either prayer or God. Public school children had to rely on either a religious community or their families if they were to be introduced to prayer. Most never were.

The United States was also becoming a more religiously diverse society. First came the sensitivity to Jews and non-believers in a dominantly Christian culture. Then came the influx of new immigrants from Asia and the Middle East from other religious traditions: Hindu, Buddhist, Muslim, Shinto, tribal and primitive religions. We had become a religiously pluralistic society.

Throughout this time of religious change, many Christian church bodies became extremely aggressive in seeking new converts for their brand of Christianity. This approach upset most people, resulting eventually in a public aversion to most expressions of religion in public life, including prayer.

The United States was also changing in other ways. The sense of neighborhood and community identity was breaking down. American urban life changed from being somewhat personal and caring to becoming detached, individualized and indifferent. Today, most Americans do not know their neighbors and do not care to. In this new atmosphere, the intimate and personal practice of prayer seems strangely out of place in most community settings. The practice of prayer has been turned over to and become the sole property of religious communities.

With this overall de-emphasis upon prayer, families are no longer motivated to pray together. They ask, *"Why should we pray? It doesn't seem to matter one way or another."* In addition, most adults lack the necessary skills for praying aloud. Less than one percent of people have ever prayed aloud for a spouse's needs. Even if there were more opportunities for praying within a community setting, few people have mastered the necessary skills for doing so.

It sounds as if it has all been settled. For various reasons, prayer has been pushed out of the life of community institutions in the United States. We are not unique. Most industrialized and urban populations live under similar conditions, with the exception of the Islamic nations, and they, too, have experienced a diminishing level of personal vocal prayer among family members. The absence of God's presence persists in communities around the world. Most of humanity lives in secular communities, devoid of the awareness of God.

So who cares? Our urban areas face the breakdown of satisfying marriage and family life, a thirty percent student dropout rate, annual increases in crime, violence, substance abuse, destructive lifestyles, depression and cancer. Our political, educational, medical, social and religious institutions have shown themselves powerless to turn things around. The quality of human life continues to deteriorate throughout America.

Who cares about prayer being returned to community life? Anyone should, who knows about the transformative power of prayer. Anyone who knows about the power and influence of huge sacred group energy fields should see the value of prayer in a community setting.

Both scientific research data and experience indicate that people gathered in prayer create a powerful sacred group energy field whose energy works to transform all persons enveloped within it. The transforming effect can mold and shape each individual with the highest moral and spiritual qualities expressed by their culture. The healing energy of prayer is information-bearing and acts intelligently to produce optimal qualities in people. Any community or group of persons who cooperate in creating a prayer-induced group sacred energy field can bathe their whole community, transforming all persons into responsible, caring and contributing members. Therapeutic Prayer introduces order into chaos, reprogramming evil with goodness and love. I know of no urban area where the citizens do not deeply desire such results.

If Therapeutic Prayer were practiced in the schools alone, its benefits would greatly increase student performance, produce children who are healthy in body, mind and spirit, and reduce violence, drug abuse and crime. Practiced in the workplace, it could reduce stress, haggling, negativity and fatigue by increasing peace, love, concern and harmony. Similar results could be predicted for every other group in the community.

Prayer is the most powerful tool known to humanity for providing an energy for healing, satisfaction and happiness. Do you want people to be loving, caring, sensitive, intelligent, creative, productive, responsible, just and healthy? Then intentionally bathe them in a prayer-induced sacred group energy field.

HOW CAN WE REVERSE PRESENT TRENDS?

To reverse present trends, we **first** need to separate prayer from religious beliefs and institutions. The PrayWell tenets stated in chapter two have already explained how prayers can be religiously neutral. We have introduced the concept and practice of Therapeutic Prayer throughout PrayWell.

The purpose of Therapeutic Prayer is to express caring and to bring the power of God into the lives of hurting people.

Some may object that prayer-created therapeutic group energy fields would infringe upon the personal freedom to be less than whole. This argument holds no weight. Free will permits those who do not wish to be changed to close their own energy fields and remain as they are.

In the context of community use, Therapeutic Prayer changes the circumstance of public prayer. The present legal perception and judgment by the United States Supreme Court that public prayer promotes religious belief would no longer apply. The use of Therapeutic Prayer cannot be understood as a community or the state seeking to establish religious beliefs. The legal argument for its constitutional use is that its purpose is virtuously therapeutic and that it does not seek to promote belief in God, but rather seek to utilize a life energy which scientifically is known to exist throughout our planet. This provides individuals, families and communities with a vital resource that therapeutically transforms human life.

Second, the United States Supreme Court has legally ruled that public prayer is illegal because it promotes the belief in God by addressing the Supreme Being. Thus, this impinges on the rights of atheistic believers who maintain that there is no God. This ruling is based upon the *belief* that God exists, not the *scientific fact* that a life energy exists. If scientific evidence were presented to the courts that the existence of life energy is a scientific fact, then it could change previous legal rulings banning public prayers. See chapter eleven for a fuller exploration of this topic.

CREATING THERAPEUTIC GROUP ENERGY FIELDS

Most religions envision their own particular religious beliefs spreading throughout the earth to bring their version of the kingdom of God to all humanity. Historically, such idealistic but aggressive religious visions have always divided people and often produced religious hostility, persecutions and wars. In today's world, the Cold War may be succeeded by religious wars. We are moving ominously toward rivalries between religions which could suddenly move us in the direction of another world war. These religious rivalries also involve national and ethnic pride, economic competition and human rights. The tenets of PrayWell are intended to build bridges of understanding and respect between diverse religious groups. The prayers in this chapter are religiously neutral and are intended to be used for therapeutic purposes in diverse settings such as are found in most communities across the globe.

If you wish to experiment with producing a large sacred group energy field through prayer, then the following knowledge will be helpful. It is crucial that your group be united by common, agreed-upon goals which all are willing to act upon. Education of individuals concerning the goals is a must. So is group action.

You must identify and recruit group catalysts to serve as leaders. These are charismatic persons. They are friendly, creative, caring, gentle persons who might not normally be considered for leadership. On the Meyers-Briggs Type Indicator, they are ENFJs. They are most likely be found among the caring professions: teachers, nurses, psychotherapists, clergy, personnel directors, and among sports coaches, caring parents and thera-peutic personalities. If you have an interest in doing this type of work, you may be a group catalyst. See chapter eight for further explanation.

The following applications are designed to be practical. They are based upon the practical needs and hopes of the people involved, the elements upon which prayer results and group energy fields have always been based.

THERAPEUTIC PRAYER IN THE EDUCATIONAL CLASSROOM

Classroom prayer creates an energy which has the power to assist in heal-ing the life hurts, angers and dysfunctions of children, to build classroom harmony and discipline and to enhance student responsibility and learning performance in school classrooms. Prayer creates a wholesome, informa-tion-bearing, therapeutic group energy field which is supportive of the needs of children, parents and teachers.

As I write, any prayer, no matter how religiously neutral, is illegal in American public classrooms. Some educators believe that this absence of prayer contributes to the ongoing deterioration of discipline and academic achievement in the public schools and to the breakdown of morality and emotional wholeness among children and youth in the home, school and community. The scientific data on the beneficial results of prayer would support this belief.

Teachers may use their best professional skills in seeking to build a sense of individual responsibility, classroom cohesiveness, academic achievement, emotional wholeness and moral maturity, but they are doomed to failure. Educational and counseling skills alone do not possess the necessary qualities for developing emotional wholeness and moral maturity. The problem lies in the absence of healing energy in the class-room. Bathing children in sacred therapeutic group energy fields is a necessary tool in achieving these goals. We need Therapeutic Prayer to restore wholeness to classrooms.

A sacred therapeutic group energy field can be achieved without using prayer or mentioning God. From the perspective of spiritual healing, emotionally and morally dysfunctional children possess unhealthy personal energy fields. This is because their energy fields lack qualities like love, joy, peace, patience, kindness, goodness, faithfulness, gentleness and self-control. Christians refer to these qualities as the fruits of the presence of God's Spirit. In other words, these qualities are the natural results of spiri-tuality.

When students are bathed in God's love, the resulting energy begins transforming them into emotionally and morally healthy individuals. This state of being is normal for all humans. The educational goal of sacred therapeutic group energy fields is to change student brain-wave patterns and energy fields, so that they contain information which produces emotional and moral wholeness. This goal is achieved through several steps.

1. CHOOSING BENEFICIAL QUALITIES

Educators first need to decide on the qualities of character and emotions beneficial for student growth and learning. Begin with the above cited qualities of love, joy, peace, patience, kindness, goodness, faithfulness, gentleness, and self-control. Add other beneficial character qualities. Then educate students in these individual qualities. As items of rational knowledge, they do not have the capacity to transform students. The education only becomes useful when these character and emotional qualities are internalized or encoded into brain-wave and energy field patterns through spiritual techniques. This only transpires while students are in an altered state of awareness. Much of the educational process needs to occur while students are surrounded in a sacred group energy field.

2. PARENTS, TEACHERS AND STUDENTS PRAYING

If a school has one thousand students, fifty teachers and one thousand parents in prayer, they form a sacred therapeutic group energy field of about one million energy units of prayer power. Such an energy field bathes not only the students but their teachers and parents in God's transforming energy. This heals the hurts and feelings of everyone involved. They could form and maintain such an energy field by offering Therapeutic Prayer several times a day. This would restore a sense of community to everyone involved. Such a Therapeutic Prayer could be very simple:

God, we thank you for the students, teachers and parents of our school. Fill us with your love and light. Provide for their needs and protect them from all harm. Heal the hurts of each person and make each whole in body, mind and spirit. Let us be one in peace and community. Amen.

3. ALTERED AWARENESS EXERCISES

These models are meant to stimulate creative thinking. Professional educators are highly capable of designing their own models. Begin with group exercises and then encourage individual practice.

A. **Playing soothing classical or easy listening music** in the background enables persons to enter an altered state of awareness. Rock and other hard beat music is counterproductive. Teachers and students can write lyrics to soothing tunes, using beneficial character traits and emotions to which they are being introduced.

B. **Group consciousness-focusing exercises** (non-religious meditation). The group impact is far stronger than individual practice because it creates a group energy field. Ten minutes of effort each morning begins equipping the brain to focus. Remember, be creative and aim to restore inner calm and tranquillity. It may take several weeks to notice any change. There are numerous choices for focusing exercises. These are slowly chanted or spoken in unison in one repetition after another, with the leader setting the cadence for ten minutes.

1. *"Aaaahhh,"* chanted.

2. The five vowels, *"A, E, I, O, U"* chanted each individually.

3. The word *"one"* spoken.

4. A term for a feeling, like *"love"* or *"peace,"* spoken.

5. Counting out-breaths in groups of four while breathing normally. 1, 2, 3 , 4...1, 2, 3, 4...1, 2, 3, 4...

6. Deep breathing exercises. Standing, students slowly take in a deep breath through their nose, filling their diaphragms on a count of eight. Hold for a count of four, exhale through the mouth on the count of eight, and hold the out-breath for a count of four.

7. Induce a light hypnotic state or other relaxed state during which the above are performed.

8. Yoga is a non-religious process. Hundreds of thousands of yoga groups meet in formerly atheistic eastern European nations. Their purpose is the discipline of the body, mind and spirit. This creates healthy energy fields and the qualities of spirituality. Internationally known yoga instructor Dr. Marilyn Rossner, a special education professor in Montreal, Quebec, has used yoga to produce significant results with children who are emotionally troubled or have learning disabilities. Yoga could also benefit juvenile delinquents and adult criminals.

C. **Use stories, movies, and videos** that express the beneficial emotions.

4. *MENTAL VISUALIZATIONS*

A. Mentally visualize specific positive and negative emotions.
B. Mentally visualize a hope, focus or need.
C. Mentally visualize a class goal.
D. Mentally visualize wholeness for a member of the class who is ill, emotionally troubled, in a bad home situation, panicky at test-time or struggling with a subject. This technique produces significant results. One style fits all situations. With the intention of helping the person, each class member mentally visualizes twin objects of any kind, then merges the objects. One object represents the person for whom there is concern. The other represents the visualizer.

5. *GROUP SPIRITUAL RITUALS*

If at all possible, have everyone hold hands. This transmits healing energy even to those who are reluctant to cooperate.

A. *A RITUAL OF EDUCATIONAL GOALS TO BE SPOKEN IN UNISON*

We are gathered to learn and grow. We seek to prepare ourselves with the resources needed to succeed in the adult world. We do not have it all together. We struggle. At times, we fail. Sometimes we are lost and uninterested and give up for awhile. Sometimes we do not feel like we belong. Sometimes the hurt from life threatens to overwhelm us. But we affirm our need to keep growing somehow beyond where we presently are.

As we gather here to learn, we agree to support each other. We agree to care about each other's pain and not add to the pain present in the world. We agree to help each other learn through encouragement and cooperation. We each agree to do our best. We agree that we are all in this together. Let us be one in affirming these goals.

B. *A RITUAL OF AFFIRMATION TO BE SPOKEN IN UNISON*

We come as individuals from many backgrounds and situations but celebrate the contributions our rich diversity produces. We affirm our fellow students in their desire to grow. We affirm our fellow students in their pain and struggles. We seek a oneness which heals and makes each of us whole. Unite us as one and may power flow from the unity binding us together. We affirm that this school and our teachers wish to help us learn the skills necessary for satisfying living. Let this be.

C. *A UNIVERSAL THERAPEUTIC PRAYER*

God, as we gather together in prayer, fill us with your presence. May each of us personally make contact with you. May this contact heal our hurts and restore us to normal. And as we pray, may your presence fill everyone in this room and create a huge energy field which encompasses us all. May your energy guide, sustain and empower us as we study. Fill us with your love, joy, and peace that we might rejoice and be happy. Amen.

These tools act to restore healthy patterns in the brain and in the energy fields, producing whole human beings. Within weeks, changes in personal qualities will be noticed. Once a fourth of the students have been changed, their energy fields begin permeating the entire classroom, accelerating the process for everyone. When all classrooms are producing healthy energy fields, their energy fields fill the whole school building and continue to transform and sustain everyone within it. When all students and teachers possess healthy personal energy fields, the process of learning is significantly accelerated and educational achievement occurs. At the same time, parents are being transformed in similar ways.

THERAPEUTIC PRAYER WHERE YOU WORK

Prayer provides an energy for wholeness in all situations. Anyplace where people work can produce stress, anger, frustration, distrust, bitterness and unhappiness. Introducing prayer to your vocational situation will change this. Therapeutic Prayer creates a sacred group energy field that bathes everyone in God's love. It acts intelligently to bring wholeness on the basis of the intentions of the pray-ers.

Before introducing any prayer activities, seek the cooperation and support of the appropriate leadership. Otherwise, these activities may be perceived suspiciously as partisan, controversial, divisive and thus, inappropriate. Prayers in the work setting must be perceived as neutral, representing the best interests of all parties involved. When prayer is used as a weapon of power or control, it ceases being prayer and might better be considered as an attempt at black magic manipulation. Emphasize to everyone that the prayers you wish to introduce are religiously neutral and their purpose is therapeutic. You wish to lower tension and stress in your work situation through therapeutic prayer. Here are some suggestions.

1. **A Prayer Chain.** Wait until someone is in crisis due to injury, illness, death, divorce, etc. Organize a Prayer Chain to pray for that person. Chapter twenty-three provides guidance for prayer chains, including procedures and prayer models. A prayer chain can personalize relationships,

providing a personal means for people to express their concern. It brings God's power into the life of hurting people. It produces group closeness and satisfaction. From this one incident, an ongoing prayer chain can develop.

2. **Special Occasion Prayers.** Prayers of celebration for promotions, retirements, weddings and new-born infants affirm the recipient and enable everyone to rejoice. Asking everyone to join you in such a prayer can be a first step in establishing prayer where you work. Models for such prayers can be found in chapter twenty-seven.

3. **Therapeutic Prayers with Which to Begin Work.** If you work with one or more persons, you might suggest a therapeutic prayer together to begin your work-day. Here are some models:

A. **Mutual Goals.** *God, we seek your guidance and support as we work here together. Enable us to be efficient and creative, cooperative and caring during our work today. We take pride in what we do and we ask you to bless us that we might become blessings to all whom we serve. Our work contributes to the welfare of our community, nation and world. It is the livelihood we each depend upon to pay the bills and put food on the table. Enable what we do to be useful, needed and profitable. God, thank you for vocations that make us feel useful and worthwhile. Protect our jobs that we might remain secure day by day, and year after year. Amen.*

B. **To Form a Sacred Group Energy Field.** *God, we thank you for the opportunity to work for _____ (name place of business). Unite us as one, as sacred and unique individuals working for common goals. We pray for the healing of every worker, that all might be whole in body, mind and spirit. Unite us as one, keep us from all harm, and provide for our needs. Enable us to be valuable in serving people. Fill us each with your love, joy and peace that our lives might be filled with your happiness and satisfaction. Unite us as one, enabling us to understand and care for each other.* (Then visualize being one with every worker.) *Amen.*

THERAPEUTIC PRAYER IN INSTITUTIONS

The residents of any institution would benefit from being bathed in a sacred therapeutic group energy field. Such institutions include medical centers, mental hospitals, prisons, juvenile detention facilities, and any other treatment facility. Staff and residents could work together. The forming of support groups as explored in chapter twenty-six would work in many institutions.

Evidence strongly suggests that violent people can be transformed into cooperative and productive citizens through Therapeutic Prayer. Chapters twenty and twenty-two provide assistance for residents in many institutional settings.

THERAPEUTIC PRAYER IN THE LOCAL-GLOBAL COMMUNITY

If there is a yearning for an improvement of the quality of life in a community, the creation of a community-encompassing, sacred group energy field may produce the desired improvements. Achieving this is not as simple as the concept might imply. Preparations include community meetings to air and discuss concerns, a community consensus on the qualities needed, specific goals and a plan for fulfilling those goals practically. Such plans might include social, recreational and commercial events, block parties and home groups.

This whole process can then be strengthened with appropriate prayers by residents during each stage. The prayers must be centered in anticipation and hope. The prayers need to be positive, with blessings for troubling elements and including the emotional and attitudinal qualities which address neighborhood needs. Such prayers create a therapeutic sacred group energy field which pervades the whole neighborhood. The information possessed by the energy field will begin acting to transform all who are bathed by the qualities inherent in the prayers.

APPLICATIONS FOR WORLD PEACE

When national interests come into conflict and tension and distrust build, war becomes a possibility. Sometimes a military conflict has already begun. People ask, *"For what should I pray?"* That depends upon what you wish your prayers to accomplish. If your purpose is peace, then do not include animosity and hatred toward your nation's current enemy. This only makes the enemy into the type of monster you feared he might become. When millions of people do this, the enemy may be transformed more powerfully into the image expressed in your prayer. If you are truly seeking peace, then send your enemy prayers of love and peace. The same is true in praying for your own country. The problem is that it takes more courage to pray openly for peace in the midst of nationalistic sentiments than it does to prepare for and fight a war.

A Prayer for Peace. *God, the creator and sustainer of all life, we come to you in prayer about the tensions existing between our nation and the nation of _____. In today's world, we know that wars destroy people and the ecology of our planet. Most wars are fought in the national interest and out of a sense of some form of social justice. Yet the world craves peace.*

We pray for our national leaders, _____, and for the leaders of the nation of _____. We ask you to fill these leaders with your love, peace and presence. Enable understanding to be negotiated so that no military operation takes place. Enable them to be responsible in recognizing the precious sacredness of every human life. We hold these leaders in oneness with you and ourselves. (Here visualize yourself being at peace and in oneness with God and these leaders.)

We also pray for the people of nation _____. Fill them with your love and peace. Unite us as fellow sacred human beings, seeking to live daily in peace with fairness for all peoples. Thank you for hearing our prayer and for the new life you bring. Amen.

When a group has successfully been transformed through prayer-created sacred group energy fields, it is time to celebrate. It is also time to spread the good news to others and to offer them help from what you have learned. This spiritual technology is just in its infancy. But it can grow to adulthood rapidly as it serves the urgent needs of people who are desperately seeking answers.

Chapter Thirty-One

Prayers for Restoring the Earth

"True dialogue between persons of different cultures is a contemporary need." ...Raimundo Panikkar*

"No man is an island, entire of itself; every man is a piece of the continent, a part of the main. If a clod be washed away by the sea, Europe is the less; ...as well as if a manor of thy friend's or of thine own were: any man's death diminishes me, because I am involved in mankind, and therefore never send to know for whom the bell tolls; it tolls for thee." ...John Donne*

"In its highest expression, spiritual religion involves a sacramental view of life, an openness to continual revelation, a recognition of a universal call to ministry, and action in accordance with a belief in the sacredness of human life." ...D. Elton Trueblood*

This is a real *"pie in the sky"* type of chapter. If you are not an idealist, stop here. If you are not a dreamer, stop here. If you are not open to creative imagination and experimentation, stop here. If you do not support the utopian goal of restoring all of planet Earth to its earlier emerald splendor, stop here. Go back and use those spiritual technologies that may prove to be the most helpful to you. But stop here, because I do not want you to dismiss the rest of this book by your rejection of what you will be reading here.

This chapter is for young adults, college students and recent college graduates, for religious and spiritual communities, for military personnel, for ecological groups and for any nation that has a community spirit. Among nations, China comes immediately to mind. This chapter is for physicists, mathematicians, engineers, clairvoyants and healers. This chapter is for those who want to go far beyond recycling trash and using organically grown food in their efforts to ecologically restore our planet. This chapter is for those who are terrified by the ultimate implications of toxic waste sites, polluted air and water, the depletion of the ozone layer and the greenhouse effect.

Even if planetary military spending were drastically curtailed and all governments began focusing new resources upon these problems, humanity remains extremely limited in what it can do at this point in history to quickly restore the health of the Earth. We appear to be doomed!

But there is a theoretical solution based upon the data of healing research. It begins with the nature of healing energy already described. The healing energy acts intelligently to restore all life to optimum health. The healing energy is also capable of intentionally acting to transform and control any form of matter or energy. In one example of this, healer Olga

Worrall was able to use her hands to change the direction of the energy flow in an atomic cloud chamber.

Healing energy is the same powerful, creative, intelligent energy force that was at work when the earliest life forms began developing on Earth. It has always been present on the living Earth. The healing energy frequency is the same electromagnetic frequency as the variable Schumann frequencies that exit from the Earth's ionosphere resonant cavity. The Schumann frequencies vary according to the day, time of month and time of year at plus or minus 7.83 hertz. All life on earth resonates with the Schumann frequencies.

That may help to account for the instinctive migratory and seasonal patterns of birds, fish, animals and plants. Because all life resonates with the Schumann frequencies of the Earth, they may be the best explanation for how all life forms are able to communicate with each other. Since the Earth is a living organism, the Earth may use the Schumann frequencies to regulate the environment intelligently, including weather patterns, the ozone layer, and the cleansing of fluorides from the atmosphere and the oceans.

Humanity's overpopulation and ballooning volume of refuse have overburdened the Earth's natural capacity to regulate its environment. Here is where humanity's uniqueness as a life form can intervene to restore the environment of Earth. Every human possesses the natural ability to utilize freely the 7.83 healing frequency -- the Life Force. The Judeo-Islamic-Christian religious tradition believes that humanity's role is to preserve the Earth and all life upon it. Environmentally that means to live in harmony with the needs of our planet. With the new picture of the healing energy's enormous potential, it becomes apparent that humanity can also recreate the environment by collectively harnessing the power of the healing energy-life force.

What if a billion people collectively formed a sacred group energy field encompassing the whole Earth through prayer, consciousness and intention? Could they collectively utilize this enormous healing energy force to restore the environment of the Earth? Squaring the power of collective planetary prayer, their energy force would amount to 1,000,000,000,000, 000,000 energy units of healing power. That would be one of the most powerful forces ever to exist on Earth.

The first step in accomplishing this is to identify and organize people who are driven to find answers through experimentation. All powerful group energy fields are formed by people who share a common strong emotion and commitment or an aroused consciousness. This we see in sports events, massive acts of violence, passive resistance movements and the group consciousness that ended the reign of Communism in Eastern Europe in 1989.

The next step is educating everyone so that a common consciousness and sense of determination are created. The educational emphasis must include a plan of action. Ideas best take form and develop power through action.

The third step is to identify group catalysts to create and maintain a group energy field. Their traits were identified in chapter eight in the profile of healers. They may not be among the people who initially decide to take action. They are not interested so much in leadership power and status as they are in caring for people.

The fourth step remains unresolved. The most powerful and intelligently-acting group energy fields that I have known occurred at large healing services. When the intention is to care through healing, the group healing energy field develops. In several small groups, we have experimented with creating group energy fields involving qualities like love or peace, by simply mentally seeking to do so. These experiments all failed. The only consistently predictable group energy fields I have seen have occurred when people were gathered for a specific action. These included support groups filled with compassion, religious rituals and healing services. Crowds at sports events naturally create such fields as they do at festivals, protest marches, riots, lynchings, wars and funerals.

All but one of these approaches must be ruled out. Since we are talking about producing a group energy field to restore the environment, that energy field must be attuned to the frequency of healing energy. The only way to do this is by having a healing service. Therefore, as unconventional as it might seem, each group catalyst must learn to practice healing both individually and in groups. Only then can they hope to produce a healing group energy field attuned to the healing frequency.

Fifth, using similar logic, everyone involved must learn to practice touch-healing and vocal prayer. This process will provide practical skills for producing and sustaining group recreative energy fields. Prayer is the primary tool for empowering such a field.

Sixth, though most group catalyst healers are capable of attuning energy, the skills of clairvoyants would be necessary for attuning and directing the group's energy. The clairvoyants must have the psi-sensitive ability to see and direct energy. Psi sensitives can be found in most groups. They must feel safe and truly useful before they will be willing to reveal themselves.

Seventh, the use of electronic technology and crystals would be helpful. The electronic technology must be able to measure reliably the electromagnetic frequencies emitted by such substances as toxic waste products, ozone and fluorides. Using specifically shaped, machine-honed quartz crystal is one way to make an energy frequency reading and facilitate the attunement of healers to the exact recreative frequency necessary to eliminate or transform harmful substances in our environment.

Eighth, small experimental test models could be developed from which one would gain knowledge, skills and strategies. After perfecting individual and group healing skills, the following test models seem appropriate.

A. Remove one ounce of oil from eight ounces of water.
B. Remove the radiation from a small sample of radioactive material.
C. Remove fluorides that have been added to air enclosed in a chamber.
D. Decrease the amount of ozone in a small sample of air.
E. Remove a toxic chemical commonly found at toxic waste sites.
F. Purify a small polluted pond.
G. Seek to change the velocity of a local wind. Or seek to create wind in an enclosed area.

H. Alter existing weather conditions.

Ninth, publicize your results in the mass media, including directions for others.

Tenth, begin organizing people of every nation to develop a planetary recreative energy field.

BEGINNING THE QUEST FOR PRAYERS IN THE COMMUNITY

Introducing the presence of God into a setting is known as "developing spirituality." On a personal basis, spirituality results in a sense of inner well-being, happiness, energy, fulfillment and focus. It produces a sense of deep satisfaction with what one is doing. In addition, it creates a sense of community and group identity, provides a sense of meaning and inter-nalizes group-created goals. This results in an awareness of group unity and common purpose. Spirituality also enhances morale, increases creativity and improves individual health and wholeness. Prayer is a low-tech tool whose costs are minimal and whose benefits are highly desirable.

Before any group energy field is created, certain foundations must be prepared. The group must agree on the common goals it wishes to achieve. Once the goals are set, an educational process can begin. Educational content focuses on a thorough understanding of the goals and their implementation in the group's life. This involves enthusiasm for the goals. It also includes the organization and process needed for praying to induce a sacred group energy field.

CREATING WORLD PEACE WITH JUSTICE AND PROSPERITY

Prominent healers throughout the twentieth century have advocated using the practice of healing to create a better humanity. None talked about the sacred or healing group energy fields discussed in chapter seven. While seeking to restore the Earth's ecology, humanity could also move to elimi-nate the root causes of hunger, disease, pollution, destructive weather, po-litical and economic enslavement, and war.

The personal experience of healing energy or life force results in a sense of whole-hearted oneness or connectedness with other persons. In a local or global setting, it can be predicted that those encompassed in prayer-induced healing group energy fields would sense a oneness with everyone else subject to that field. Conflicts generated by differences of class, race, ethnicity, nationality and religion would disappear. People would see each other as sacred, unique and precious. Compassion, coop-eration, fairness and harmony would pervade human communities. Should a global network of healing group energy fields be put in place, these would be the side-effect. The consciousness of all humanity could change. If this should happen, a new era of world peace, freedom and prosperity would be the natural result.

PREPARING FOR A POSSIBLE NEW SPIRITUAL REALITY

For more than a generation, there have been prophecies, predictions and forecasts from religious and psychic sources that sometime between now and the year 2012, dramatic events are going to occur which will affect all life on earth as we presently know it. The predictions include possible changes to the planet Earth herself, such as a change in the earth's axial tilt and mammoth natural disasters, destructive weather patterns, disease plagues, and the deterioration of social, financial and political institutions. Humanity has little choice but to display a skeptical wait-and-see attitude. But just suppose the earth changes do occur. How would one go about coping with them?

If millions of people are already involved in the ecological restoration of the planet through healing prayer and group healing energy fields, these millions would be qualified to teach others how to alter and maintain the environment through prayer, healing skills and consciousness.

As always, the greatest crisis would involve the emotion of fear itself. People become fearful and angry about changes over which they have no control. The people of the industrialized nations may lose much of what they have considered to be vitally important to their security, status and happiness. The actions resulting from human panic might cause more destruction than the natural changes that would occur. Yet, as they say, life will go on, **if** we have a faith and hope that life will be good again and **if** we cooperate peacefully with each other.

Among the predictions are warnings about a change in the spiritual vibrational frequencies of the planet Earth. This would purportedly result in most of humanity becoming more aware of God's Spirit, other spiritual entities, emotional empathy and mental telepathy. Under such circumstances, it would be crucial to realize that in this new reality, thoughts, emotions and prayers would have immensely more powerful effects on physical reality than they presently do. We would very likely be able to change physical reality through mental, emotional and spiritual acts of will. It would be an exciting new world to explore, if humans were able to sense each other's thoughts and emotions, as well as those of animals and plants.

This would require a level of honesty and integrity never before known to humanity. It would also cause us to become deeply aware of the total Earth environment, with a new awareness of our relationship and responsibility to all life. Under those circumstances, it would be practical to accept the reality of change, learn new skills and ways for adjusting and find the means for happiness and satisfaction within these changes.

We could face such a crisis with calm confidence and be filled with generous love and peace. The supposed reasons for such change are the purification and restoration of Earth, creation of a new awareness and way of life for all humanity, and establishment of a better world where peace, prosperity and justice will benefit all humankind. Skills in prayer, healing and spirituality could become keys to meaningful survival.

Let us deal specifically with one persistent prediction. A changing of the energy frequencies of earth will lower the walls between various vibrational dimensions of reality. Among other things, this will place us in a heightened awareness of spirit beings like ghosts (earthbound spirits), familiar spirits, deceased loved ones and interdimensional entities. If this should occur, remain calm. These new entities may prove to be a nuisance but it is unlikely that they are capable of physically harming human life. In calmness, send them love. Let your thoughts and prayers be focused upon cooperation and friendship. If this should happen, we might need to accommodate ourselves to the long-term relationship required by a shift in energy frequencies.

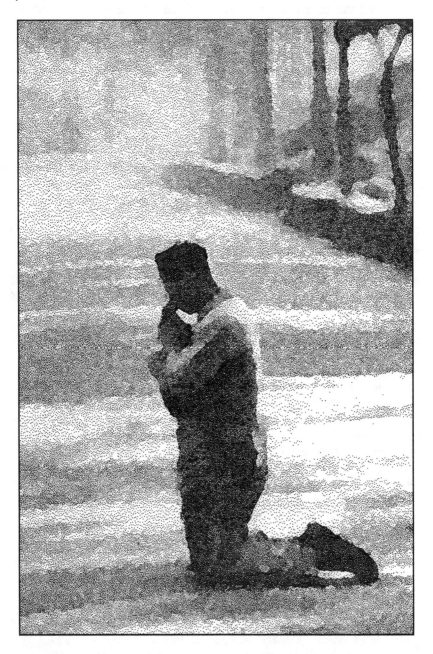

Figure 18. *This lone praying person is typical of the billions of human beings who daily turn to God for help, seeking to bring the power of God into the life of the world. What if a billion persons could join together in prayer for common purposes that express the deepest yearnings of humanity? The energy of their planetary prayer induced group energy field could restore the earth's ecology, limit the damages of nature and produce a Golden Age of peace with justice.*

Chapter Thirty-Two

The Future of Alternative Medicine

"If we have ever made any valuable discovery, it has been owing more to patient attention, than to any talent." ...Isaac Newton

"In science the credit goes to the man who convinces the world, not to the man to whom the first idea occurs." ...William Osler

"I think the greatest discovery will be made along spiritual lines. Here is a force which history clearly teaches has been the greatest power in the development of man. Yet we have merely been playing with it and have never seriously studied it as we have the physical forces.

"Someday people will learn that material things do not bring happiness and are of little use in making men and women creative and powerful. Then the scientists of the world will turn their laboratories over to the study of God and prayer and the spiritual forces which as yet have hardly been scratched. When this day comes, the world will see more advancement in one generation than it has seen in the past four." ...Steinmetz

---

Therapeutic healing and other forms of alternative health care are being used more frequently in the United States. *The New England Journal of Medicine*[1] reports that one-third of Americans used at least one form of alternative or unconventional therapy in 1990.

But the big issue for alternative medicine is health insurance coverage for their patients. In 1990, 425 million visits were made to alternative thera-pists compared with 388 million visits to primary care physicians. Yet, of the 800 billion dollars spent on health care, only 13.7 billion dollars was paid to alternative therapists. That is 1.7 percent of the health care dollar. The average charge per visit for alternative medicine was $27.60. Of that amount, only twenty percent was covered by health insurance.[2]

Can alternative health care providers make a living under these condi-tions? Can a health center providing uninsured holistic health services financially survive?

Alternative medicine takes more time to provide than conventional medicine. I work part-time in a wellness center and spend about ninety minutes with each patient, providing wellness counseling, touch-healing prayer, relaxation therapy, and hypnotherapy. All of this is paid for cash-out -of-the-pocket by the patient. It cannot provide a vocational living for an alternative health care practitioner. The only way alternative medicine can be more available to serve the public is through coverage by private and public health insurance policies.

HEALTH INSURANCE PROMOTES SICKNESS, NOT HEALTH

Dr. Elmer Green of the Menninger Clinic states that no part of the Clinton health care plan for America promotes health. *"In America we have what is euphemistically called 'health care,' but it is actually a Sickness Business, organized for the greatest good of a colossal medico-pharmaceutical complex and its stock holders.*

"And we, passive medical consumers, are held in thrall by smooth advertising of new 'miracle cures' and hyping of multi-million dollar medical technologies. Unfortunately, we are pawns in the medico-pharmaceutical battles that have little to do with the quality of our life, but instead reflect marketplace competition for the eight hundred billion dollars we spend annually for sickness."[3]

Green proposes that we promote health, cut costs and improve the quality of life by teaching youth mind-body self-regulation skills. This, alone, could prevent about fifty percent of all sickness.

Where does the health insurance industry stand on these issues? Green states that the greatest obstacle to *"health"* training comes from hospitals and insurance companies who do not want to reduce medical costs. The present system provides them with huge profits and enormous salaries. They see no personal benefit in promoting health or alternative medicine.

Dr. Green provides clinical evidence that mind-body self-regulation through biofeedback training has permanently cured six thousand alcoholics but Blue Cross/Blue Shield of Kansas will not reimburse this therapy, even though its own medical committee voted for reimbursement.

These policies will only change when the insured demand it. In the meantime, alternative health care providers have developed their own insurance coverage plans in several communities.

THE CONCERNS OF THE MEDICAL COMMUNITY

I would like to be able to walk into a medical center just the way a pharmaceutical representative or a medical specialist does and, with simplicity and directness, say to physicians, *"These are the ways that touch-healing Therapeutic Prayer can benefit your patients. These are the cost savings you can realize with specific patients. Can we sit down together and develop a plan to put this therapy to work with patients in your medical center?*

The first barrier for doing this is that touch-healing is not included in the standard operating procedures of conventional (allopathic) medicine. To include touch-healing in medical center procedures would require the approval of their board of directors and several committees. Therefore, we might best gain entrance to medical centers through medical center doctors.

The brings up the second barrier, the rejection by traditional doctors of touch-healing as a helpful medical tool. Spiritual healing contradicts everything doctors learned in medical school about the basis of health and treatment. It shocks their personal and professional sensibilities. In their minds, this conjures up images of superstitious nonsense and health fraud.

The third barrier to integrating touch-healing with traditional medicine is the shame and embarrassment felt by the general public toward the use of spiritual healing as a legitimate medical tool. Health care professionals believe they would face ridicule from the public, their patients, their peers and licensing agencies, and so they react with resistance and fear. The New England Journal of Medicine article on unconventional medicine refutes all these arguments. The fact is that when people have illnesses that do not respond to conventional medical treatment, they will seek any alternative that offers possible help.

The fourth barrier involves the religious connotations associated with prayer and healing. The argument goes somewhat like this: *"Clergy are already praying with the sick, so we do not need healers using Therapeutic Prayer or Therapeutic Touch. If you want to pray with the sick, come in and voluntarily do it on your own, like everyone else."*

My response is this: *"You do not understand. We are talking about something new, a completely new vocation -- the professional healer whose special skills take years of development and who can consistently and significantly contribute to a patient's recovery, health and general well-being."*

The fifth barrier involves money at several levels. Throughout the centuries, healing prayer has been offered to the sick, free of charge, by both clergy and laity. When you are dealing with well-educated professionals who work full-time at their vocation -- physicians, nurses, accountants, engineers, *and healers* -- financial reimbursement for services rendered is normal and essential.

Because of the general skepticism about healing results, paying a healer according to agreed-upon end results objectively addresses this major concern. One way of doing this is to pay the healer a percentage of the patient care costs saved by the successful practice of healing. This approach has several advantages. It would financially weed out ineffective healers who had passed through the certifying process. It would also force health care professionals to keep clinical statistical records of healings. This promotes objective integrity and trust in every one involved. It also provides the evidence needed to justify the use of professional healers.

Perhaps the scientific data presented here in <u>PrayWell</u> will provide the objective data needed to begin addressing all five of the above listed barriers and open the doors to the practice of professional touch-healing. Any doctor open to cooperating with professional healers only need provide a few patients who exhibit the medical conditions listed in chapter six.

For example, try touch-healing on arthritis, which is resistant to medical treatment. Provide the healer with five arthritic patients and give the time needed in a private setting. Assess the effectiveness of treatment. Then, make your decision about using a professional healer in your office. Or, ask the healer what medical conditions respond most readily to her treatments and provide the patients for the clinical tests.

CAUTION! Be fair. Do <u>not</u> sabotage the clinical tests. The presence of one hostile witness can negate all healing efforts by untuning the frequency of the healing energy or by creating harmful tension in the healer.

Perform the clinical tests quietly and privately. Use volunteer patients. Even patients who are skeptical but open will provide valid results. Some healers, myself included, do work quite well even in a hostile setting.

THE VALUE OF TOUCH-HEALING FOR DOCTORS

Every physician has patients whose conditions are resistance to traditional medical treatment. A doctor's personal compassion should prompt the use of professional healers who can help the acutely, chronically and terminally ill. From the standpoint of self-interest, the doctor should consider employing the skills of a professional healer whose successes will result in healthy patients and will boost the reputation of the office and practice.

THE PRACTICE OF PROFESSIONAL HEALING

Respect for the vocation of professional healer could come upon America very quickly and unexpectedly. It is already happening in isolated instances throughout America as doctors and healers begin working together. A few hospitals already employ healers through the pastoral care office. A more practical approach is for a healer to independently contract with doctors to work with their patients. A hospital healer could also be a nurse or a physician.

One healer could work with forty or more patients a week. Areas of care where we know healers could make major contributions are surgical units, intensive care, coronary care, trauma, orthopedics, oncology, burn units, pediatrics, and nurseries for premature and handicapped infants. Some healers might be able to accomplish genetic restructuring on newborns with birth defects. The AIDS virus may respond to healing efforts. Keeping accurate records of clinical data would be essential to justify the effort, expense, and publicity.

Large hospitals would best be served by a team of four healers, who would form a group energy field link to enhance their healing flow. They could also offer specialties such as diagnosis, treatment approaches for stymied medical researchers, regeneration of organs and other tissue, curing schizophrenia, and restoring functioning to the brain-dead through the skills of catalyst, attuner, sensitive, and healer.

For two decades I have wanted to work in a medical research center, practicing touch-healing, carrying out research and teaching others to heal. I believe my dream will become a reality within a few years.

TAKING ON THE PROFESSIONAL IDENTITY OF A HEALER

Every vocation develops professional standards, identity and respect through such mechanisms as certification, state licensing, education, training or apprenticeships, associations, dress codes and emblems. Healers, themselves, are not eager to develop professional standards, viewing it as an impossible task.

How do we measure competency in touch-healing? Because someone has completed a course in a healing technique does not make him or her a healer. As earlier noted, anyone can learn to transmit energy, but the energy may not necessarily be attuned to the healing frequency or the energy may not be powerful enough to produce the needed therapeutic results. The abilities of healers also vary. Some healers may only be competent in regenerating tissue, or healing viral infections, or healing emotional trauma. Acknowledging these realities enables us to develop professional standards.

State Licensing. Many vocations are licensed and regulated through state boards composed of practitioners of the vocation. Most health care professionals are licensed by state boards. A strategy to license healers would best be developed through a national effort by healers. First, healers and scientists need to gather together to develop the criteria and technology needed to license healers. Second, a national network would have to be established to work towards legalizing healing in all the states in the United States. The most forthright way is to lobby for healer licensing state boards. If you are interested, contact me at P.O.Box 618, Wadsworth, OH 44281.

Healer identification. It would be helpful for healers to be immediately recognizable. Doctors, nurses and priests established their professional identity and status in previous generations through distinctive clothing immediately recognizable by the public. You knew their profession as they worked with the ill. You knew they contributed to the health of the ill. Three identifying approaches for healers immediately come to mind.

First is clothing. Healers could wear a distinctively designed shirt or smock. The color gold comes to my mind. The most elegant design might be a golden Ghandi-cut smock.

Second is a distinctive identification emblem, different from those of other institutional personnel. The shape of a healing hand or of praying hands would be appropriate.

Third, and most difficult, is to find a means for causing the emblem to glow when a healer is in a mode to transmit healing energy. This might be achieved through an electronic device that both picks up the 7.83 hertz frequency and somehow calibrates the power of the healing flow to various levels of illumination.

The rationale for such identification includes several factors. Healers need to build a professional status for the sake of establishing their own sense of identity and self-worth and to earn the public's respect. If that status does not derive from the priestly role supported by religious institutions, then uniform clothing and a distinctive emblem are a first step. Having worn a clerical collar into medical centers, I know that wearing special clothing builds professional identity and confidence, helps one receive the cooperation of the staff, and provides recognition and respect for one's vocation. When healing efforts produce dramatic results, the good word gets around.

The consumer also needs a visible means of objectively perceiving that something is happening during the healing encounter. To see the healer's symbol alight during the transmission of healing energy would instill confidence in the reality of the healing experience.

THE FUTURE OF HEALING RESEARCH

Medical researchers will have their own goals for healers, but healers, too, have their research agendas. As a healer, I want tools for examining energy fields and exploring energy frequencies. I want to know how long I must spend with a patient to produce optimum healing results. I want to explore the correlation between personality type, disease and healing results.

For example, I have been working with patients who have Chronic Fatigue Syndrome, mostly women. Of the dozen women I have worked with in the past two months, all appear to possess the same personality type on the Meyers-Briggs Type Indicator. Coincidentally, this personality type fits the profile of healers. Could this disease be related to the tendency of latent healers to be victims of energy vampires and ruptured energy fields? I can only suspect this. Exploring this could help cure an estimated one million Americans who suffer with Chronic Fatigue Syndrome.

THE MULTIDISCIPLINARY HEALING RESEARCH CENTER

Richard Gerber, MD, in his book <u>Vibrational Medicine</u>, proposes a multi-disciplinary healing research center. The key issue in healing is experimental validation. His vision is stated here:

"What is truly needed is a multidisciplinary healing research center which can study the elements of the model I have elaborated upon within this book. I have long envisioned a kind of Mayo Clinic of healing research which could study the many dimensions of healing phenomena within an academic research setting. Such a center would be staffed by medical personnel from all fields of study...but also by acupuncturists, healers, herbalists, clairvoyant diagnosticians, engineers, chemists, physicists, and a host of others. This would be an interdisciplinary team which could design experiments to measure the subtle energies of human function and observe how they are effected by different modalities of healing.

"Within the center would be all manner of existing diagnostic technologies, from brain-wave mapping and magnetic resonance imaging to more unconventional techniques such as electroacupuncture monitoring. A wide variety of resources would be brought to bear in trying to understand the basic nature of healing and the potential effectiveness of the healing modalities presented within this book and elsewhere within this developing field."

SPORTS MEDICINE

When my favorite National League Football player went down with a season-ending injury, my first reaction was to contact him and offer touch-healing. I quickly sobered up, remembering the many non-responses to other attempted contacts with professional athletes from the Cleveland area.

Sports injuries are the easiest things to heal, with touch-healing increasing the normal healing rate by two to a hundred times. Tear up a knee, bruise your shoulder, or break a leg, and with touch-healing you can be back on the field in a fraction of the normal time. Any team that begins using touch-healing will have a tremendous advantage over other teams. Trainers who work with the players must practice some forms of energy medicine. They can quickly be trained in the practice of touch-healing. The most likely candidate for initiating reform would be the team owner. Send a copy of <u>PrayWell</u> to your favorite team's owner, along with a cover letter of explanation.

REJUVENATING SENIOR CITIZENS

The movie that best dramatized the effects of healing energy was *"Cocoon."* The extraterrestials from another star were yellow-glowing energy creatures who wore an artificial skin in order to pass as humans. We, too, are energy creatures, but our energy does not glow to the extent of these movie extra-terrestials. The swimming pool in *"Cocoon"* fascinated me the most. Residents of the neighboring nursing home jumped into the pool and were rejuvenated in it, becoming many physiological years younger.

We already possess the technology to fill a swimming pool with healing energy, but it is unlikely to be utilized for many years. We do have other resources for older adults. Touch-healing can alleviate the symptoms of arthritis. The hypnosis described in chapter eighteen can reduce physiological age by fifteen to twenty years. These therapies can be practiced by older adults upon each other.

THE FUTURE OF HEALING IS IN YOUR HANDS

How do we change public opinion about the value of touch-healing prayer? Change occurs when enough people lose their shame and embarrassment about touch-healing prayer to the extent that they begin talking about it. If you are open to the possibilities offered by touch-healing prayer, you can change public consciousness by taking action in several ways.

1. If you are helped by touch-healing, tell others about your experience, just as you would tell others about how helpful your physician has been. You have the support of many other consumers with 425 million visits to alternative therapists by Americans in 1990.

2. Tell your physician and other health care professionals of your touch-healing health care treatment.

3. If you have any means for influencing the health care industry, seek to promote changes in attitudes and practice among physicians, medical centers and insurance carriers.

4. Send a letter to your newspaper's editor about your experience.

5. Invite your alternative therapist to speak to a community group.

6. If <u>PrayWell</u> has been helpful in shaping your own understanding and attitudes, give a copy to your health care professionals, mass media reporters, the person in charge of your health insurance coverage, friends, and loved ones.

PERIACTIN -- A POSSIBLE CURE FOR CANCER

I found no logical place for this article throughout this book, so I am tagging it on to the end of this chapter on alternative medicine.

Biologist Bernard Grad found evidence that the simple, inexpensive antihistamine, periactin, can help victims of cancer. In the early stages, it can cure cancer. Suggesting this approach to friends, he received their reports. Within two weeks, Periactin shrank cancerous tumors so that they disappeared in persons with cancer of the breast, bronchia, prostate, pancreas and brain.

He found investors for further research and contracted with Dr. Ramesh Singh Chouhan of Pondicherry, India to conduct two years of trials on women subjects with cervical cancer using periactin, generically known as cyproheptadine.

The clinical study was entitled, "Cyproheptadine in the Treatment Of Carcinoma Cervix," by Ramesh S. Chouhan, MB, ChB, Bernard R. Grad, PhD, and Roman Rozencwaig, MD

Cyproheptadine (periactin) has been reported to play a useful role in the treatment of some cancers. For example, of 13 available marketed drugs claimed to produce symptomatic benefit against the excessive secretion of serotonin in the malignant carcinoid syndrome, cyproheptadine was reported to be the most helpful. Cyproheptadine has long been known as an appetite stimulant, due to its anti-serotinin action in the brain. More over, cyproheptadine has melatoninergic properties, producing melatonin that is reported to have regenerative and anti-aging potential.

In the clinical studies, four milligrams of cyproheptadine was taken once daily in the evening for up to 99 weeks by 42 patients with cervical cancer to counteract their anorexia, body weight and anemia. Six of these patients were also treated with surgery while the remaining 36 received cobalt treatments. In the control group, 25 were treated with surgery and 35 received cobalt treatment. The treatment group as a whole was in more advanced stages of cancer (Stage III) than the control group, being more underweight and anemic.

After 99 weeks, survival rates for those taking cyproheptadine were 83% for those treated by surgery alone and 52% of those receiving cobalt treatments alone. This was about 20% higher than the control group that had begun the study at a healthier baseline. Those on cyproheptadine who died lived significantly longer with a higher quality of life than their counterparts in the control group. The life qualities included being more positive, less depressed and calmer.

In the early stages of cancer, cyproheptadine (periactin) offers hope for the complete remission of all symptoms. Caution is still merited. If I were diagnosed with cancer, I would use all available traditional and holistic treatment approaches, in addition to cyproheptadine (periactin). If delaying treatment was not harmful, I would take cyproheptadine (periactin) for a month before any treatment and then assess the results.

As an antihistamine, a heavier daily dosage of 12 milligrams of cyproheptadine (periactin) is normal. For cancer, Chouhan recommends one 4 milligram tablet a day taken each evening within an hour of sunset (darkness) with the user in a darkened room from 11 p.m. until morning. This is because the action of cyproheptadine (periactin) takes place during the night hours. Alcohol should not be consumed while using it. Chouhan and Grad recommend that cancer patients take it the rest of their lives.

The side-effects of cyproheptadine (periactin) may include drowsiness for the first few days. If this becomes a problem, take half a tablet. Cyproheptadine (periactin) may also induce sleepiness and produce emotional calm. I used cyproheptadine (periactin) to quit smoking. It greatly reduces withdrawal symptoms and the craving, as well as producing emotional calmness and inner confidence. It may yield the same effective results with other addictive-compulsive chemicals.

In the United States, cyproheptadine is a prescription medicine. In Canada, it is sold over the counter. A 100-day supply of cyproheptadine cost me $13 or about $50 a year.

Whether cyproheptadine (periactin) will ever be clinically tested in the United States is questionable. It costs over a million dollars to do the clinical studies on any new drug approved by the Food and Drug Administration. No one can make the profits from this drug necessary for the clinical studies. Its recommended use for cancer would also diminish a whole multibillion dollar industry devoted to the treatment of cancer.

Chapter Thirty-Three

Talking To the Author

"Never go to a doctor whose office plants have died." ...Erma Bombeck

"The man who has no imagination has no wings." ...Muhammed Ali

"When you're all alone reading, you wish the author that wrote it was a terrific friend of yours and you could call him up on the phone." ...J.D. Salinger

---

I was so excited following the reading of <u>Vibrational Medicine</u> that I had an immense urge to talk to the author, Dr. Richard Gerber, MD. It was early one Saturday evening. I phoned a colleague in the metropolitan area where his book said he lived. She readily found the phone number of his suburban residence.

I immediately called Richard Gerber, expecting him to be cool to a weekend overture that invaded his privacy at home. Dr. Gerber answered the phone in a welcoming voice and his warm tone did not change throughout our half-hour conversation. We animatedly lost ourselves in the sharing of our mutual interest, spiritual healing.

Finally, I became self-conscious and asked, *"Did I interrupt you in the midst of something?"* Dr. Gerber responded, *"I almost forgot! We invited two couples over for a barbecue and they are waiting for me on the patio. Thanks for calling. It was my pleasure!"*

This is not an invitation for you to phone me for a casual conversation. I hope to sell thousands of copies of <u>PrayWell</u> and my home phone can only handle a few calls. What I *would* like to do is establish a link with readers. I am asking for your help. Because I have self-published, I can break the usual book mode by including this chapter. I want interactive communication with my readers. Here are some of the ways that we can work together.

YOU CAN CONTRIBUTE TO THE NEXT EDITION OF <u>PRAYWELL</u>

I view <u>PrayWell</u> as unfinished. It needs improvement. I welcome your suggestions for improving the next edition. At times you surely responded to <u>PrayWell</u> critically, saying to yourself,

"He could have expressed this idea better by..."

"This is wrong. It does not match my understanding. I would like to influence him to have a different approach on this issue."

"He should have added this...."

"He should have known about and included this scientific study."

"He omitted a type of prayer that I need."

"I could have written a better prayer than that."

"I would like to contribute my own ritual of affirmation or rite of passage."
"Weston should have included _____ in his book."

Your contribution must not be copyrighted by someone else. If you, your-self, copyrighted the material, include written permission for me to use it. Please avoid historic prayers. What you contribute and is used will be acknowledged as yours wherever it is used, unless you state that you wish it to be used anonymously. Your contribution may be used in a future edition of PrayWell, in other writings and in speeches I deliver.

Wherever your contribution is finally used, I am willing to pay for your valuable help. (Yes, I am aware that you might wish to make a free contri-bution of your creativity. If so, clearly state, *"This is my free contribution to the work of Walter L. Weston and I do not now nor will I ever seek financial compensation for it."* Then sign your name and the date.) Those contribu-tions I do not use will not receive remuneration.

Though I am requesting creative contributions in specific areas, feel free to submit ideas for any area. Here are my specific requests.

I am looking for more scientific data that you think will improve PrayWell. The person submitting the data will be paid $100 if the data is used.

Second, I am looking for new healing techniques. The person sub-mitting the healing technique will be paid $100 if the data is used.

Third, I am looking for practical applications of group energy fields for transforming groups of people or renewing the environment. The person submitting the data will be paid $100 if the data is used.

Fourth, I am looking for prayers that improve on the present ones in PrayWell. The person submitting the prayer will be paid $50, if the prayer is used.

Sixth, I am looking for Rituals of Affirmation. The person submitting an affirmation will be paid $100 if the affirmation is used.

Seventh, I am looking for Rites of Passage. The person submitting a rite of passage will be paid $25 each, if the rite is used.

Eighth, I am looking for any contributions you can make to im-prove Pray-Well. An appropriate fee will be established for any used con-tribution.

Mail your creative contributions to:

Walter L. Weston, P.O.Box 618, Wadsworth, OH 44281

or FAX it to 1-800-886-5735

YOU CAN HELP GATHER DATA ON HEALING PRAYER

I am establishing a _PrayWell_ Registry of Healings. I am asking readers to send me detailed reports of their healings. These reports will be on two levels: medically documented and medically undocumented. The PrayWell *"Registry of Healings"* will establish a data base needed to verifying that

Therapeutic Prayer works and to provide patterns of effective approaches for specific medical conditions. Please provide the information requested on the form on the next page.

COMPUTER AND FAX NETWORKING

I have been a dissatisfied member of two computer on-line services because neither had a special interest group devoted to touch-healing. If you are knowledgeable about such computer telephone links, I am interested in the best one that could offer an **international** special interest group devoted to touch-healing, subtle energy and spirituality. Contact me if you can help. I would be delighted to include information on such a computer on-line service in my next edition of <u>PrayWell</u>. This would be the beginning of an interactive touch-healing network.

Another level of touch-healing, subtle energy and spirituality networking could be accomplished through FAX transmissions. Through FAX we could compile lists of names for regional, national and international touch-healing associations and communications and then share them with local coordinators. For now, I would be willing to coordinate the beginnings of such a FAX network. To respond to either of these ideas, FAX or phone me at 1-800-886-5735.

HELP PROMOTE TOUCH-HEALING

Let us take touch-healing out of the closet of its shame and embarrassment. This is the time to go public. Change occurs when enough people lose their shame and embarrassment about touch-healing prayer to the extent that they begin talking about it. If you are open to the possibilities offered by touch-healing prayer, you can change public consciousness by taking action in several ways.

1. If your practice of touch-healing or prayer has been helpful to someone or any form of touch-healing or alternative medicine has helped you, tell others about your experience, just as you would tell others about how helpful your physician has been. You have the support of many other consumers with 425 million visits to alternative therapists by Americans in 1990.

2. Tell your physician and other health care professionals of your touch-healing health care practices or treatment.

3. If you have any means for influencing the health care industry, seek to promote changes in attitudes and practice among physicians, medical centers, insurance carriers, and those who pay the premiums.

4. Send a letter to your newspaper's editor telling about your experience.

5. Invite your alternative therapist to speak to a community group.

PRAYWELL -- *REGISTRY OF A HEALING FORM*

Name of person reporting_____Phone _____
Address_____ZIP_____

This is a report of ___a self-healing or ___ the healing of another.

Name of the person healed: _____Phone_____
Address _____ZIP_____
Age ___ ; Sex __M __F; Social Security No._____

Name of person doing the healing: _____Phone_____
Address _____ ZIP_____
Age ___ ; Sex __M __F; Social Security No._____

Name of condition healed _____
Date onset of condition _____ Date professionally diagnosed_____
Professional making diagnosis: Name_____Title_____
Address_____ Phone_____

Details of healing approach used:_____
_____
_____

Healee's signed statement: *The symptoms of my condition were alleviated by (date)_____.* Comments_____
_____Signature _____

Professional's signed statement: *The symptoms of the above stated
condition were alleviated by (date)_____. I determined this by _____*
_____.

Comments _____
Signature _____Professional Title_____

Complete story of the condition and the healing in your own words:
(If needed, use the back and other sheets of paper.) _____
_____
_____
_____
_____
_____
_____
_____
_____
_____
_____

Mail to: The Healing Registry, P.O.Box 618, Wadsworth, OH 44281

7. If <u>PrayWell</u> has been helpful in shaping your own understanding, attitudes and practice, give a copy to your health care professionals, mass media reporters, the person in charge of your health insurance coverage, book editors, friends, and loved ones.

POCKET BOOKS OF THERAPEUTIC PRAYER

A few readers have suggested needing specific sections containing only Therapeutic Prayers. A Montreal reader offered to translate into French only the prayers in <u>PrayWell</u>. Another reader wanted me to produce a booklet containing only the Therapeutic Prayers in Part Two. Several intuitives see a time when people are walking around with small <u>PrayWell Pocket Books of Prayer</u> in their pockets and purses, each containing portions of <u>PrayWell</u> prayers.

All of my own efforts to experiment with such formats have seemed inadequate. I am looking for readers who may have creative expertise in such matters. If you think you can be of help, please let me know.

HELP PROMOTE <u>PRAYWELL</u>

I have self-published <u>PrayWell</u> and could use your help on promotion in several ways. If you have access to book editors or the media, do what you can to help. I do telephone interviews for book editors and radio stations.

If you have a favorite bookstore, tell the manager that you liked <u>PrayWell</u> and ask the manager to stock it. Have the manager call me at 1-800-886-5735 to make an order, or call me and I will contact the manager.

If you would like to order extra copies for others, you can get them at discount through me at these prices.

1 book at $19.95 US (I do not want to undercut book store sales.)
2 - 4 books at $18.00 US a copy including shipping and sales tax
5 - 9 books at $16.50 US a copy including shipping and sales tax
10 books or more at $15.00 a copy including shipping and sales tax

Send your order with your check, Master Card or Visa Card number to: Walter Weston, P.O.Box 618, Wadsworth, OH 44281. (Checks and credit cards must clear their sources before any shipment.) Thanks for your support.

HEALING REQUESTS

The present evidence is that I am not competent in healing through absent prayer. Therefore, I refuse to offer individual absent prayer for the sick, believing my consent would offer false hope and be a needless waste of time for all parties involved.

My strength as a healer is in the process of touch-healing prayer. Most illnesses require a series of interactive counseling and healing sessions occurring over a period of time lasting weeks and sometimes months. Overnight healing of most diseases following one contact-prayer is possible, but extremely unlikely at our present level of understanding. It is likely that one or two full days of contact-prayer with a completely co-operative client who earnestly desires to get well would initiate and significantly enhance the healing rate of any illness.

But always remember, you, yourself, may be the best resource for touch-healing help. Accepting the role of bringing the power of God into the life of the world through touch-healing prayer requires one of the biggest shifts in self-images a person can make. The only qualifications for doing it are a loving concern and the confidence that goes with experience.

I have effectively used healer-charged containers of water or cotton towels as the only mode of absent treatment. My experience is that healer-charged cotton towels effectively remove the symptoms of arthritis, skin diseases, benign breast lumps, trauma injuries and grief. I have no evidence that other conditions respond to my healer-charged towels. I charge twenty-five dollars for the towel, healing time and postage. I reduce or eliminate this fee for those who cannot afford it.

I charge a fee for my time. I am willing to travel when I believe my presence has a good possibility of producing healing results. You need not look to me as your best or only resource. Resources in your community are available. Your own touch-healing prayers are the best resource for the process of healing your loved ones.

INQUIRIES BY GROUPS AND PROFESSIONALS

I am interested in working personally with therapeutic group leaders who wish to integrate healing prayer into the format of their meetings. I am also interested in helping any professional group wishing to use any concepts or practices of PrayWell in their work. I enjoy teaching and interacting. I would welcome lectures to self-help groups, associations, professional groups, college students, medical groups, and sports leadership. Workshops teaching competent skills in healing and prayer for participants need to provide eight to sixteen hours of group time to be effective. At all such events, I would be available to practice healing as time permits.

I am also available to work with health care professionals. I prefer co-operating with medical research centers but will work with any general hospitals/medical center. I am willing to be a test subject, but reserve the right to be involved in the format plans. My primary personal goal is to work on the staff of a medical center as a professional healer, researcher, and teacher.

INDEX

PROMOTING HEALING AND SPIRITUALITY

QUOTATIONS

RELIGIONS, WORLD'S GREAT

RESEARCH

RITES OF PASSAGE

FOOTNOTES for Praywell

CHAPTER THREE

[1] Hass, H., Fink, H., and Hartfielder, G., "The Placebo Problem," *Psychopharmocology Service Center Bulletin,* Vol 2, July, 1963, pp. 1-65.

[2] Truax, C.B. and, R.R., "For Better or For Worse," in *Recent Advances in the Study of Behavioral Change in the Proceedings of the Academic Assembly in Clinical Psychology,* 1963, p. 118.

[3] Grad, Bernard, "The 'Laying on of Hands:' Implications for Psychotherapy, Gentling, and the Placebo Effect," *Journal of the American Society for Psychical Research,* Vol. 61, No. 4, Oct., 1967, pp. 301-2.

[4] Grad, Bernard, "Some Biological Effects of the Laying on of Hands," *Journal of the American Society for Psychical Research,* Vol. 59, No. 2, April, 1965.

[5] Grad, Ibid.

[6] Benor, Daniel J., "Survey of Spiritual Healing Research," *Complementary Medical Research,* September, 1990, Vol.4, No. 3, pp. 9-34.

[7] Wirth, Daniel P., "The Effects of Non-Contact Therapeutic Touch on Full Thickness Dermal Wounds," *Subtle Energies,* Vol. 1, No. 1, pp. 1-19.

CHAPTER FOUR

[1] Swartz, S.A; Demattei, R.J.; Brame, E.G. and Spottiswoode, J.P., (1986) Infrared Spectra Alteration in Water Proximate To the Palms of Therapeutic Practitioners, Final Report, The Mobius Society, 4801 Wilshire Boulevard, Suite 320, Los Angeles, CA 90010.

[2] Grad, Bernard, The Healing of Induced Goiters in Mice Experiment, Parapsychology: Its Relation to Physics, Biology, Psychology and Psychiatry, ed. Gertrude R. Schmeidler, The Scarecrow Press, Inc, Metuchen, NJ., 1976.

[3] Miller, Robert, Methods of Detecting and Measuring Healing Energies, Future Science, ed. White and Krippner, Doubleday, 1977.

[4] Grad, Ibid.

[5] Krieger, Dolores, Therapeutic Touch, 1979.

[6] Beck, Robert, "New Technologies Detect Effects of Healing Hands," *Brain/Mind Bulletin*, Vol 10, No 6, p 3, 9-30-85.

[7] Zimmerman, John, Brain/Mind Bulletin, 1985.

[8] Zimmerman, John, "Laying on of Hands Healing and Therapeutic Touch: A Testable Theory," an unpublished paper, June, 1988.

[9] Green, Elmer E., Ph.D., Park, Peter A., M.S, Guyer, Paul R., B.A., Fahrion, Steven L., Ph.D., & Coyne, Lolafaye, Ph.D., "Anomalous Electrostatic Phenomena in Exceptional Subjects," *Subtle Energies*, Volume Two, Number Three, 1991, pp. 69-91.

[10] Puharich, Andrija, a medical doctor healing researcher in lecture in Montreal, May, 1985. Dr. Puharich worked with the U.S. Navy physicists and stated that this data was classified top secret at that time.

[11] Brennan, Barbara Ann, Hands of Light, A Guide To Healing Through the Human Energy Field, Bantam Books, 1988.

[12] SPINDRIFT, INC, P.O.Box 5134, Salem, OR 97304-5134 Begun by a group of Christian Science Practitioners and now including others across the United States, Spindrift conducts scientific experiments on prayer and mental effects.

[13] Krieger, Dolores, Therapeutic Touch, 1979.

[14] Zimmerman, John, Laying-on-of-hands Healing and Therapeutic Touch: a Testable Theory, Boulder, Colorado, June, 1988, an unpublished paper.

[15] Poulas, Lee, <u>Miracles and Other Realities</u>, along with lecture in Montreal, May, 1992.

[16] Miller, Robert, "The Positive Effect of Prayer on Plants," Psychic, April, 1972.

[17] Grad, Bernard, "The 'Laying on of Hands:' Implications for Psychotherapy, Gentling, and the Placebo Effect," *Journal of the American Society for Psychical Research*, Vol. 61, No. 4, Oct, 1967, pp. 301-2.

[18] Solvin, GF, Psi Expectancy Effects on Psychic Healing Studies with Malarial Mice, *European Journal of Parapsychology*, 1982; 4(2); 160-197.

[19] Becker, Robert O., MD, <u>Body Electric</u>, 1985.

[20] Becker, Robert O, MD, <u>Cross Currents</u>, Jeremy P. Tarcher/Perigee Books, the Putnam Publishing Group, 1990.

[21] Becker, Ibid.

[22] Becker, Ibid.

[23] Cerutti, Edwina, <u>Mystic with the Healing Hands</u>, Harper & Row, 1975.

CHAPTER FIVE

[1] Brennan, Barbara Ann, Hands of Light, <u>A Guide To Healing Through the Human Energy Field</u>, Bantam Books, 1988.

[2] Ibid, Brennan

[3] Gerber, Richard, <u>Vibrational Medicine</u>, Bear & Company, Santa Fe, NM 87504-2860, 1988.

[4] Rose-Redwood, Dr. Daniel, Robert Nash is Turning Science Fiction into Science, Pathways, Fall, 1989.

[5] Rose-Redwood, Ibid.

[6] Barbara Ann Brennan, <u>Light Emerging</u> - The Journey of Personal Healing, Bantam, 1993.

CHAPTER SIX

[1] Steffy, Joan and Vilenskaya, Larisa, "Some Comparisons of Psychic Healing in the USSR, Eastern and Western Europe, North America, China, and Brazil," PSI RESEARCH, June, 1984.

[2] Ibid.

[3] Barbara Ann Brennan, <u>Hands of Light</u>, 1988.

[4] Becker, Robert O, MD, <u>Cross Currents</u>, Jeremy P. Tarcher/Perigee Books, the Putnam Publishing Group, 1990.

CHAPTER EIGHT

[1] Michael, Chester P., and Norraisey, Marie Christian, <u>Prayer and Temperament</u>.

[2] Zimmerman, John, Brain/Mind Bulletin, 1985.

[3] Green, Elmer E., Ph.D., Park, Peter A., M.S, Guyer, Paul R., B.A., Fahrion, Steven L., Ph.D., & Coyne, Lolafaye, Ph.D., Anomalous Electrostatic Phenomena in Exceptional Subjects, Subtle Energies, Volume Two, Number Three, 1991, pp. 69-91.

[4] Beck, Robert, New Technologies Detect Effects of Healing Hands, Brain/Mind Bulletin, Vol. 10, No. 16, p. 3, Sept. 30, 1985.

[5] Zimmerman, Ibid.

[6] Zimmerman, Ibid.

[7] Grad, Bernard, The 'Laying on of Hands:' Implications for Psychotherapy, Gentling and the Placebo Effect, *Journal of the American Society for Psychical Research*, Vol. 61, No. 4, Oct, 1967, pp. 301-2.

[8] Jackson, Edgar N., <u>The Role of Faith in the Healing Process,</u> Winston Press, 1982, p. 46.

[9] Meek, George W., Editor, <u>Healers and the Healing Process</u>, The Theosophical Publishing House, Wheaton, IL, 1977. pp. 41-44.

[10] Beck, Robert O, MD, <u>Cross Currents</u>, Jeremy P. Tarcher/Perigee Books, the Putnam Publishing Group, 1990.

[11] LeShan, Lawrence, <u>The Medium, the Mystic, and the Physicist</u>, Bantam.

[12] Dossey, Larry, <u>The Power of Prayer: Old Approach/New Wonders</u>.

[13] LeShan, Ibid.

CHAPTER TEN

[1] Green, Elmer, "Alpha-Theta Brainwave Training," Lecture at Montreal symposium, May, 1993

[2] Brennan, Barbara Ann, <u>Hands of Lights: A Guide To Healing Through the Human Energy Field</u>, Bantam Books, 1987.

[3] Zimmerman, John, Laying-on-of-hands Healing and Therapeutic Touch: a Testable Theory, Boulder, Colorado, June, 1988, an unpublished paper.

[4] Brennan, Barbara Ann, <u>Light Emerging</u> - <u>The Journey of Personal Healing</u>, Bantam, 1993.

[5] Ibid, Zimmerman.

[6] Ibid, Brennan.

[7] Ibid, Brennan.

CHAPTER ELEVEN

[1] Grad, Bernard, "Some Biological Effects of the Laying On of Hands," *Journal of the American Society for Psychical Research,* Vol 59, No 2, April, 1965.

[2] Grad, Ibid.

[3] Benor, Daniel J., "Survey of Spiritual Healing Research," *Complermentary Medical Research*, September, 1990, Vol.4, No. 3, pp. 9-34.

[4] Wirth, Daniel P., "The Effect of Non-Contact Therapeutic Touch on Full Thickness Dermal Wounds," *Subtle Energies*, Vol. 1, No. 1, pp. 1-19.

[5] Swartz, S.A; Demattei, R.J.; Brame, E.G. and Spottiswoode, J.P. (1986), Infrared Spectra Alteration in Water Proximate To the Palms of Therapeutic Practioners, Final Report, The Mobius Society, 4801 Wilshire Boulevard, Suite 320, Los Angeles, CA 90010.

[6] Grad, Ibid.

[7] Grad, B., The Healing of Induced Goiters in Mice Experiment, <u>Parapsychology: Its Relation to Physics, Biology, Psychology and Psychiatry</u>, ed. Gertrude R. Schmeidler, The Scarecrow Press, Inc., Metuchen.

[8] Krieger, Dolores, <u>Therapeutic Touch</u>, 1979.

[9] Beck, Robert, New Technologies Detect Effects of Healing Hands, Brain/Mind Bulletin, Vol. 10, No. 16, p. 3, Sept. 30, 1985.

[10] Beck, Ibid.

[11] Zimmerman, John, Laying on of Hands Healing and Therapeutic Touch: A Testable Theory, an unpublished paper, June, 1988.

[12] Puharich, Andrija, medical doctor and healing researcher, in lecture in Montreal, May, 1985. Dr. Puharich worked with the Naval physicists and stated that this data was classified Top Secret at that time.

[13] Grad, Ibid.

[14] Grad, Bernard, "The 'Laying on of Hands:' Implications for Psychotherapy, Gentling, and the Placebo Effect," *Journal of the American Society for Psychical Research*, Vol. 61, No. 4, Oct, 1967, pp. 301-2.

[15] Solvin, G.F., Psi Expectancy Effects on Psychic Healing Studies with Malarial Mice, *European Journal of Parapsychology*, 1982; 4(2); 160-197.

[16] Solvin, Ibid.

[17] SPINDRIFT, INC, P.O.Box 5134, Salem, OR 97304-5134. Begun by a group of Christian Science Practitioners and now including others across the United States, Spindrift conducts scientific experiments on prayer and mental effects.

[18] Krieger, Dolores, Therapeutic Touch, 1979.

[19] Miller, Robert, The Positive Effect of Prayer on Plants, Psychic, April, 1972.3

CHAPTER TWELVE

[1] MacNutt, Francis, The Power To Heal, Ave Maria Press, 1977.

[2] Wu, Dr. Joseph Wen-Teng, The Concept of Spirit in Chinese Medicine, Integral Chinese Therapy Center, 107-1956 West Broadway, Vancouver, B.C., Canada V6J 1Z2, May 1, 1993.

CHAPTER SIXTEEN

[1] Shealy, Norman C., MD, PhD, and Myss, Caroline M, MA, The Creation of Health, the Emotional, Psychological, and Spiritual Responses that Promote Health and Healing, Stillpoint Publishing, 1993.

[2] Ibid.

CHAPTER EIGHTEEN

[1] Green, Elmer, "Alpha-Theta Brainwave Training," Lecture at Montreal symposium, May, 1993.

[2] Green, Elmer, Ibid.

[3] Green, Elmer, Ibid.

[4] Norris, Patricia, Current Conceptual Trends in Biofeedback and Self-Regulation, Eastern and Western Healing Approaches, Edited by Anees Sheikh, John Wiley & Sons, 1989.

[5] Wadden, T.A. & Anderton, C.H. (1982). The Clinical Uses of Hypnosis, *Psychological Bulletins*, 91(2).

[6] Norris, Patricia, Ibid

CHAPTER TWENTY-THREE

[1] Bird, Randolph C., MD, "Positive Therapeutic Results of Intercessory Prayer in a Coronary Care Population," *Southern Medical Journal*, July, 1988, Vol 81, No 7, pp. 826-829.

CHAPTER TWENTY-NINE

[1] Eliade, Mircea, Birth and Rebirth, New York, Harper, 1958.

CHAPTER THIRTY-TWO

[1] Eisenberg, David M., MD; Kessler, Ronald C., PhD; Foster, Cindy, MPH; Norlock, Frances E, MPH; Calkins, Davic R., MD; and Delbanco, Thomas L., MD. "Unconventional Medicine in the United States." *The New England Journal of Medicine*, Jan. 28, 1993, pp. 246-283.

[2] Ibid.

[3] Green, Elmer, "The Necessity for Promoting Health," paper for the Lieffer report.